PENGUIN CANADA

THE WELLNESS OPTIONS GUIDE TO HEALTH

A journalist and veteran patient, Lillian Chan was born in Hong Kong. Canada has been her home since 1975 and she now lives with her family in Toronto. She has over thirty years experience in journalism and editing, and has established unique editorial directions for several award-winning publications, including *WellnessOptions* magazine and the Chinese edition of *Maclean's* magazine. She has served as a Governor and Deputy Chairperson of the Board of Governors at Simon Fraser University, and as a board member of the North–South Institute.

Having experienced different physical illnesses and emotional turmoil in her life, Lillian has come to realize that it is possible to attain optimal well-being, both in health and in sickness. She has discovered the value of life, including its many difficulties and joys. Because Lillian benefited from different medical and health disciplines, she wishes to share and explain these perspectives.

The WellnessOptions Guide to Health

Integrating Western, Natural and Oriental Approaches to Well-Being

Lillian Chan

PENGUIN
CANADA

PENGUIN CANADA

Published by the Penguin Group

Penguin Books, a division of Pearson Canada, 10 Alcorn Avenue, Toronto, Ontario, Canada M4V 3B2
Penguin Books Ltd, 80 Strand, London WC2R 0RL, England
Penguin Putnam Inc., 375 Hudson Street, New York, New York 10014, U.S.A.
Penguin Books Australia Ltd, 250 Camberwell Road, Camberwell, Victoria 3124, Australia
Penguin Books India (P) Ltd, 11, Community Centre, Panchsheel Park, New Delhi – 110 017, India
Penguin Books (NZ) Ltd, cnr Rosedale and Airborne Roads, Albany, Auckland 1310, New Zealand
Penguin Books (South Africa) (Pty) Ltd, 24 Sturdee Avenue, Rosebank 2196, South Africa

Penguin Books Ltd, Registered Offices: 80 Strand, London WC2R 0RL, England

First published 2003

10 9 8 7 6 5 4 3 2 1

Manufactured in Canada.

National Library of Canada Cataloguing in Publication

Chan, Lillian, 1949–

    The WellnessOptions guide to health : integrating western, natural and oriental approaches to well-being / Lillian Chan.

Includes bibliographical references and index.

ISBN 0-14-301376-9

    1. Self-care, Health. I. Title.

RA776.95.C43 2003   613   C2003-901874-1

Visit Penguin Books' website at **www.penguin.ca**
Visit the *WellnessOptions* website at **www.wellnessoptions.ca**

To those who wish to feel well, in sickness and in health

Contents

A Road Sign to Wellness Options *1*

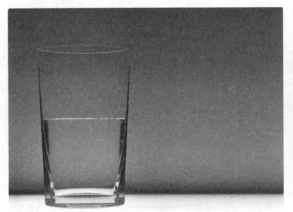 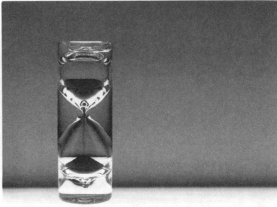

Part I

New Avenues to Wellness *13*

1. Thinking Well, Feeling Well:
   The Wellness Mentality *15*

2. Integrating Wellness Options
   for Optimal Living *21*

Part II

**Everyday Wellness Options
for Health Conditions** *31*

3. Who Are We?
   Our Relationship to Our Bodies *33*

4. How Are You?
   Feeling Bad, Feeling Good *51*

5. How Are You Doing as
   the Years Go By? *73*

6. What Is Your Body Telling You?
   Understanding Pain *97*

7. How Are You This Morning?
   Sleeping Well *125*

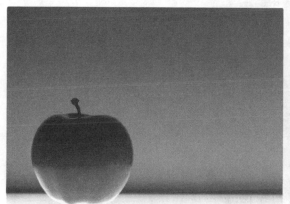
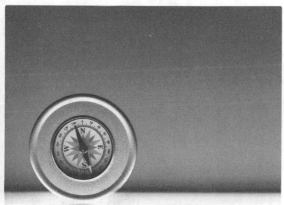

Part III

Forging Your Own Path to Wellness:
Healthy Lifestyle Practices *149*

8. Gourmet Wellness:
   The Tao of Food and Nutrition *151*

9. Our Bodies in Motion:
   Forward to Wellness *193*

10. From Daily Hassles
    to Spiritual Fitness *223*

Appendix

How to Evaluate Health
and Wellness Information *245*

Acknowledgments *260*

About the *WellnessOptions* Team *261*

Endnotes *262*

Index *273*

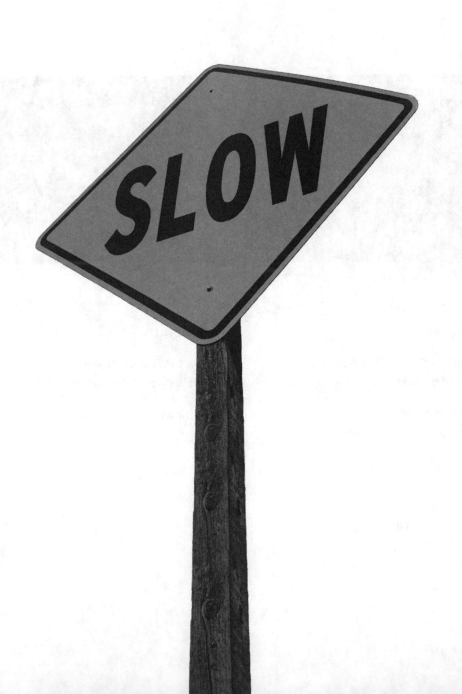

A Road Sign to Wellness Options

Years ago, a 19-year-old girl, bursting with youth and vitality, a top student with a sparkling future, was stricken with cancer. The news landed like a bombshell, and once the initial shock had passed, she was overcome with anger that the world was so unfair, that she was so powerless and unable to control her own destiny. What possible meaning could there be in life?

On a moonless, windy night as she sped down the road on her motorcycle, thinking of her plight, the anger kept growing in her until, rounding a curve, she saw the "SLOW" sign. She gave herself over to the consuming rage, sped up, and charged toward the sign. Girl, bike, and sign flew into the air. The lights of a thousand homes glittered and twisted below, and in one brilliant instant, she realized she did not want to die.

"I'll keep my eyes open," she thought, "to see how I die!"

She embraced the darkness rushing toward her with arms stretched wide. A dull thumping sound followed as she landed with a taste of grass, mud, and blood mixed in her mouth. It was a strange homecoming after reaching such great heights. She looked up, relieved to see the stars from the right perspective. Then everything went black, and all she could hear were the fading sounds of people running.

The girl woke up in hospital and asked for a Coke. She savored every sip; it was simply the most marvelous beverage on earth. How could she have failed to notice this before?

On the day she was allowed to go home, she looked out the taxi window and realized for the first time that not all the leaves on the trees were the same. Never before had she seen so many shades of green. It fascinated her, and she smiled.

Everybody has to die. Nobody can overcome death.

What is there to overcome?

"I'll stay feeling well. Even when I die, I'll die feeling well," she decided.

> When a moment is framed and frozen in memory and in essence as a complete, fully lived and experienced moment, it becomes eternal.

A Chinese proverb describes how helpless and out of control one feels when struck with a disease: "A general fears most not an advancing cavalry a million strong but the grinding torture of sickness." Most of us accept the inevitability of a sickness and resign ourselves to the suffering with despair or annoyance. We may blame it all on bad genes, invading germs and viruses, lousy weather, contaminated foods, departing spouses, the world, or the gods. Most of the time, we place the blame on anything but ourselves.

Seeking medical relief is usually the next thing to do. But how well do we do that? In my own case, I had ascribed magical life-dictating powers to my doctors for years. I expected them to be saviors. When I visited a fortune teller, I would provide precise birth information and then expect to be told about my future. But I would only half-believe what I was told. When I visited my doctor, however, I would just go with a few verbal descriptions of symptoms vaguely remembered, and I'd spend less time on the visit. Based on that brief appraisal, I expected to be told how my life was, what my health problems were, how they could be fixed. I believed completely that I would be able to walk away from the doctor with some magic potion that would restore my health immediately.

When I was sick, it didn't even occur to me at the time that there were options. But I discovered the feeling of wellness, and that was a start. I got lucky on that moonless, windy night. Certainly there were consequences, such as having to pay a hefty fine for the ruined SLOW sign. But what that fall taught me was that I could actually cope with my life-threatening illness much better when I was *feeling* well. Even more profound was the question: If I can feel well in sickness, what would it be like to feel well in health?

The realization that struck me might have been born out of desperation to hang onto something simple yet profound in order to make sense of life and death. Or I might have been shocked out of my element by the discovery that being un-sick was obviously not enough. Even when I was in an apparently healthy state, I could be developing well-hidden problems that would reveal themselves only when they spun out of control. In any event, I was alerted, and since then, I've been able to adopt what I would call the *wellness mode*: an awareness of the need for optimal living and well-being. Wellness is more than health; being well prepares you to combat sickness when it comes.

I have come to understand that there are three levels of "health":

→ **Healing.** The art of medicine is the art of sickness management. It's the art of treatment and healing.
→ **Un-sick.** The state of remaining healthy, or un-sick. Medicine also helps prevent disease.
→ **Optimal living.** Even when we are un-sick or healthy, we are not necessarily well. Going through the motions of avoiding disease is not the same as optimal living.

Maybe it's only when we are facing death that we realize the value of life including its many difficulties. And from there, we come to realize life's many potentials and joys.

My own experience had demonstrated this reality. Something had been quietly going wrong for some time without my knowing about it. I hadn't been well even before the cancer manifested itself. On the other hand, when I was recovering from the accident, even though the cancer was still there, I was feeling quite well. This made me realize that the *sense and feeling* of optimal well-being are attainable both in sickness and in health.

Health, as defined by the United Nations World Health Organization (WHO), is not just the absence of disease, but a state of complete physical, mental, and social well-being—a resource for optimal living. Health is not a goal. It is a process. It is not meant to be an attainable goal; it is what we strive for and work toward in our everyday living. Perhaps it is even a process we can enjoy—like experiencing good food, good sex, or a good night's sleep!

Optimal well-being is based on the greatest possible sense of harmony and contentment that can well up from within you, the sense that you and everyone else and everything else is fine. This leads to optimal living—to living to the fullest and maximizing your potential.

All of us have the right and the ability to choose to be well, in sickness and in health. We are also free to choose *how* to be well. As Canadian bioethics expert Guy Bourgeault has put it: "There is no life except in living ... expressed through matter."[1] With the knowledge that science gives us about life energy, we can make everyday lifestyle choices that give us maximum energy. What is there to stop us?

Many obstacles, in fact. Some we inherit, some we let others and the environment impose on us, but most we create for ourselves. It is easy to get lost on the journey to optimal well-being. It is like a journey up a magnificent mountain. There are dark valleys where we go astray, and there are high places where we can feel as if we're on top of the world, enjoying panoramic views. As I started out, I had no directions, roadmaps, or compass. All I had was a mindset, limited theoretical knowledge about health and well-being, and an all-powerful feeling that I could feel so *well*—when the world was so colorful, and the Coke tasted so good .... The feeling that I could feel so well and the knowledge that it is possible to feel so well have given me hope and therefore have sustained me and saved me time after time.

Once you decide that you want to stay feeling well, regardless of your genetic predisposition and the dictates of your environment, you have an

All of us have the right and the ability to choose to be well, in sickness and in health. We are also free to choose how to be well.

optimal living mindset. You are in *wellness mode*, ready to embark on the journey to optimal well-being. Even in sickness—especially in sickness— it is both possible and important to establish a sense of well-being.

As on any journey, thousands of pathways can be taken to reach the same destination. Even the same person taking the same journey in different seasons or with different companions might follow completely different routes. So many things can affect the outcome at every step of the way.

Gaining knowledge about health and wellness is obviously necessary. But wisdom is also required, as life's dynamics affect our balance in everyday living. We need to do more than access information; it's also vital that we assess the information we gather and use it to make wise choices that have a positive effect on our sense of well-being. We can choose to feel well, we are free to choose *how* to be well, and the choices we make every moment have a continuing impact on our well-being. That is the essence of WellnessOptions. That was the seed sown in my mind the moment I realized in mid-air that I didn't want to die. But I did not systematically organize my thoughts and feelings until more than 20 years later.

The girl went in for surgery, and was on Chinese herbal medication, acupressure, and a strict diet for more than five years. She could eat anything for lunch, but could have only vegetables for dinner. She felt really well for a long time.

Then she got too used to feeling well. The danger seemed to be over, and she started to let life events, people, and other priorities take over her life again. Wellness was taken for granted.

Many things happened: graduation, employment, relationships, marriage, motherhood. Instead of enjoying everything that came her way and being thankful (staying in the wellness mode), she slowly got back into the old habit of letting life's demands overwhelm and overwork her. And as soon as she forgot that life, health, and wellness are part of a continuum that needs constant tending, good choices and awareness slipped away. It's difficult to remember when or how, but somehow, gradually, the wellness mode and the inner self both took a backseat and slowly faded away.

And then her life was no longer full of the feelings of living.

Most of the time we do not notice that we are being propelled up the magnificent mountain of life by something called time. It is not

Even in sickness— especially in sickness— it is possible and important to establish a sense of well-being.

Wellness was taken for granted ... she forgot that life, health, and wellness are part of a continuum that needs constant tending.

mountain climbing and it doesn't feel like climbing, but moment by moment and step by step, we keep going up the path to new places. There are schedules and expectations to meet every day: feeding, sleeping, playing, thinking, working, imagining, wishing, loving, hating, and regretting. There is always another appointment, another preoccupation, another demand, another avenue to explore. So we tread on through everyday life, somehow assuming that it is permanent. We are only occasionally and vaguely conscious of the process of living that is still taking place. Until the day we do not feel well enough to move on anymore.

When did it start to happen again? When did she start not to care enough to take care? All of a sudden, the full impact of 20 years of mindless choices and wasted wellness chances hit home.

This time it was abrupt; she lost 10.4 kilograms (23 pounds) in two weeks. It started with vomiting; she couldn't keep anything down. Then she was told that she had a lump in her pancreas 3.5 centimeters (1.4 inches) in diameter. It was likely cancerous.

For a long time she'd thought she had everything: a top-student son, a loving husband who was always supportive, a nice house in a good neighborhood, two chow-chow dogs, and nine fish. Then the husband wanted a divorce and the lump demanded attention.

When had things started to go wrong? How could her whole world fall apart at the snap of a finger?

I didn't go for surgery. I didn't think I'd be able to withstand the physical trauma. But most of all, I didn't want to go under anesthetic for two reasons: I was found to be sensitive to certain anesthetics when I went through a cesarean section for my son's birth; I was also afraid to lose any more control of my life and therefore didn't want to be put under.

Instead, I went for acupuncture, massages, and herbal formulas from a famous Chinese herbalist who specialized in poisons. I was not a person of religion, and to prepare for death I only made my will. At one point when I was despondent, my brother gave me a chant to sing. I didn't know what it was all about and didn't care to find out until much later, but it sounded soothing, and I associated it with the feeling of wellness that I had found and lost.

So I sang it often and used it as a reminder that I could choose to feel well at any time. In fact, I taped my own chanting and from then on played the tape whenever I chanted. This was like singing along when you turn up your Walkman. I couldn't listen to music because it made me cry, so I went for the chanting.

The sound drowned out all thoughts, and I would go on for hours just so I would not have to think. It kept me calm. Looking back, something of a psychological, emotional, or even spiritual nature must have been taking place, even though I didn't understand it at all.

It took another three months before I got back to solid food, and I had to follow a very strict individualized diet prescribed by my herbalist for more than six years. But I lived.

Again, I was extremely lucky. As a scrupulously logical person who values reasoning above all else, it was difficult for me to try anything not clinically understood or not tested thoroughly. Some health disciplines and wellness practices, such as Chinese traditional medicine and spiritual fitness, would escape me. Now I have learned to respect all approaches and have at least opened my eyes and my mind.

Years later, I discussed this incident with a pancreas specialist, who told me that the problem couldn't possibly have been cancer because the survival rate for pancreatic cancer is almost nil. But it was just semantics anyway. I'd been throwing up and losing weight at such a rapid rate that I wouldn't have lasted long no matter what. So I told him I'd never know for certain, but I had stayed feeling well, and that was all that mattered.

There are things I wish had been different. For example, I wish my doctors—Western, natural, and Oriental—had been able to share information and work together on my case. But such cooperation was not a common part of health practice at the time. It would also have been helpful if someone had coached me on how to tell my friends gently that I was dying.

Another frustration was that even though, as a professional journalist, I had an enormous amount of information at my fingertips, I still found it difficult to make informed and wise choices about my own health and wellness. I realized that all of us would benefit from learning more about our bodies and about how to feel well. This would help us make healing and healthy lifestyle choices from the options available and to find out what works best for us. We need the help of reliable and credible professionals to interpret and validate the information we discover, but it's also vital to take responsibility for ourselves, in order to apply those interpretations to our own situations. This does not have to be an odious task! Life is here to nourish us and to give us joy. Learning and living wellness is a wonderful experience.

Five years to the month after the pancreas incident began, my best friend in high school, with whom I had lost contact for 32 years, found out where I was by chance. We met, and two years later we were married.

In one of our last pieces of correspondence before we'd lost contact, he asked me which field I thought he might work in well. My reply was "biochemistry and psychiatry." He went on to become a clinical biochemist, worked at a teaching hospital, and did pharmaceutical research. When he showed me the letter containing that line I had written so long ago—which I had totally forgotten—I felt touched and thankful. Fortunately, I had said the right thing, and he had done well in his chosen field.

We are so often unaware of how we affect people around us—how sometimes a word of encouragement or a word of condemnation can totally change the direction of another person's life, and how that might come back to benefit or to haunt us years later.

My husband's medical knowledge and background, his friends and connections in the health-care field, and his confidence in me were exactly what I needed to complete the concept of health that I had begun to understand. These things allowed me to develop a systematic working model of how a wellness options approach might be applied in everyday life.

As I began to lead a relatively healthy and happy life, we decided to engage all our resources to start a wellness magazine with no professional or product-specific agendas. The magazine that we have now created, *WellnessOptions*, works on the principles of combining disciplines, asking simple questions about wellness conditions, and providing well-researched, credible information that can be applied to everyday life. The *WellnessOptions* concept has worked so well for me that we hope it becomes a helpful tool for other people. It's our way of saying thank you to the magnificent mountain that is Life.

How to Use This Book

Part I, "New Avenues to Wellness," explores why *WellnessOptions* is a helpful approach and shows how to apply it, using the immune system as an example. In a step-by-step presentation, we offer some recent scientific research about allergies and immune disorders, in order to show how each health aspect affects the others and how greater integration of medical disciplines can lead to better wellness.

In Part II, "Everyday Wellness Options for Health Conditions," we provide information roadmaps for five of the most common wellness conditions: body image, mood, aging, pain, and sleep. What are our coping options? It's often a daunting task to create places for wellness in our busy days, so we've tried to make the job easier by presenting and explaining a number of choices.

In the section on sleep (Chapter 7), for instance, we raise questions such as: What do we know about sleep as a wellness condition? What are the Western, natural, and Oriental treatment approaches to insomnia? What "sleep-smart" strategies can you bring into your life?

Of course, our guidelines are not comprehensive, since each of these conditions deserves volumes. We present them here only as demonstrations of how the integrated *WellnessOptions* approach may be applied in general. As we are all similar in some ways and uniquely different in others, the information provided in this book is intended as a guideline and reference only. Anything that you learn here will have to be adapted to your individual situation, and in some cases, checked with medical professionals.

Each chapter in Part II can be looked at separately or in a different sequence. (For easy access to different chapters and sections, cross-reference notes have been provided in the margins.) Nevertheless, all wellness conditions are ultimately interrelated, and they affect each other like the workings of different musical instruments in an orchestra. Understanding a condition from multiple perspectives is the basis for mastering it. So the more you learn about various conditions, the more you will understand the value of the life invested in you and the sense of well-being you can attain or enhance.

Part III, "Forging Your Own Path to Wellness," is about nutrition as well as physical, mental, emotional, and spiritual fitness. In Chapter 8, we discuss gourmet wellness, food and diet trends, and the easy "Tao of Food and Nutrition." In Chapter 9, "Our Bodies in Motion," we look at activities that can be adopted for body wellness. We all know that we should exercise, but we don't always follow through. Why is that? How can we change the situation? What easy daily routines can we follow from the Western, natural, and Oriental perspectives?

> All wellness conditions are ultimately interrelated, and they affect each other like the workings of different musical instruments in an orchestra.

> Understanding a condition from multiple perspectives is the basis for mastering it.

In the last chapter of Part III, "From Daily Hassles to Spiritual Fitness," we look at how fully lived moments can be expanded into the integrated totality of optimal living.

Finally, in the Appendix, "How to Evaluate Health and Wellness Information," we present guidelines to help you make your way through the masses of sometimes conflicting health and wellness information that is available.

I'm closing this chapter about my health journey and the beginnings of the *WellnessOptions* project with a note of appreciation. We would have started the *WellnessOptions* magazine sooner, but I went through another major surgery, so we launched it in November 2000. It was the anniversary of the day I'd met my high-school best friend once again. My thanks go to him and to all who have believed in *WellnessOptions*, including Cynthia Good, former publisher of Penguin Books Canada, who approached us with this book idea. I'm also grateful to all whom I have had the good fortune to encounter: loved ones, friends, strangers, events, things … including the SLOW sign I mowed down so long ago.

I didn't mean to destroy it. But we shared a moment of eternity leading to *WellnessOptions*.

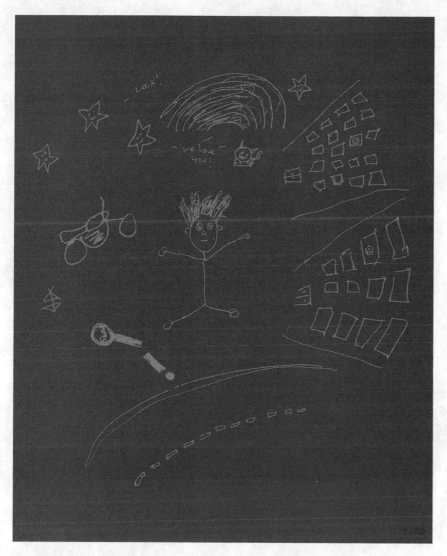

The slow sign and I shared a moment of eternity leading to **WellnessOptions.**

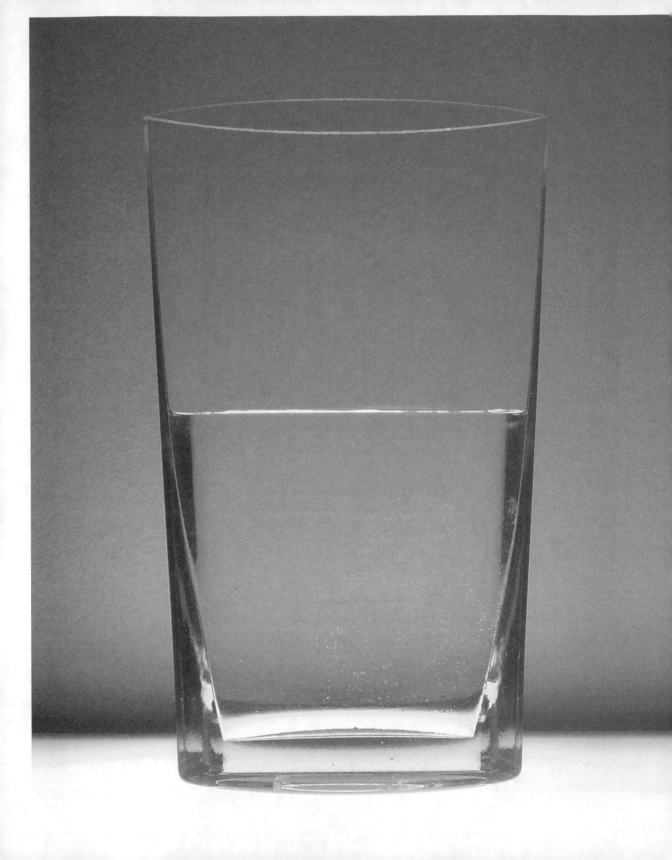

Part I

New Avenues to Wellness

Life is a glass half full
To be full-filled
To be spilled
Day after day

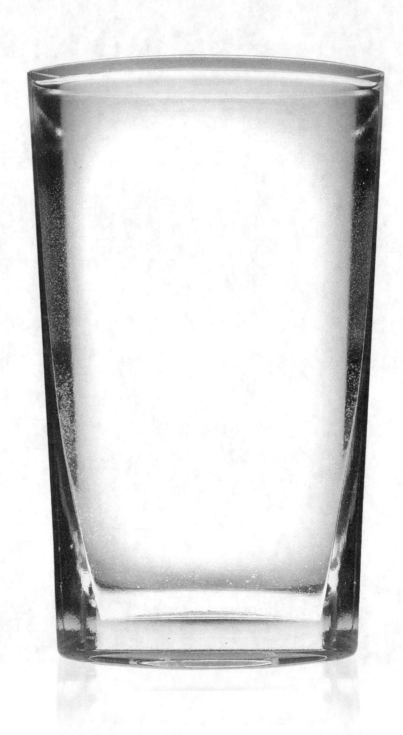

1 Thinking Well, Feeling Well: *The Wellness Mentality*

The mist of familiarity obscures from us the wonder of our being.
—Percy Bysshe Shelley

Full-filled

"There is nothing to be seen more worthy of wonder than man," said Italian Renaissance author Pico della Mirandola at a time when Western civilization was becoming more aware of the intricate workings of the human mind and body. Ironically, that era, which produced such masterly understanding of the human form, also set the pattern for the objective, mechanistic view of our bodies that has dominated modern science. A compartmental approach, while inspiring thousands of medical discoveries and saving countless lives, has sometimes led us further away from appreciating life as a whole and from remembering how "fearfully and wonderfully" we are made.

Works of Art in Progress

Information increases awareness; awareness leads to appreciation. Appreciation, in turn, provides incentives for seeking more information.

A little knowledge of how exquisite you are may help you value the life that is invested in you—and inspire you to do more for your health and well-being. There are an estimated 75 trillion cells in your body, all organized into a web of interlocking systems, diligently working together so you can live, grow, function, and enjoy. We are all living, sleeping, walking wonders.

We are poetry in motion, works of art in progress. Even the satisfaction of simple animal hungers such as eating, drinking, and having sex are transformed in us and by us. We enter realms of emotion and association, capturing the essence of heaven or hell and everything in between. At its most beautiful, physical gratification transcends the five senses and captures the totality of a moment, where time, atmosphere, and experience are all woven into a fully lived compendium of savoring, absorbing, embracing, expressing, and creating. And when these joys are later recalled, they inspire new expressions and creations. Eternity can be captured in a single moment.

Although we live in the here and now, our appreciation of the moments, the wonders that surround us—the wonder that is us—is often muted by the urgent obligations of the day. Sometimes our perception is obscured because we do not have enough information, and this prevents us from appreciating the walking wonders that we are, and all the wellness possibilities in our lives. Information is only one of the keys to this heightened understanding and appreciation of life, but it is an important beginning.

Take, for example, your immune system. Like a well-trained militia, it is an extremely complex mechanism—flawlessly designed, meticulously organized, beautifully orchestrated, and intensely poised for action. It has a threefold task: to guard the borders of your body by killing, expelling, or rendering harmless any foreign microorganisms that try to invade; to patrol and police the internal territories, eliminating dissidents at the first sign of deviance; and to identify and accept cells that conform and behave normally.

Your immune system is made up of many subsystems, each with its own specific functions: setting off alarms, trapping enemies, presenting them for identification, processing information, memorizing data, triggering responses, defending, killing, or cleaning up after battles. It can tell the difference between a foreign body (called an *antigen*) and its mirror image when they are put side by side. It can't be easily fooled. The army serving this system has foot soldiers, helpers, messengers, and many specialized task force units. These units even share the same biochemical language codes so they can communicate among themselves and with the brain. They receive signals, understand commands, and pass along intelligence efficiently and effectively when the body is in a healthy and peaceful state, as well as during battles against sickness.

But in a time of misfiring, few harmful foreign microorganisms can match the efficiency of your own perfect immune system in killing you so violently. It is your most faithful and protective guardian angel. It is also your shadow and your most deadly foe. Such a powerful protector needs to be treated with care and respect. But how often do we think about what we are doing to our immune systems? Or better still, how often do we do something good for our immune systems? How often do you thank yourself for the living you are doing and how often do you thank your cells for working so hard that you can enjoy life?

Your Immune System: Friend or Foe?

Although the human body is protected by a sophisticated immune system, that powerful guardian can also become dangerous. A person who is highly sensitive to a particular allergen, for instance, may go through the following stages if not rescued in time: restlessness, followed by sneezing and coughing, an increased heart rate, shortness of breath, and gasping for air. The blood vessels then dilate, blood pressure drops to dangerously low levels, air passages become constricted, and the person's lungs become inflated. Death can occur within a short time.

Foreign allergens that are normally harmless—such as food, an insect's sting, or airborne particles—can trigger this deadly response, known as anaphylaxis, in a person susceptible to a particular allergen.[1]

"Live neither in the
past nor in the future,
but let each day absorb
your entire energies."
–Canadian physician
 William Osler
 (1849–1919)

The process of living starts at birth and continues throughout our lives, but it is never the same on any two days. You can start to make a difference on just about any day you choose, at any age. A little appreciation goes a long way. There's value in each present moment if you appreciate yourself and the day at hand. Live today for the rest of your days.

Developing Your Wellness Attitude

So how can you develop a wellness attitude that maximizes choices and perspectives in your day-to-day life? I can give you an example from my life that illustrates the point.

We need to drink enough water for health. For me, drinking enough water was a major wellness problem. I know I have a duty to my body to drink water, but I grew up in Hong Kong, where drinking water had to be imported to the island and during an era when water was not disinfected. We even had to boil the water we used to brush our teeth. As a result, I have always hated the taste—or should I say non-taste—of plain water.

I will never be able to follow a strict diet of drinking enough plain water to be well. I want to be well, but if I force myself to follow this strict regime, I will not be very happy and that would contradict the spirit of optimal living. Because of this dilemma, I started to create recipes that use water as the main ingredient, adding rose petals, jasmine flowers, orange blossoms, ginger, cinnamon, a splash of juice or tea ... anything that gives the water some zip and flavor and that is also good for my health. Now drinking enough water is no longer a duty—it has become a pleasure.

For examples of water recipes, see Chapter 8, "Gourmet Wellness."

I choose to be well and then I choose how to be well. Now I drink plenty of water, but only water that I enjoy. It is now my own daily wellness option and part of my optimal living. Creating and enjoying water recipes demonstrates the essence of the *WellnessOptions* approach to health.

WellnessOptions is the conscious decision and effort to:

→ choose well-being and optimal living;
→ choose how to be well, in sickness and in health;
→ seek reliable health information;
→ develop a sense of appreciation;
→ learn about healing options and lifestyle choices;
→ expand medical and health perspectives;
→ integrate different health aspects (physical, emotional, social, environmental);
→ maximize what's best for you (physically, psychologically, practically);
→ replace dogmatic disciplines with balanced wellness strategies;
→ live and enjoy wellness, today and always.

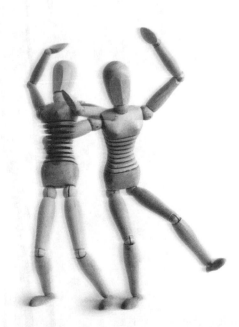

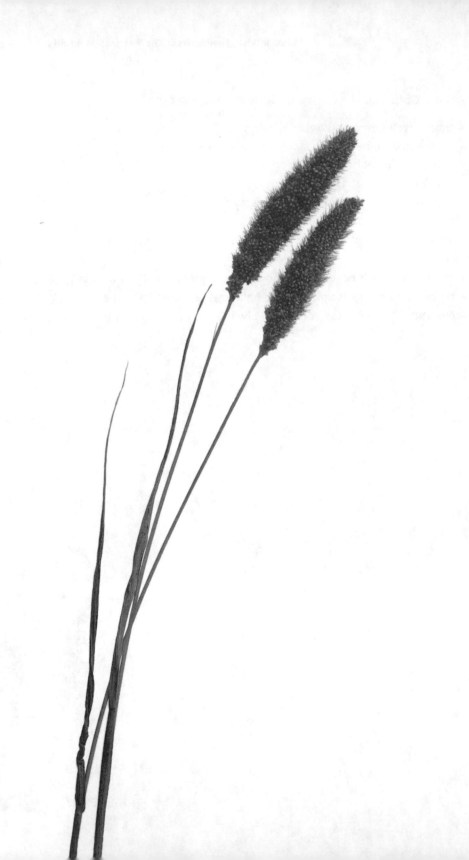

2 Integrating Wellness Options for Optimal Living

We have met the enemy and he is us.
—Walt Kelly's *Pogo*

Sometimes we work against our own interests, putting unnecessary stress on ourselves, and this always takes a toll on our overall health and sense of well-being—physical, mental, and emotional. There has actually been a long-standing belief that the state of a person's mind or heart can in some way control the body's immunity and therefore the state of health. In fact, for centuries, the healing arts in both Europe and Asia were based on the notion that disease was caused by a general imbalance of many aspects of our health. Only with the rise of modern medicine, and its mechanistic view of physiology, were life and health seen to be purely physical and chemical processes that took place in compartmentalized body parts. And conventional Western medicine is still often practiced under the assumption that the head and heart are separate entities.

"When we've broken down living systems to molecules and ... analyzed their behavior, we may kid ourselves into thinking that we know what life is, forgetting that molecules have no life at all."
—Albert Szent-Gyorgyi, Nobel Prize–winning biochemist

But even during the days when this mechanistic view was coming into its own—toward the end of the 19th century—some conventional medical experts realized that there was more to health than just working parts. The world-renowned Canadian physician William Osler (1849–1919), for instance, is reputed to have said that it is just as important to know what is going on in a man's head as in his chest when predicting the outcome of his tuberculosis. And D.H. Lawrence, a contemporary of Osler, wrote in his poem "Healing":

I am not a mechanism, an assembly of various sections.
And it is not because the mechanism is working wrongly, that I am ill.
I am ill because of wounds to the soul, to the deep emotional self.

The strands of this thinking are becoming stronger today, as many physicians are taking more multidisciplinary, integrated approaches to life and wellness. The accumulating medical evidence has begun to reveal that different aspects of our being work together in amazingly complex ways to affect our health. Each aspect also has an impact on the others, creating a web of interplay that needs to be taken into account when we are looking for cures and healthier lifestyles.

That Allergy: An Integrated Event!

An allergic reaction is in every sense an integrated event. Research on allergies has shown us intriguing correlations: delicate balances can trigger either a proper immune response or an allergic reaction, which is a response that occurs when the immune system overreacts to a substance that is normally harmless.

In the Western world over the past two decades, there has been a great increase in the numbers of people who are sensitized to different allergens, creating an explosion of allergies and allergic diseases. This explosion is one of the most fascinating phenomena in medicine. About 40 to 50 percent of all children in the developed world, including North America, Australia, and Western Europe, now develop some type of allergic disease before they reach puberty. No other medical condition currently exists that comes close to matching allergies in their galloping rate of prevalence. What has led to this crisis?

Research has shown an inverse relationship between rates for infectious diseases and rates for allergies—that is, the more infections, the fewer the allergies. Interestingly, birth sequence is also related to allergy risk, with first-born children being at the highest risk. Researchers in Australia, Scandinavia, North America, and the United Kingdom have discovered that our immune response first started in the allergic mode, so the allergic response is actually the default setting.

Within the immune system, there are two types of specialized cells called T-cells produced by the thymus, the command center of the immune system, which resides in the thorax. They are the TH1 cells in normal mode, which produce the protective immune response, and the TH2 cells in default mode, which produce the allergic response. There is a delicate balance between the two, and our Western lifestyle is a major factor in preventing the allergic mode from being switched to normal.[1] Strange as it may seem, we need an external "force," such as a bacterial infection, to switch the immune system from its default setting to a normal setting. If infections occur regularly—especially early in life—the immune system deviates from the default allergic mode, and allergies do not develop or have less opportunity to develop.

An allergic reaction is in every sense an integrated event.

Immune Balance

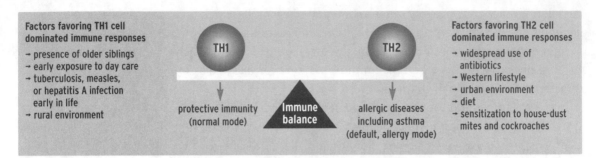

Factors favoring TH1 cell dominated immune responses		Factors favoring TH2 cell dominated immune responses
→ presence of older siblings → early exposure to day care → tuberculosis, measles, or hepatitis A infection early in life → rural environment	TH1 TH2 protective immunity (normal mode) Immune balance allergic diseases including asthma (default, allergy mode)	→ widespread use of antibiotics → Western lifestyle → urban environment → diet → sensitization to house-dust mites and cockroaches

An imbalance between TH1, the protective immune response in normal mode, and TH2, the allergic response in default mode, leads to allergies. Numerous factors, including genetic predisposition, diet, environment, repeated exposure to allergens, overuse of antibiotics, and early childhood infections, affect the likelihood of developing an allergy.

Ironically, some attempts to improve health in the Western world have made us more prone to allergies. Exaggerated cleanliness and widespread overprescription of antibiotics have made it more difficult for children to come down with bacterial infections, so their immune systems have fewer occasions to switch from default allergic to normal response. By the same token, first-borns have less chance to be exposed to infectious diseases from other children, and this makes them more susceptible to allergies.

Parts of the physical environment may also affect us even when we have no direct contact with them. *The New England Journal of Medicine* reported in 1998 that a patient who received a liver-kidney transplant from a donor with a peanut allergy also developed a peanut allergy. This suggested that direct exposure to an allergen (the triggering substance) is not necessary for an allergy to develop.[2] Similarly, about 85 percent of children who are allergic to peanuts have a reaction the first time they ever eat them. There is evidence that they may have developed the peanut allergy when they were in their mothers' wombs—possibly because their mothers ate too many peanuts during pregnancy. A child can develop the same allergy when being breast-fed if the mother has consumed a significant quantity of peanuts.[3]

What is true of peanuts also seems to be true of cats! After researchers from the University of British Columbia and University of Toronto surveyed residents on the island of Tristan da Cunha, they concluded that direct exposure to cats is not necessary for a person to develop sensitization to cat allergens and therefore an allergy to cats.[4]

Tristan da Cunha is a remote island in the Atlantic Ocean. It lies about 2,000 kilometers (1,240 miles) from the nearest mainland point, and no cats have lived on the island since a disease exterminated them in 1974. Tristan da Cunha cannot be reached by air, and a maximum of six ships visit the place each year. Only 1 home out of the 20 tested (from a total of 100 homes on the island) had cat allergen present in house dust. But researchers found that 6 of the 51 residents who were born after 1974 were allergic to cats. Apparently, even a minuscule amount of allergen hidden somewhere in the environment from 20 years before was able to cause an allergic reaction.

However, no environmental factor can affect a person who has no genetic predisposition to an allergic response. No matter what the environmental stimuli may be, some people have genes that dictate normal responses and others have genes that favor allergic responses. Many of the genes that lead to or away from allergies are now being identified.[5]

Mind over Allergy?

Robert Good, an American pioneer in psycho-immunology, reports that human subjects under hypnosis can be made to choose to react either positively or negatively to an allergen, and this may cause an allergic skin response on either arm. A group of British researchers has reported essentially the same findings.[6]

How Stress Affects the Immune System

Noted Canadian stress researcher Hans Selye was the first to demonstrate that stress has a direct impact on the immune system.[7] He proved that exposure to various stressors shrinks the thymus (the immune system's command center) and causes a substantial decrease in the number of lymphocytes (white blood cells, including T-cells, that spearhead the immune response). Since then, intensive studies have confirmed that stress is also associated with suppressed immune responses.

New studies in psycho-immunology—the interdisciplinary field concerned with the interactions between brain hormones and the immune system, as well as their health implications—have revealed that immune changes associated with stress are activated through the nervous system and the endocrine system. The brain is connected to all parts of the body by nerves and sends nerve impulses to influence the activities of all parts of the body. It also produces thousands of different kinds of chemicals and releases them into the bloodstream to circulate throughout the body, affecting our actions and reactions. The immune system itself produces hormone-like molecules that are very much like some of the chemical molecules the brain produces. This allows the brain and the immune system to carry out molecular communications in a common biochemical language. Medicine is just beginning to unravel this dialogue, but it is clear that the connection is a two-way street.

More research will be needed before we can discover exactly how the psycho-immuno connection works and how we can take advantage of this link to treat allergies. But for now, the best way to prevent an allergic reaction is to avoid the substance that triggers the allergy. Other lifestyle factors, such as diet and nutrition, exercise and sleep, all strengthen or weaken the immune system and may provide some relief or make the allergy worse. It has been suggested, for example, that certain foods high in histamine—including cheese, tuna, some wines, and most nuts—should be avoided by people with allergies, and that foods such as colored vegetables, onions, and garlic, which inhibit histamine, may help. The more we learn about allergies, the more we discover that everything in our lives has a bearing on how the immune system works and on the likelihood of our being free of allergies. A complexity of intersecting circles and paths affects who we are and how we feel today. To develop new preventive strategies, coping therapies, and a wellness lifestyle, it's important to understand and address many different aspects separately and together.

The more we learn about allergies, the more we discover that everything in our lives has a bearing on how the immune system works and on our overall well-being. It's important to understand and address many different aspects separately and together.

Integrating Medical Disciplines and Health Perspectives

Fortunately, we live in an age when researchers and medical practitioners are more open to examining the multiple factors that affect our health. And because of globalization, we are also able to learn about more perspectives and options than ever before. How do different wellness perspectives affect us? How do we begin to integrate them?

New perspectives expand our scope and help us see things differently. If, for example, you picture a man going away in the desert, you may dress him and the environment in a thousand and one ways. He may be a lone ranger riding into the sunset—a hero. Or he may be in exile, walking away with a donkey as night falls—an outcast. Your mind can fill in the blanks with all the details, complete with music and colors, even though the viewed object is the same—*a man going away in the desert*. Just as there could be many options to help this man in the desert feel better, there are also numerous methods of tending our bodies. Sometimes it isn't a matter of which perspective is better; it's a matter of which method suits you as an individual physically, emotionally, mentally, and practically.

A few years ago, an editorial adviser for the *WellnessOptions* magazine was called back from an overseas trip. His wife had fallen into a deep coma after developing life-threatening complications from a severe case of flu, and she was being kept alive on life support. The adviser, a Cambridge-trained doctor, had studied and practiced acupuncture for many decades. When he learned of his wife's condition, he set to work to revive her using laser beams (contemporary Western technology) and needles (traditional Oriental technology). The acupuncture and laser beams stimulated the flow of blocked energy in her body, and within hours, his wife began to respond. Within weeks, she was recovering at home.

Had it not been for the technology of life-support systems, the adviser would almost certainly have arrived too late to use a complementary technology to save his wife. This is only one powerful example of how a life can be saved by the integration of different medical disciplines and health practices.

But is it possible to integrate different medical disciplines harmoniously within the health-care system as a whole? In King County, Washington State, steps have already been taken to combine the streams of conventional and natural medicine, with the backup of U.S. federal and

Sometimes it isn't a matter of which perspective is better; it's a matter of which method suits you as an individual physically, emotionally, mentally, and practically.

state funding. The King County Natural Medicine Clinic combines the resources of Bastyr University, the local naturopathic medicine college, the Seattle–King County Department of Public Health, and the Community Health Centers of King County and the City of Kent. It may be one model for future integrated health care in North America and around the world. Today, many medical schools in North America have established research centers for integrative medicine and are offering academic programs in different health disciplines.

If you draw on many wellness disciplines and pay attention to different factors affecting your wellness, you benefit from diverse sources of wisdom.

Bodies, Cars, and Everyday Wellness

A lot of car owners take their vehicles seriously, and take care of them. We think of them as necessities—everyday conveniences that we depend on. Usually, we don't wait till they break down before we take them in for repairs or tune-ups. We happily learn about our cars' condition; we keep track of mileage and service schedules. We naturally accept the work and effort as part of having a car. If we treat our cars this well, why do we often wait until our bodies break down before we pay attention to them?

Our driving behaviors—starting and stopping impatiently, turning sharply, speeding angrily—not only reflect what condition we are in; they also affect our cars' present and future performance. Likewise, the ways we sit, stand, walk, react to stress, and use our bodies for work and play are important, but often neglected, factors that affect our well-being.

In terms of health communication, you are the focal point and your doctor, dentist, hairstylist, family, and friends form circles that overlap around you. Since you are the focal point, you can also be a point of influence, not just being affected by these systems, but exerting influence as well. You can take charge, moving information back and forth between the circles, creating positive change in your own immediate and more remote wellness environment.

"Draw Willingly from Any Source"

William Osler's book *The Principles and Practice of Medicine* was published in 1892, and for the next 30 years it was considered to be an authoritative medical text. Surprisingly, though it was published when much non-Western traditional medical knowledge was being ignored in Europe and North America, the book included this endorsement of multiple medical traditions: "The great minds," Osler wrote, "the great works transcend all limitations of time, of language and of race ... the full knowledge cannot be reached without drawing on supplies from lands other than one's own ... one should draw willingly from any and every source with an open mind and a stern resolve to render unto all their dues."[8]

In fact, communication links between the circles are essential. At a simple and crucial level, you need to tell all your health practitioners what medications you are taking. Seemingly harmless cross-medication such as taking Aspirin together with willow bark can lead to an overdose and a serious health risk, since willow bark contains acetylsalicylic acid, the main ingredient in Aspirin.

Expanding medical and health perspectives and then integrating wellness options maximizes wellness potentials for optimal living. The *WellnessOptions* process is a simple step-by-step one: be aware that you can choose to be well and how to be well; be informed of your health and wellness choices; develop a sense of appreciation; and practice integrating:

1. all aspects of your health, including physical, emotional, psychological, social, and environmental;
2. different medical and health perspectives;
3. treatment options and everyday healthy lifestyle practices;
4. communications among health circles around you, such as exchanges of health information between your doctor and your dentist.

The purpose of it all is not simply to practice health measures. The aim is to feel as well as you possibly can, by enjoying the process of living and maximizing all its potentials every moment.

Each chapter in the next section, "Part II: Everyday Wellness Options for Health Conditions," is devoted to one wellness condition, explaining it from different medical perspectives and listing some treatment options as well as preventive lifestyle measures for related disorders.

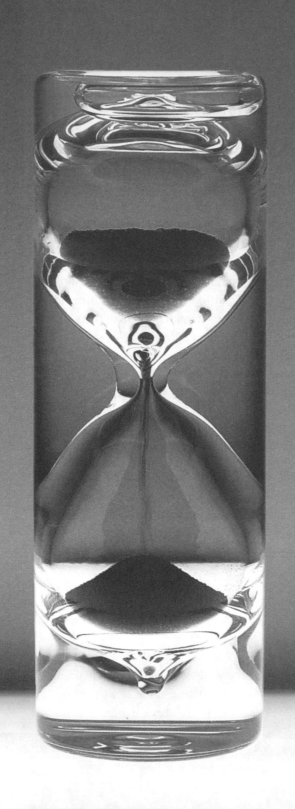

Part II

Everyday Wellness Options for Health Conditions

*Life is a continuum
And health a process
Every day,
At every age*

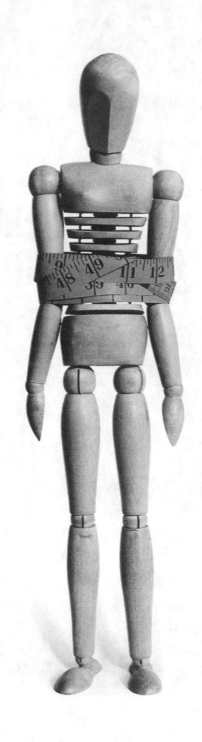

3 Who Are We?
Our Relationship to Our Bodies

Mirrors reveal only what we think we see or what we want to see.
Who we believe we are always changes our processes of living.

Body perfect, and perfectly bound

It is perhaps universally agreed that because we do not see ourselves, we need some kind of reflection, either from mirrors or from others, to give us a sense of who we are. But much like making the right decisions in life, trying to see a clear image reflected either from the mirror or from others has evolved into a rather complex affair. From simple acceptance of rippling-pond or blurry bronze-surface images, our perception of ourselves has gone far beyond a crystal-clear exchange. It has evolved from "what you see is what you get" to an intricate combination of anticipation, conditioned expectations, and multiple perspectives.

Even though we think our mirrors do not lie, those dangerous, faithful agents of reflection do not often present an accurate picture. Usually, they reveal only what we *think* we see or what we *want* to see. And who we believe we are always changes our processes of living. Sometimes these perceptions can create almost insurmountable obstacles. Since self-awareness is the fundamental point of reference to wellness and optimal living, our relationship with our body can have a profound impact on our health and well-being.

> Usually mirrors reveal only what we **think** we see or what we **want** to see. Sometimes these perceptions can create insurmountable obstacles.

Is That Me in the Mirror?

Our relationship with our bodies is complex. We love our bodies, we hate our bodies, and we focus on them to distract ourselves from other things. Sometimes we hide behind a body that takes attention away from the person we are and sometimes we blame all our problems on our bodies. And then there is the whole affair of how others see us: How do we want them to see us? How do we think they see us? And how do we expect them to see us? In a world that bombards us with information and images telling us who we are and who we should be, can we ever be who we really are? Does the mirror ever reflect our real selves?

When I was 13, I suddenly gained about 18 kilograms (40 pounds) in a matter of months. I grew from 43 kilograms (95 pounds) to 61 kilograms (135 pounds) without adding an iota to my height of 1.54 meters (five foot one). I was horrified. I became more and more withdrawn, locking myself in the bathroom for hours at a time, talking to this person in the mirror, trying to make some sense of her sudden change in appearance. When I became furious with her balloon-shaped face, I would turn on the hot water and steam up the room. She looked much better through the mist. This situation lasted for a couple of years, until I couldn't hide her behind the steam anymore. Then I started a campaign to change her. I could not accept that balloon-shaped face as my own.

During this process, I was helped most by information. I kept a notebook with me at all times and recorded my calorie intake throughout the day. As the total approached my target, I stopped eating. When I gave in, I would make a note and reduce my intake the following day. I became obsessed with calorie calculations. Perhaps I just traded an obsession with food for an obsession with calorie counting—but it worked! I got back down to 45 kilograms (100 pounds) in about a year and stayed there for a long time.

But I thought I was fat for a long time too. It would take another six years, and a life-and-death battle with illness, before I learned to look in the mirror and see me and like what I saw—flaws and fat and all. I found out that it's only when we change on the inside that we also change on the outside. After all, appearance is only the manifested representation of what and who we are.

> It's only when we change on the inside that we also change on the outside.

What is body image? Media experts and a great many non-experts have been debating this issue for years. Some researchers define body image as our direct perception of our physical appearance. Others describe it in terms of our thoughts, feelings, and attitudes about our body. For example, Peter Slade, a clinical psychologist at the Medical School of Liverpool University, England, defines body image as a "loose mental representation of the body's shape, form and size, which is influenced by a variety of historical, cultural and social, individual and biological factors, which operate over varying time spans."[1]

The debate over definition is likely to remain unresolved, but the emphasis on body-image perception in our society grows stronger all the time. According to Marius Griffin, author of *Building Blocks for Children's Body Image*, it is believed that a person's basic body image is developed by the age of six.[2] For some people, that image is set at a very early age as being less than desirable, and as life goes on, media and advertising images only reinforce the negative view. In North America, and in most developed countries, attaining the *perfect* body seems to be, more than ever, the perceived pathway to success, happiness, and total fulfillment. Both men and women have become obsessed with their looks, their weight, and their general attractiveness. The message that life canbegin only when we become thin has become a powerful one.

Because of this obsession, plastic surgery is now a commonplace procedure as we aim to increase, lift, or reduce breast size; reshape noses; redefine jawlines; and remove fat. According to Walter Erhardt, President of the American Society of Plastic Surgeons, "Cosmetic surgery has increasingly become accepted as a reasonable and, in fact, a desirable component of the total spectrum of methods people use to achieve the look they've been striving for." And, he says, "both women and men are choosing cosmetic procedures to maintain or enhance their looks."[3]

We have become a visual society, constantly bombarded by electronic and billboard advertising—an endless stream of images that is causing our sense of self-worth to migrate from the internal to the external. This flurry of visual stimuli imposes impossible standards of the "ideal" body on our psyches, reinforcing the idea that our own appearance is not measuring up. But do the people behind the ad machines really have the authority to tell us what's attractive? From an evolutionary point of view, attractiveness would have to come from genetic indicators of fertility and survivability programmed into our brains over the centuries, and the media images don't necessarily match up with the evolutionary ones. Are they really attractive or have we only been told that they're models of beauty and handsomeness?

Should I Look Like That?

How have the media played a role in perpetuating the body-image obsession and what are the consequences? A study of 4,294 commercials on American network television revealed that 1 out of every 3.8 commercials sends out some sort of "attractiveness message," telling us what is or is not acceptable.[4] This translates into 26 percent, which doesn't seem disproportionately high, but there is nothing in the remaining 74 percent to counterbalance the commercials that promote attractiveness stereotypes. And even with a minority of advertisements sending out attractiveness messages, the theme is reinforced through continuous repetition.

The Perfect Body?

Two features that receive the most attention in attractiveness studies are based on body measurements: the body mass index (BMI) and the waist/hip ratio (WHR). The body mass index is a measure of body size expressed as weight in kilograms divided by height in meters squared (kg/m^2), and the waist/hip ratio, an indicator of body shape, is measured by dividing waist size by hip size. To find out what female body types are most attractive to men, psychologists developed a series of drawings or photographs of women representing a range of WHRS: normal, underweight, and overweight.[5] Men and women were then asked to rank the photos or diagrams according to attractiveness. A number of such studies concluded that the waist/hip ratio was the major determinant of female attractiveness, the optimum WHR being 0.7—that is, a waist/hip ratio of 24.5 to 35 or 30 to 43, for example.[6] When males of several different cultures on different continents were surveyed, it was found that in all cases, they had a strong preference for females with a low WHR (0.7 to 0.8).[7]

Some evolutionary psychologists suggest that the preference of males for such females arose during the course of evolution.[8] Since evolution results from adaptations that enhance survival and ensure reproduction, this preference ought to reflect such an adaptation, and in fact, there is evidence that women with waist/hip ratios of 0.8 or more have reduced fertility. In addition, obesity in women, which can result in a higher waist/hip ratio and an elevated body mass index, is associated with a higher incidence of type 2 diabetes, infertility, gall-bladder disease, heart problems, and stroke.[9] A low waist/hip ratio may therefore be a signal that a female is likely to be more fertile and generally healthier—and this may explain why males are often more attracted to such types.

Some psychologists disagree with this interpretation, however, suggesting that men prefer women with low waist/hip ratios because they've been conditioned by stereotypical images portrayed in the West on television and in movies and magazines.[10] One study that took place in

BODY MASS INDEX (BMI)				WAIST TO HIP RATIO (WHR)		

BMI takes into account weight and height to gauge total body fat. It can be calculated as:

$$\frac{\text{body weight in kg}}{\text{height in meters x height in meters}}$$

or

$$\frac{\text{body weight in lbs x 703}}{\text{height in inches x height in inches}}$$

$$\frac{\text{waist circumference}}{\text{hip circumference}}$$

Those over 1.0 for both sexes are at a higher risk for fat-related illness, such as high blood pressure, heart disease, and diabetes.

BMI	WHO*/U.S.	CANADA	ASIA PACIFIC	AGE	17–18	40+
Normal	18.5-25	20-25	18.5-23	Male	0.9	0.98
Overweight	25-30	25-27	23-25	Female	0.8	0.9
Obese	over 30	over 27	over 25			

*World Health Organization

Peru seemed to confirm this viewpoint. In order to measure the effects of the media on perceptions of attractiveness, the study was done with a group of three hundred Matsigenka people in Peru who were isolated from Western influence. When men of this group were shown images of females, their judgment for attractiveness was based first on weight and then on waist/hip ratio, but for WHR, they favored a tubular shape, rather than a curvaceous one.[11]

Another study surveyed men of the Hadza tribe of Tanzania, a society of hunter-gatherers. When images of women of different weights and WHR were presented, the men's choice of attractiveness was based on weight alone, and heavier women were preferred. When the test images showed women of constant weight but varying WHR, they rated women with WHRs of 0.9 to 1.0 as the most attractive.[12] American university students shown the same images chose figures with WHRs of 0.7 as the most preferred. This led the authors of the study to suggest that what makes a female attractive depends on the society. In a foraging society such as that of the Hadza, women must use more physical energy to fulfill their roles, so having more fat may suggest that they would make good mates.

When other studies were done showing body pictures but with an attractive face on one set and an unattractive face on the other, facial attractiveness, which has little to do with fertility or survivability, had the edge over WHR.[13]

Another indicator of attractiveness is fluctuating asymmetry (FA), which refers to the fact that there are often slight differences in shape and size between the left and right sides of the body. In one study, computer-generated images of bodies with perfect symmetry were compared to photos of real female bodies with their faces covered.[14] When a normal asymmetrical body image was put beside a perfectly symmetrical image, both male and female judges selected the symmetrical image as being more attractive.

Clearly, a low waist/hip ratio is not a universal standard of attractiveness for women—but what about men? In a British study of male physical attractiveness, females were asked to judge pictures of 50 men who represented a range of three body measurements: BMI, WHR, and waist/chest ratio (WCR).[15] The results showed that women were most attracted by particular WCRs—a measure of upper-body shape and an indicator of physical strength. Even a small difference in WCR would

While body size is a major factor in female attractiveness, body shape seems to be more important in making men attractive to women.

result in a significant difference in men's attractiveness ratings. Men with broad chests and shoulders and narrow waists were preferred, while BMI and WHR were of little importance. So while body size is a major factor in female attractiveness, body shape seems to be more important in making men attractive to women.

Looking only at these studies, we might conclude that men and women are attracted to each other only because of physical factors. Sometimes, sex appeal even seems to be a matter of the brain computing attractiveness using a genetic-based program related to a woman's survival and reproduction abilities. But historical and social components also come into play—making different body shapes and sizes attractive in different eras. It has been suggested that the frail, pale, and sickly look cultivated by many British and North American women of the Victorian period corresponded with their weakness in political and economic spheres. Paradoxically, however, contemporary women, who now make up a large part of the workforce and hold significant political roles, are considered to be most attractive when they are thin—a look still usually equated with frailty and weakness.

The Things We Do for Appearances

Individual preference is often overshadowed in Western society by external, visual influences based on a "look" that we have been told is appealing, through media and advertising bombardments. Unfortunately, our measures of attractiveness, right or wrong, also affect many judgments we make in life—going beyond our preferences for mates. One research group from Michigan State University examined 68 studies on the subject of attractiveness.[16] Conducted over 40 years with more than 5,000 subjects, the studies found that, for the most part, good-looking people were rated as being more capable than their less attractive peers. Thinness, one of the major components related to attractiveness in the studies, was often associated with success, control, and higher socio-economic status. With this much value being placed on looks—not just in sexual terms but also in relation to social position—it is little wonder that people in Western society are willing to sacrifice a lot to acquire physical attractiveness.

One body image study reported in *Women's Own* magazine in Britain indicated that 1 in 12 women (i.e., 8 percent) would give up a limb for the perfect body image, 15 percent would part with their entire spouse, and 30 percent would give up their life savings.[17] What is more, earlier

A 4,000-reader survey published in **Psychology Today** revealed that 15 percent of women and 11 percent of men would trade more than 5 years of their lives to achieve their weight targets.

results of a 4,000-reader survey published in *Psychology Today* showed that 15 percent of women and 11 percent of men would trade more than 5 years of their lives to achieve their weight targets.[18] *Five years of their lives.* Although it is widely believed that obesity can lead to a number of health problems, this statistic brings to light a dangerous undercurrent in the obsession with weight that goes far beyond any concern about health. In fact, in some cases, weight obsession itself can be detrimental to overall health and well-being.

Body Image Disorders and Extremes

Eating Disorders: Anorexia Nervosa and Bulimia Nervosa. The first medical case history of anorexia nervosa was published in 1689 by an English doctor, Richard Morton, but it was not until 1868 that Sir William Gull gave it this name, which means "nervous loss of appetite."[19] Those suffering from anorexia lose visible amounts of weight, eat very little, claim that they are not hungry, and diet when they are not overweight. Women with anorexia nervosa may also lose their menstrual cycle. Signs of bulimia nervosa (binge eating, then dieting) include frequent fluctuations in weight, purging such as vomiting and laxative use, and frequent fasting or excessive exercise. Bulimia was classified as a distinct disorder by the American Psychiatric Association in 1980.

Although men and women who suffer from eating disorders are similar in many ways, most females with anorexia or bulimia will diet and purge to lose weight, while men are more likely to engage in compulsive exercise. A 1999 study also found that men develop eating disorders later than women: men at age 20, on average, and women at age 17, on average.[20] A number of researchers have found evidence indicating that men with eating disorders are more likely to be involved in an occupation or sport in which weight control affects performance, such as wrestling, jockeying, rowing, gymnastics, running, dancing, or weightlifting.[21] In an issue of the *American Journal of Psychiatry,* Woodside and colleagues from the University of Toronto also concluded that men with eating disorders are more likely than other men to suffer from psychiatric illnesses, such as depression or anxiety, and to report feeling unhappy in their lives.[22] The same is true of women with eating disorders.

In the past two decades, there has been a significant increase in the number of men seeking help for serious eating disorders such as anorexia

> Although men and women who suffer from eating disorders are similar in many ways, most females will diet and purge to lose weight, while men are more likely to engage in compulsive exercise.

Bible Story May Include First Report of Anorexia

The biblical story of Hannah, the mother of the prophet Samuel, may describe the first documented case of anorexia nervosa and its associated infertility. In an article in the January 1998 issue of *Fertility and Sterility*, physician Isaac Schiff, chief of the Vincent Memorial Obstetrics and Gynecology Service at Massachusetts General Hospital, points out that Hannah was so unhappy about her inability to conceive that she did not eat.[23]

and bulimia nervosa. An editorial in the April 2001 issue of the *American Journal of Psychiatry* suggests that the prevalence of eating disorders among men in the United States may be as high as 16 percent.[24] Among men, homosexual orientation seems to be a risk factor for the development of an eating disorder or body dissatisfaction. While 2 to 6 percent of North American men are homosexual, gay males account for an estimated 26 to 33 percent of all male eating-disorder patients in the United States. Numerous studies have also demonstrated that gay men have a higher rate of dieting, bulimic symptoms, and body dissatisfaction than heterosexual men[25]—probably because the male gay subculture places so much emphasis on the ideal of a lean and muscular body.

The Adonis Complex. While women usually believe they are too fat, men often believe that they are too small or scrawny and obsessively pursue "bigness." Massachusetts psychologist Roberto Olivardia and his colleagues coined the term "muscle dysmorphia" to describe this pathological preoccupation with muscularity.[26] The condition was later called the "Adonis complex" after the Greek god renowned for his beauty. Men with muscle dysmorphia worry that they look too small, even though they may actually be quite hefty. In addition to exercising compulsively, even to an unhealthy extreme, they frequently use and abuse anabolic steroids, which can have negative physical and psychiatric consequences. Most men with this disorder say that the preoccupation with their bodies and exercise regimes has led to intense psychological distress, severe problems at work, and problems in their relationships. They also seem to be more likely to have current or previous psychiatric illnesses, including mood disorders, anxiety, and eating disorders. But it is difficult to treat muscle dysmorphia because men often do not admit they have a problem. Once a person admits their condition, however, they may be helped by cognitive behavioral therapy.

> While women usually believe they are too fat, men often believe that they are too small or scrawny and obsessively pursue "bigness."

A Man Like GI Joe

Over the past 30 years, the bodies of male action-figure toys have changed in ways that seem to reflect changing ideal body images. In fact, one study has found that GI Joe and *Star Wars* figures have become so lean and muscular that no man could achieve that ideal today "without massive doses of steroids."[27]

When a Good Part Looks Bad. Apotemnophiles want to have one or more of their normal, healthy limbs removed in order to gain a sense of "wholeness." They feel the limb is not a part of them, and in rare cases, apotemnophiles have persuaded surgeons to perform amputations. Some have even attempted removal themselves.[28] Despite the identification of this condition more than two decades ago by Johns Hopkins University psychologists Taylor and Money, few scientific studies have been conducted on the problem, and it is yet to be classified as psychiatric.[29]

Straight and Narrow. Physician Steven Bratman, author of the book *Health Food Junkies,* coined the term "orthorexia nervosa" (from the Greek *orthos,* meaning straight or correct) to define a new type of eating disorder.[30] "Orthorexics" puritanically stick to a diet that may consist of a very narrow range of health foods. For instance, they may eat only raw beans for a while.

It might seem strange to classify an obsession with seemingly healthy food as a disorder. But physiologically necessary nutrients such as calcium and protein might be missing from an orthorexic diet, leading to anemia and osteoporosis. And on the psychological front, it's unhealthy to demonstrate an intense obsession with obtaining and preparing healthy foods to the degree that social activities are avoided and anxiety results from being unable to follow a strict regimen. Fixating on food may be a way for a person to avoid dealing with deeper emotional issues.

Diet Magic and Off-the-Shelf Weight Management

Fixating on food may be a way for a person to avoid dealing with deeper emotional issues.

Over a 30-year period—from 1959 to 1988—the female body ideal as represented in the centerfold of *Playboy* magazine became thinner and thinner and thinner. This influenced, or perhaps reflected, the standard that North America set for women. A study of *Playgirl* magazines from 1973 to 1997 revealed the opposite side of the coin.[31] It analyzed the heights and weights of male models, which followed a pattern of more "dense" and muscular bodies, with progressively less fat.

With women trying to look thinner and men attempting to build up their muscles and get rid of fat, it's not surprising that diet magic is for sale everywhere and all the time. Walk into almost any bookstore and you will find entire sections devoted to weight management. Cruise the Internet and you will be bombarded with site advertisements for diet supplements and quick tips on how to "eat for looks." Turn on the TV, watch the "beautiful people" strutting their stuff, and you'd think weight management was as easy as drinking a delicious chocolate shake once a day. Dieting is a multimillion-dollar industry that hooks into everyone's desire for a "quick fix."

But how effective are these diets, and what are the benefits and risks associated with them? Contrary to the advice of most registered dietitians, a lot of fad diets overemphasize one particular type of food. The guiding principle of good nutrition is to eat a balanced diet, including choices from all the major food groups. Because no one type of food has all the nutrients necessary for good health, some fad dieters risk nutritional deficiencies.

If fad diets don't appeal, over-the-counter diet aids are ready and waiting. Another entire industry built on body-image problems is the selling of remedies and various treatments often touted as "magic solutions." These should all be examined carefully and in some cases approached with extreme caution.

> Because no one type of food has all the nutrients necessary for good health, a fad dieter risks developing nutritional deficiencies.

Emotional Issues: Cause or Effect?

Eating disorders and their related health risks reflect a disorder in society as a whole—our unhealthy obsession with body image. In a supposedly advanced civilization, shouldn't spiritual enlightenment take precedence over appearance as a sign of human evolution? Our reliance on, and obsession with, our body image as a source of personal fulfillment and standard of judgment for social status points in the opposite direction. Why have we taken this route as a society? Perhaps because we often look to the outside world and others for acceptance, respect, and love. And these all seem to be conditional upon our compliance with artificially imposed standards of body image and attractiveness. We strive to meet the expectations of the stereotyping news media in order to feel fit for companionship and caring.

Living in a society that often says, "You are not good enough," we put pressure on ourselves to be beautiful and thin and lose our ability to simply enjoy living as human beings.

The Bottom Line

During the past two decades, the prevalence of "overweight" children has doubled among U.S. children and almost tripled among adolescents.

Besides enhancing body image, sensible weight management does bring important health benefits. Recent results of the Framingham Heart Study (research supported by the U.S. National Heart, Lung, and Blood Institute or NHLBI) that were reported in the August 2002 issue of *The New England Journal of Medicine* showed that for each increment of one point in the body mass index (BMI), there is a 5-percent increase in heart-failure risk in men and a 7-percent increase in women.[32] The effect of BMI on heart failure is independent of age, sex, smoking status, alcohol consumption, or the presence of diabetes or even heart-valve problems. Compared to individuals with normal weight, the risk of heart failure (a condition in which the heart cannot pump enough blood through the body) is double in obese women and 90 percent higher in obese men.

"Overweight" and "obesity" are defined in the table on page 37.

   In spite of these obvious ill effects, obesity and weight problems are so common in North America that they have become a serious health issue. Claude Lenfant, director of the U.S. National Heart, Lung, and Blood Institute, puts it this way: "Obesity has reached epidemic proportions in the U.S., and it is increasing." In 2001, an estimated 61 percent of adult Americans between the ages of 10 and 74 were either overweight (34 percent) or obese (27 percent), and 48 percent of Canadians were reported to be either overweight (19 percent) or obese (29 percent). In the United States, an estimated 50 million people were obese. An estimated 13 percent of American children aged 6 to 11 were overweight, and 14 percent of adolescents aged 12 to 19 were also overweight. During the past two decades, the prevalence of overweight children has doubled among American children and tripled among adolescents. Weight management at any age is an important component of wellness and health. But fad diets and medications are far less likely to produce healthy, balanced, and long-term results than proper, regular nutrition and exercise.

Cosmetic Surgery

Eating disorders and other conditions that result in severe health problems are definitely regarded as pathological behaviors. But when it comes to concerns about body image, the line between acceptable care and obsession is sometimes blurry. Take cosmetic surgery, for instance. More and more people are going under the knife to improve their appearance. Does that mean we care more about our bodies or is body image a growing social obsession?

An article in the *British Medical Journal* has noted that patients who request cosmetic surgery are usually "normal individuals but with a heightened consciousness about their looks."[33] Liposuction, breast augmentation, eyelid surgery, facelifts, nose reshaping, and tummy tucks top the list for women, while men tend to go for nose reshaping, skin laser treatment, and hair transplants. And these procedures are expensive. According to a Canadian price list posted on the Web site of a cosmetic surgery center in Ontario, a new set of cheekbones costs about $3,000, a facelift will set you back between $5,000 and $9,500, and liposuction procedures carry a price tag of $1,500 to $4,000.[34] But the expense has not stopped consumers from heading into operating rooms to look better. According to U.S. national plastic surgery statistics, almost 2.7 million reconstructive and cosmetic procedures were performed in 2001, and certified plastic surgeons performed operations on more than 1.3 million Americans—an increase of 227 percent from 1992 figures.[35]

If concerns about looks are any indication, the number of cosmetic surgeries will continue to grow. A recent survey of 30,000 people found that 93 percent of women and 82 percent of men care about their appearance and work to improve it. In this 1997 study, researcher D.M. Garner found body dissatisfaction to be "increasing at a faster rate than ever before among men and women."[36]

Is it a good idea to go for cosmetic surgery if you are persistently unhappy about your appearance? This is a personal decision, but it should not be made without considering all foreseeable consequences. As a reference, here are three examples of operations that had satisfactory results—but were not without complications.

Case 1: Breast Reduction. The patient, now 26 years old, first thought of breast reduction when she was 17. At the time she decided to go for surgery, she was 18, weighed 50 kilograms (110 pounds), was 1.57 metres (five foot two) tall, and had trouble fitting into a size 38C bra. The procedure lasted four hours, required 175 stitches, and three months of very painful recovery. Severe swelling and bruising also brought on short-term depression. In the longer term, there was some severe scarring, though the patient felt relief from the back pain experienced before the operation. A year and a half later, a benign tumor was removed from her left breast, and doctors have expressed concern that this may have been linked to the procedure, but this is not conclusive.[37]

"Cosmetic surgery is often a trade-off between good results and potential for problems."
—Robert Yoho, physician, **A New Body in One Day**

Cosmetic Surgery Preferences: He wants, She wants

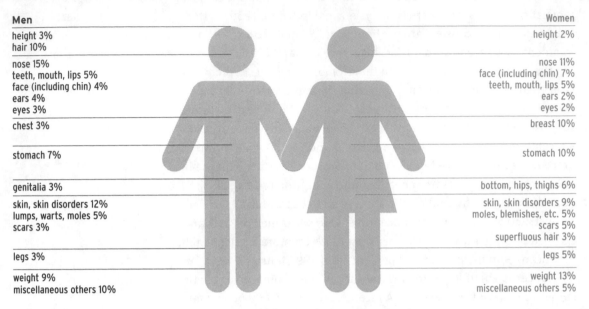

Men	Women
height 3%	height 2%
hair 10%	
nose 15%	nose 11%
teeth, mouth, lips 5%	face (including chin) 7%
face (including chin) 4%	teeth, mouth, lips 5%
ears 4%	ears 2%
eyes 3%	eyes 2%
chest 3%	breast 10%
stomach 7%	stomach 10%
genitalia 3%	bottom, hips, thighs 6%
skin, skin disorders 12%	skin, skin disorders 9%
lumps, warts, moles 5%	moles, blemishes, etc. 5%
scars 3%	scars 5%
	superfluous hair 3%
legs 3%	legs 5%
weight 9%	weight 13%
miscellaneous others 10%	miscellaneous others 5%

Data from Harris and Carr, "Prevalence of Concern about Physical Appearance in the General Population," British Journal of Plastic Surgery 54 (2001), 223.

Case 2: Facelift. The patient involved in this operation was 52 years old and had been unhappy with the effects of aging since her 40s. After the operation, her face was swollen, bruised, and very sore. During her three-week recovery, she hid behind dark glasses and went overseas. In her case, no long-term complications were reported.[38]

Case 3: Breast Enlargement. Now 53 years old, this patient first thought of breast enlargement when she was in her 20s. She had breast-implant surgery when she was 41. The patient felt that the procedure was not painful, but shortly after her surgery, news broke about a possible link between silicone implants and breast cancer (since disputed). So the patient had the silicone implants removed and replaced with saline implants, which she found to be too hard and unnatural. She then had those replaced with smaller saline implants. In retrospect, she wishes she had done more research—especially on advances in implant options.[39]

Cosmetic surgery can provide the quick fix that many of us are longing for, but at a substantial cost, both financially and physically. Robert Yoho, physician, who has a cosmetic surgery practice in California and is co-author of the book *A New Body in One Day*, confirms this caveat: "A doctor who claims that he never has [complications] is either inexperienced or a liar. Cosmetic surgery is often a trade-off between good results and potential for problems. Patients should understand the facts and plan for the best and the worst possibilities. If you feel as though you couldn't possibly survive a long hassle with a difficult recovery, you should not have cosmetic surgery."[40]

Unconscious Attractions

In the end, though, there may be no universal standard for attractiveness. Looking like a Miss or Mister Universe may not bring Mister or Ms. Right into your life after all. Perhaps individual preference has always been the real, natural determinant, with individual personality and chemistry playing key roles. For example, there is evidence that the nose may play a greater part than we might think in determining who is attractive to us. It did for Napoleon Bonaparte. In a famous love letter, he once beseeched Josephine not to bathe because he was on his way home. And, in fact,

> The nose may play a greater role than we might think in determining who is attractive to us.

Sniffing Out a Mate: Body Odor Attractions

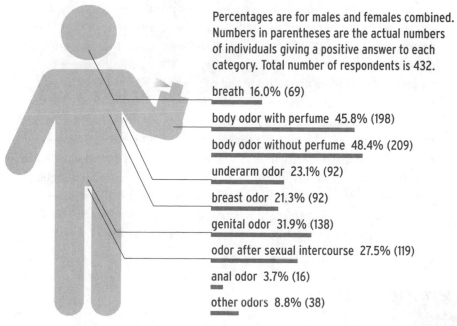

Percentages are for males and females combined. Numbers in parentheses are the actual numbers of individuals giving a positive answer to each category. Total number of respondents is 432.

breath 16.0% (69)

body odor with perfume 45.8% (198)

body odor without perfume 48.4% (209)

underarm odor 23.1% (92)

breast odor 21.3% (92)

genital odor 31.9% (138)

odor after sexual intercourse 27.5% (119)

anal odor 3.7% (16)

other odors 8.8% (38)

Data from I. Ebberfeld, Botenstoffe der Liebe (Transmitters of Love; 1998).

studies have shown that body odors are forms of communication, and have a significant effect on human attraction and sexual arousal.[41] In essence, body odor (BO) is the result of molecules released as waste by trillions of bacteria as the bacteria feed on fat products eliminated from our skin. The key component of BO is (E)-3-methyl-2-hexenoic acid.

But Napoleon was not the only one to understand this earthy encouragement to love. In her book *Botenstoffe der Liebe* (*Transmitters of Love*), German researcher Ingelore Ebberfeld reports that 76 percent of respondents surveyed in Germany (273 women and 159 men, aged 15 to 84) were sexually stimulated by specific body odors. Both men and women agreed that body odor without perfume is the most stimulating, and body odor with perfume ranked second. For men, genital odor (43.4 percent) ranked third, while women put body odor after intercourse (26 percent) in third place.[42] Ironically, we spend a fortune eliminating body odor—scrubbing, deodorizing, and disguising it with costly scents.

As important as our noses are, some chemical messages bypass them altogether. Some molecules, referred to as *pheromones*, trigger certain patterns of animal behavior, including sexual attraction, when they are detected by an organ in the nasal cavity called the vomeronasal organ (VNO). We do perceive pheromones, and are affected by them even though we are not conscious of them as smell.[43] Sometimes, these unconscious effects are subtle yet sophisticated. Researcher Claus Wedekind and his team at the University of Bern, Switzerland, discovered that the more dissimilar men's genes known as MHC were to their own, the more women seemed to be attracted to the men's body odor.[44] MHC stands for a group of genes called *major histocompatibility complexes*, which are unique to each person. It's the function of this group of genes to recognize and reject everything that is "non-self." This subconscious recognition of dissimilarity in MHC is thought to be associated with mate selection, which is often determined by the fact that dissimilar genetic traits combine to create evolutionary advantages. Unlike other studies, these have shown that the complex process of human attraction and sexual arousal may in fact be an extremely individual affair.

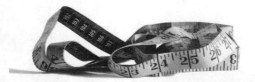

Live a life without having to measure up to a tape.

Putting the "Self" Back in the Image

Simone de Beauvoir once said that "to lose confidence in one's body is to lose confidence in one's self." But what do we really lose first? Is it confidence in the body or confidence in the self? We are the ones who form our perceptions of our bodies. Depending on what we think of ourselves, we can look in the mirror and see someone entirely different from the person we really are. Perhaps we should stop gazing at the looking glass to check for appearances and discrepancies from the status quo. Perhaps we should take that moment in our morning routine to see how unique our nose is and appreciate how it has taken human evolution 3.5 billion years to give us a sense of smell!

We also bear striking similarities to everyone else on the planet: most of us feel compassion, empathy, love, and joy. We are all human. The beauty of our souls, the biological ingenuity in our bodies, and creativity in our minds are what make us who we really are. Faces and bodies are roadways between others and ourselves. To judge these roadways in terms of media-promoted body images is to disregard the self.

Yet, who is immune to the temptation of judging others by their looks? As we are confronted with the everyday injustices that occur because of this judgment, we have to wonder if a better balance can be reached. Placing too much value on the importance of body image is artificial and pretentious, but denying the effect of that image on our day-to-day well-being is also unrealistic. We would perhaps be happier if we could find our own balance between the two extremes—aware of and caring for our bodies as part of ourselves, but not accepting the unrealistic and even damaging norms imposed by a media-hyped society.

In an age when so many methods are available to give us a new look, our choices are not really about what we can or cannot change on the outside. The important options are: What do we *need* to change, both inside and out? Into *what* do we change? *For what and for whom* do we change? And at *what price*—in dollars, health, and wellness? After all, what is more important: Your body? Your body image? Or you? Who is in control?

The simplest logic is this: the body houses you, you and your body are inseparable, and together, you project an appearance. The body image reflected in your mirror represents what you are and how well you are physically, emotionally, mentally, and spiritually. Loving that image and the totality it represents is the basis of well-being and optimal living.

> Faces and bodies are roadways between others and ourselves. To judge these roadways in terms of media-promoted body images is to disregard the self, but denying the effect of body image on our day-to-day well-being is unrealistic.

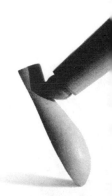

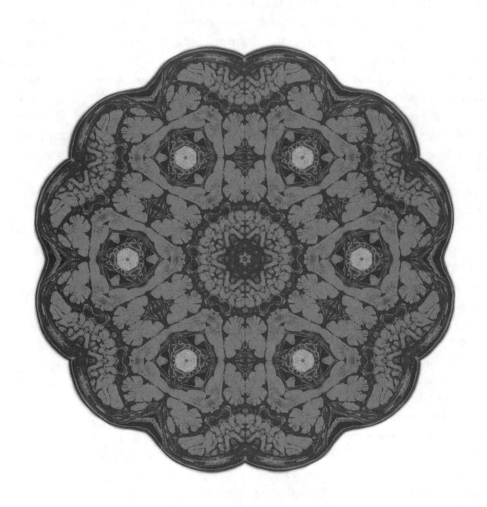

4 How Are You?
Feeling Bad, Feeling Good

Let me think: was I the same when I got up this morning?
I almost think I can remember feeling a little different.
But if I'm not the same, the next question is, Who in the world am I?
—Alice in Lewis Carroll's *Alice's Adventures in Wonderland*

Kaleidoscopic image of a colorized brain scan

The diversity and intensity of our feelings can be wonderfully fulfilling or frenetically frightening. As they ebb and flow, our moods can also be confusing—both to the people around us and to ourselves. Good and rewarding feelings encourage us to repeat certain activities, while bad feelings serve to warn us against what we need to correct in our lives. Both positive and negative feelings are natural parts of life and necessary for our survival. A constant stream of feelings mirrors what goes on inside of us and outside of us, and reflects the relationship between the two. When a certain feeling is sustained for a while, it is defined as a mood.

Let's take a look at a simple, everyday life incident to see how fleeting feeling can be in nature and what a good or bad feeling may consist of.

It was a quiet morning. My 16-month-old son had just finished his bottle and was playing contentedly in his playpen. I was totally absorbed in the magazine I was reading. We were both in a pleasant mood.

Then he held onto the rail and stood up. The abrupt movement jolted me. This was the first time he'd stood up unaided. Usually he just sat or moved around in his walking chair—he had never even attempted to crawl. The pediatrician had assured us that one day he would start walking, so there was no need to worry. After many months of anxious longing, the walking day seemed finally to have arrived. I was so happy!

Kneeling down next to the playpen, I watched him intensely. I would capture every movement and every moment of this first walk. He caught on to my excitement and started to jump up and down. I said, "Good! Good! Good!" and after I repeated it 20-odd times, he was still jumping up and down. I started to coach him: "Okay, walk now ... It's okay, you can walk now." I got up and paced back and forth, trying to show him how to walk. He stopped jumping and looked at me, confused.

I bent down and tried to move him along the rail to make him walk. After a few frustrated attempts, he started to cry, and my heart sank. As I picked him up, it suddenly dawned on me: I couldn't, for the life of me, remember when I started to walk. Healthy babies always walk when they are ready. It was really my problem, not his. I held him close and told him everything was fine.

After a while, we returned to our respective activities and the neutral state of calmness. About two months later, he got up one day and started to walk. I didn't have to teach him.

What are some of the feelings involved here? Within a matter of minutes, this mother covered many elements of the feeling spectrum: quietness, surprise, anticipation, excitement, elation, anxiety, confusion, disappointment, impatience, astonishment, guilt, love, calm. It's almost miraculous that her feelings and moods went back to a neutral state after all that upheaval.

What are some of the contributing elements to the mood changes?

→ genetic predisposition (determining how readily, how easily, and how deeply we feel)

→ conditioned predisposition (a learned inclination to restrain feelings or to feel freely)

→ physiological condition (e.g., people are always more easily agitated when they aren't getting enough sleep)

→ neurological activities (perception, processing, and response procedures taking place in the brain and the central nervous system)

→ psycho-sociological factors (the interplay of emotional, psychological, and social influences)

→ cultural expectations (learned standards of what is acceptable and satisfactory with regard to knowing and expressing feelings)

→ interpersonal relationships (e.g., feelings aroused by family members are different from those evoked by strangers, even if the triggering event is similar)

→ environmental factors (e.g., feelings expressed in a home setting may differ from those expressed in other social or physical settings)

→ external events, which trigger certain emotions[1]

Genetics seem to play a key role in determining our feelings. But even simple variables such as what we eat, whether we are exposed to enough sunlight and are active during the day, and whether we have had enough sleep all have an effect on us, and the list goes on and on.

> Genetics play a key role in determining our feelings.

A Good Mood: What Is Its Physiological Basis?

As neuroscience unravels the mystery of the brain, we are beginning to understand the physiology of the brain and how it helps determine good moods and depression. The circuitry that underlies good feelings and rewarding responses starts far down in the brain stem. It then goes upward to the brain control center—the nucleus accumbens—and from there nerve impulses project upward and outward to the emotional

What we eat and drink affects our brain chemistry, which, in turn, alters our appetite and nutritional state—and this has a profound influence on our daily moods.

brain center and ascend to the frontal cortex, the brain area associated with memory and thinking.

It is estimated that the human brain contains about 100 billion nerve cells, or neurons. The cerebral cortex (the two hemispheres of the brain) alone contains more than 30 billion nerve cells, an equivalent of 100,000 neurons in each cubic millimeter. These neurons are connected through an intricate electrical and chemical intercommunication network. Between neurons, there are tiny gaps called synapses. It's estimated that the neurons in the cerebral cortex can establish about 60 trillion synapses, which means each neuron is capable of establishing about 2,000 synapses.

Brain chemicals called neurotransmitters are stored at our nerve endings, and when needed or stimulated, they are released and act as messengers. By crossing the gaps, or synapses, between neurons through an electrical-chemical-electrical sequence, neurotransmitters carry messages from cell to cell along nerve fibers. Changes in the availability and concentration of neurotransmitters working in the gaps have a direct impact on the carrying of brain chemical messages and therefore a direct effect on mood.

The most important brain chemicals for feelings and mood are the neurotransmitters known as norepinephrine, dopamine, and serotonin.

Norepinephrine is responsible for mood changes, alertness, and stamina. Dopamine is a feel-good brain chemical that regulates muscle movement, attention span, and motivation and is associated with eating, sex, and many other pleasurable states. Serotonin controls sleep, appetite, pain sensitivity, and the processing of sensory perceptions such as touch and sight. Imbalances and low concentration levels of these messengers can result in a range of mood disorders and behavioral problems. But fortunately, discoveries about the workings of the brain have taught us that there are things we can do—or stop doing—in ordinary everyday life to improve mood and decrease feelings of depression.

Most anti-depression medications and remedies work on the basis of either increasing the release of these neurotransmitters or blocking their re-uptake. The end result is increased availability or concentration of certain neurotransmitters in gaps between brain cells.

Feel-Good Physiology

Neurotransmitters are the major brain chemicals stored in nerve endings. They are released when needed or stimulated. By crossing the gap between brain cells (neurons), they send chemical messages from cell to cell along the nerve fibers.

Changes in the availability of neurotransmitters working in the gaps between nerve cells have a direct effect on mood. When nerve impulses stimulate the release of stored neurotransmitters into the gap, some of them are attached to the next neuron and they pass along a signal or message. Others are re-absorbed back to storage (the re-uptake process). A deficiency of feel-good neurotransmitters and their stimulation can result in depression.

More feel-good neurotransmitters can be produced with food or drugs. Or the re-absorption (re-uptake) of feel-good transmitters can be blocked, leaving more of them working in the gaps to stimulate their adjacent brain cells.

The same basic model applies to all three major feel-good neurotransmitters that regulate mood and behavior: norepinephrine, serotonin, and dopamine (the "reward" neurotransmitter).

All addictive substances also work on the same model, leading to increased availability of dopamine in the synapses. This, in turn, increases rewarding stimulation of the brain. Heroin, for example, increases dopamine release, and cocaine inhibits its re-uptake. In both cases, this artificially enhanced dopamine activity produces mood elevation and euphoria. As the body becomes accustomed to the intensity of the reward feeling, greater and greater amounts of addictives are needed to produce the same pleasurable effects. Attempts to stop bring on more craving as withdrawal symptoms take place.

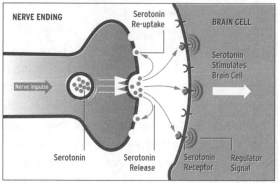 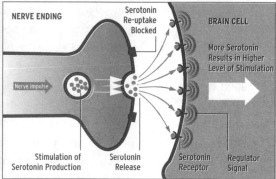

Left panel: Represents a synapse where neurotransmitters work to pass along signals. Nerve impulses stimulate the release of stored serotonin into the gap. Some of the serotonin attach to the adjacent neuron and transmit signals. Some of the serotonin is reabsorbed back to storage. A deficiency of serotonin and its stimulation can result in depression.

Right panel: Shows the effects of some drugs in correcting a deficiency of serotonin. More serotonin can be produced through dietary means or drugs. Or, certain drugs known as selective serotonin re-uptake inhibitors (SSRI) can block the re-uptake of serotonin, leaving more serotonin available to stimulate the adjacent brain cell.

Lifestyle Factors Affecting Mood

LIFESTYLE HABITS	PHYSIOLOGICAL AND/OR PSYCHOLOGICAL EFFECTS	RECOMMENDATIONS
Cigarette Smoking	Increases cortisol, reduces production and the availability of serotonin	Limit or stop
Alcohol	Depresses the central nervous system, reduces neurotransmitter levels, disturbs sleep, and causes blood sugar problems	Set limits; do not overdrink
Caffeine	At intakes exceeding 10.5 U.S. grains per day, caffeine is linked to depression	Monitor intake; set limits
Carbohydrates and Simple sugars	Disrupts blood sugar control and reduces insulin sensitivity	Set limits of intake
Exercise	Physical activity reduces symptoms of anxiety and depression	Combine strength training with regular aerobic activity

Our Lifestyles: How They Affect Mood

What we eat and drink affects our brain chemistry, and this, in turn, alters our appetite and nutritional state. Nutritional deficiencies and diet imbalance can lead to, or perpetuate, bad feelings and depression. People who follow diets extremely low in carbohydrates, for example, may be depleted of brain chemicals such as the feel-good neurotransmitter serotonin and the amino acid tryptophan, which is needed to synthesize neurotransmitters.[2] These people may be at risk of depression.

Cigarette smoking is also linked to depression because of its effect on brain chemistry. The nicotine in cigarettes increases the production of cortisol from the adrenal glands. These elevated levels of cortisol depress a key enzyme in the body responsible for the synthesis of "feel-good" serotonin. Besides reducing the production of serotonin, high cortisol levels make the brain less sensitive to the serotonin that is available.[3]

See Chapter 8, "Gourmet Wellness," for more on food and mood.

Like cigarette smoking, alcohol contributes to depression for a variety of reasons. It depresses the central nervous system (CNS), and increases the amount of circulating cortisol, reducing the availability and concentration of all neurotransmitters needed to ward off depression. Alcohol also affects blood sugar control and can cause episodes of hypoglycemia (low blood sugar), which might put additional pressure on an already stressed central nervous system.[4]

The impact of caffeine consumption on mood is not as clear-cut as the effects of cigarette smoking and alcohol consumption. In small quantities, caffeine can be stimulating, allowing for better concentration and greater alertness, but daily consumption of more than 700 milligrams (10.5 Imperial grains) of caffeine (about five cups of coffee) is linked to depression.[5] Considering that caffeine can be obtained from a variety of sources (coffee, tea, and soft drinks), it is best to monitor intake closely.

Activity and the lack of it have also been linked to mood changes. Regular activities and physical exercise can decrease anxiety and depression.

Bright light also has a profound impact on mood. About 25 percent of the world's population suffers from some degree of the mild version of a winter depression known as seasonal affective disorder (SAD), and about 5 percent suffer from the more severe form. "Winter blues" is not an imaginary illness. It can affect anyone, but women sufferers outnumber men two to one, and young people are also at risk. The average age of onset is 23, but SAD can also affect children and young people between the ages of 9 and 19 years at a prevalence rate of up to 5.5 percent. People who work night shifts are vulnerable to the disorder.[6] Two causes for SAD have been suggested. One links the problem to melatonin, a substance produced by the pineal gland in the brain that promotes sleepiness. Bright light causes the gland to stop producing this substance, but on dull winter days, especially indoors, there may not be enough light to trigger this wake-up process.[7] Strong evidence has also linked exposure to bright light with the increased production of serotonin. Although many neurotransmitters are associated with depression, serotonin is the only one implicated in depression that shows a distinct seasonal pattern of metabolism in normal humans. In temperate climates, our bodies' serotonin levels are generally lowest in winter and spring and highest in summer and fall.[8]

Depression is an episodic illness, which is especially disabling because its onset is gradual. It may take years before a person realizes he or she is suffering from depression.

Seasonal Affective Disorder (SAD) Symptoms

Sleep disorders	hypersomnia but still fatigued, cannot get out of bed, need naps during the day
Cravings	for carbohydrates, which lead to weight gain
Feeling depressed	despair, misery, persistently sad, anxious, empty, guilty, unable to complete normal tasks, and feelings of hopelessness; some people become suicidal
Family and social problems	avoidance of social situations, irritability, loss of libido, loss of pleasure in previously enjoyable activities
Chronic lethargy	too tired to cope, every simple thing seems to need an effort
Physical symptoms	body aches and pains, joint pain or stomach problems, lowered resistance to infection
Behavioral problems	especially in young people, declined creativity, frequent mood changes, anxious and irritable; irritability may even turn into eruptive violence

It seems that the more we learn, the more we discover how many factors affect our lives and the way we feel: heredity, lifestyle, environment, economics, what we eat and drink, who we are with, how we were treated, when it rains, when the sun comes out. Everything has a bearing on how our feel-good system works. Because of this complexity, diseases associated with the feel-good system, such as clinical depression and addiction, are among the most elusive and challenging problems to medical science.

Depression as a Mood Disorder

Mood disorders are called affective disorders because they involve, in addition to mood, other symptoms generally affecting our overall sense of well-being.[9] Our vitality, self-esteem, motivation, sex drive, and appetite are all affected by any mood disorder.

Depression, the most common mood disorder, exacts a heavy human and economic toll. It is the leading cause of disability worldwide, affecting 121 million people. According to the United Nations World Health Organization (who), depression is expected to be the second-most-debilitating disease in the world after heart disease by the year 2020. As this trend continues, depression will become one of the leading causes of death, taking more lives than traffic accidents, chronic lung disease, or aids.[10] Surprising as it may seem, depression is more disabling than hypertension, diabetes, chronic lung disease, or arthritis. Only acute heart disease in general requires more hospitalization days than depression.[11] Approximately 80 percent of suicides are related to mood disorders, and more than 90 percent of all suicide is related to depression and substance abuse. About 15 percent of patients with recurrent major depression kill themselves.[12]

No one understands exactly how or why some people become depressed when others do not. Current thinking suggests that some people have a genetic predisposition to the condition.[13] Anyone can experience depression, however, through life-event stresses such as the loss of a loved one, financial struggles, job changes, a difficult relationship, or health problems. Sometimes apparently insignificant influences such as diet, sleep, or seasonal changes can also precipitate a depressed state.

Mental Disorder Statistics

According to Statistics Canada, during a 12-month period from 1999 to 2000, the total of all Canadian hospitalizations for mental disorders came to more than 9 million days. Depression and manic depression, the most common types of mental disorder, affect more than 3 million Canadians. Depression can occur at any age, but it is 4 to 5 times higher among those aged 18 to 44, with about 40 percent of depressed patients in their 20s.[14] An estimated 80 percent of suicides are associated with mood disorders, and youth suicide rates worldwide are increasing so alarmingly that youths under 25 are now the highest suicide risk group in 30 percent of all countries. Youth suicide rates are highest in Russia, followed by Lithuania and Canada. Most suicides in Canada are among males aged 25 to 44.[15]

Symptoms and Concurrent Disorders

Depression is an episodic illness, which is especially disabling because its onset is gradual. It may take years before a person realizes he or she is suffering from depression. The disorder can deceive both patient and medical professionals because no specific localized symptom announces its arrival. Life events or other medical conditions may also camouflage symptoms, and the illness may take on many confusing forms.

Depressed people often feel slowed down, disinterested in life, sad, or irritable, and they have feelings of emptiness, hopelessness, and worthlessness. They may yell at people or get frustrated by situations they would normally not find upsetting. Sleep and appetite problems are common, and they may have difficulty in concentrating, thinking clearly, or remembering things. Depression may also manifest itself in the form of physical problems such as headaches and indigestion, and severe cases of depression can result in psychotic symptoms, including hearing voices or paranoia. Many sufferers attempt suicide. If several of the above symptoms last for more than two weeks and if they interfere with normal life functioning, professional treatment is required.[16]

Types of Depression and Symptoms

DYSTHYMIA
Chronic depression, a less-severe form but symptoms linger for a long time. Usually able to function normally, but consistently unhappy.

- → Difficulty sleeping
- → Loss of interest in general
- → Loss of energy or fatigue

- → Difficulty concentrating, thinking, or making decisions
- → Changes in appetite

- → Observable mental and physical sluggishness
- → Thoughts of death or suicide

- → Excessive feelings of guilt or worthlessness

SEASONAL AFFECTIVE DISORDER
Occurs each year at the same time, usually starting in fall or winter and ending in spring or early summer. More serious than just "the winter blues" or "cabin fever."

- → Fatigue
- → Increased need for sleep
- → Decreased levels of energy

- → Weight gain
- → Increase in appetite
- → Difficulty concentrating

- → Increased desire to be alone
- → Weight loss
- → Trouble sleeping

- → Decreased appetite

BIPOLAR (MANIC-DEPRESSIVE) DISORDER
People swing from feeling overly happy and joyful (or irritable) to feeling very sad (or overly unhappy).

Manic periods:
- → Overly happy, hopeful, and excited
- → Change suddenly to being angry and hostile
- → Restless
- → Talk rapidly

- → Lots of energy and need less sleep
- → Make grand plans
- → Show poor judgment
- → Headstrong, annoying, or demanding
- → Easily distracted

- → Abuse drugs and alcohol

Depressive periods:
- → Feel empty, sad, or hopeless
- → Cry often
- → Lose interest in things they usually enjoy

- → Unable to think clearly, make decisions or remember things
- → Sleep poorly
- → Low energy
- → Abuse drugs and alcohol
- → Become focused on death
- → Attempt suicide

ANXIETY DISORDERS
Intense, often unrealistic and excessive state of apprehension and fear. (Panic Disorder, Social Phobia, Obsessive-Compulsive Disorder.)

- → Blood pressure rises
- → Racing heart
- → Rapid breathing, nausea
- → Signs of agitation and discomfort

PANIC DISORDER; AGORAPHOBIA
Periodic attacks of anxiety or terror, often unexpected, uncontrolled, and without reason. Attacks can last 15 to 30 minutes with frequency varying from every week to every few months.

- → At least four of the following symptoms and four or more attacks within a four-week period:

- → Fast heart beat
- → Extreme sweating
- → Shortness of breath
- → Shakiness

- → A choking sensation
- → Dizziness
- → Nausea
- → Numbness

- → Hot flashes/chills
- → Chest pain
- → Fear of dying
- → Feeling of losing control

EATING DISORDERS
Most common types are anorexia nervosa and bulimia nervosa, emotional illnesses resulting in harmful eating habits. Most common among teenage girls and women. Frequently occurs among teenage girls and young women, often along with depression and anxiety disorders.

- → Rapid weight loss over several weeks or months
- → Dieting even with very low body weight
- → Intense fear of gaining weight or getting fat

- → Watching every bite of food
- → Eating in secret
- → Unusual interest in food
- → Exercising very often
- → Becoming very depressed or anxious

- → Infrequent or absent menstrual periods
- → Wanting to be perfect or being highly self-critical
- → Eating large amounts of food all at once, and then vomiting

- → Common to purge, or empty themselves, through vomiting and abuse

POST TRAUMATIC STRESS DISORDER (PTSD)
Result of exposure to situations where severe physical harm either occurred, or was threatened. Includes experiencing or witnessing war situations, natural disasters, rape, mugging, physical abuse, and sexual abuse.

- → Symptoms of PTSD are often triggered by an object or event that reminds the person of the trauma
- → Flashbacks, nightmares, or terrorizing thoughts

- → Emotional numbness
- → Sleep disturbances
- → Irritability
- → Feelings of intense guilt
- → An excessive startle reaction to loud noise

- → Substance abuse
- → Headache
- → Stomach and immune system problems
- → Chest pain and dizziness
- → In order to be diagnosed

with PTSD, symptoms must last for more than one month
- → PTSD generally begins to show up within three months after experiencing a trauma, although this is not always the case

What Does It Feel Like?

The following excerpt from an interview with a person coming out of four years of depression and alcohol addiction may give a glimpse of what that dark world is like:

Ups and downs of gigantic proportions ... in the end, the only thing that turns out to be predictable is my own cycle of depression. A sense of powerlessness looms and turns into a slippery slope of heavy, dark sludge. I always know when it begins.

Exhaustion ... all cravings turned into void—a great big absorbing maw of blackness and instant despair. Sobbing is near, but even that is beyond happening.

About 32 percent of all mood disorder patients and a higher percentage of depressed people are also substance dependent or abusers. And there is growing evidence that concurrent addictions worsen the treatability of depression and vice versa. Many medical illnesses are also associated with mood disorders. Studies have linked depression to heart disease, and patients are two to four times more likely to die from a heart attack or stroke when depressed.[17]

The list of health conditions associated with depression goes on: autoimmune disease, hormonal system disorder, stress, migraine headaches, chronic pain, diabetes, chronic fatigue syndrome, and fibromyalgia. These conditions may lead to depression, and depression can also worsen them.

Chronic administration of several classes of medications for gastric ulcers, hypertension, arthritis, pain and inflammation, Parkinson's disease, as well as some anti-cancer and hydrocortisone drugs may also lead to a major depressive episode.[18]

Western Anti-Depression Medications

In Western medical practice, physicians may prescribe anti-depressant and anti-psychotic medications that target one or more of the neuro-transmitters serotonin, dopamine, and norepinephrine. However, neuroscientists now realize that depression is caused by far more complex events than simple disturbances in a single neurotransmitter. It is more likely that depression is caused by disturbances in any one or more of many neurotransmitters, each affecting the others like musical instruments of an orchestra playing a symphony.[19]

> Depression may be caused by disturbances in any one or more of many neurotransmitters, each affecting the others like musical instruments of an orchestra playing a symphony.

If you are taking anti-depression medication, it's important to be very cautious about cross-medication problems.

The most popular class of anti-depressant medications is made up of selective serotonin re-uptake inhibitors (SSRIs) such as Paxil, Zoloft, and Prozac. SSRIs block the reabsorption of serotonin into nerve-ending storage, ensuring that parts of the brain are well bathed in whatever serotonin is available. It can take about one month before an anti-depressant is fully effective, and it may take up to two months before a sufferer feels significantly better.[20]

Since relief is not immediate, medication should not be terminated for lack of improvement after a few days. Stopping certain anti-depressants abruptly can also cause withdrawal symptoms. Even after improvement or disappearance of the depressive symptoms, continued medication may be necessary in order to prevent relapse or recurrence of symptoms. Those who have recovered from depression are also at a higher risk of recurrence during the first couple of months after initial therapy.[21]

If you are taking anti-depression medication, it's important to be very cautious about cross-medication problems. Many over-the-counter drugs—especially cough and cold products—may contain ingredients that interact with anti-depression medication, so it's vital to consult a pharmacist or doctor before you take other medicines or remedies in combination with anti-depression drugs.

If one specific medication does not work, many other effective anti-depression medications can be combined until an appropriate and effective regimen is found. More than 80 percent of people with depression will respond well to anti-depression medications and can return to normal lives.[22]

Natural Remedies

Natural medicine provides some hope for patients with mild to moderate depression who do not want to take conventional anti-depression medications. The natural path includes herbal remedies and dietary supplements such as St. John's wort (*Hypericum perforatum*), DHEA (dehydroepiandrosterone), L-5-hydroxytryptophan (5-HTP), SAM-e (S-adenosylmethionine), Ginkgo biloba, and Omega-3 oils. However, these produce different side effects, ranging from nausea and vomiting to dizziness, gastrointestinal upset, and fatigue—and they should never be taken in combination with prescription medications. A further caveat: any natural remedy not regulated by law is not governed by official product standards either. Also, pregnant women should seek medical advice before using any of these remedies. Because the effects of these remedies have not been studied in pregnancy it is important to avoid them when planning, or during, a pregnancy and during breast-feeding.

Finally, these remedies are not useful for severe depression. Depression is a serious health condition that needs to be fully evaluated by medical professionals before decisions are made about treatments. So if you are suffering from this problem, you should consult a doctor before making any choices concerning medications—natural or otherwise.[23]

Natural remedies most often used for mild to moderate depression are:

→ *5-HTP.* Derived from the seed of the African plant *Griffonia simplicifolia*. Up to 70 percent of an oral dose of 5-HTP may be converted to serotonin. It may also raise endorphin levels. The most common side effects are mild nausea, heartburn, and gastrointestinal symptoms.
→ *SAM-e.* May increase levels of serotonin and dopamine and may also improve the binding of neurotransmitters to receptors. However, this medication should never be administered to patients with bipolar disorder, since it may precipitate a manic episode. Side effects can include nausea and vomiting.
→ *St. John's wort.* A popular herbal anti-depression medication for mild to moderate depression; may increase levels of serotonin and dopamine. But this medication should not be combined with conventional anti-depression medications. Health Canada has issued a warning regarding potential interaction between St. John's wort and many prescription medications, including digoxin, warfarin, theophylline, and oral contraceptives.[24] Common side effects include photosensitivity, gastrointestinal upset, dizziness, dry mouth, constipation, fatigue, and some allergic reactions.
→ *Ginkgo biloba extract.* Used as a herbal medication for mild depression by increasing blood flow to the brain. Side effects include gastrointestinal upset and headache. Health Canada has reported on adverse drug reactions associated with warfarin, including increased coagulation time, subcutaneous hematoma, and intracranial hemorrhage.[25]

Therapies

Tomorrow hasn't come. Worries do not create feelings of wellness. But directions steer you on with hope.

Psychotherapy. Individual psychotherapy (talk therapy), group therapy, or family therapy may help improve personal relationships and reduce stress. Often, two or more treatments such as medications and psychotherapy can be combined to create the most effective outcome.

Talk therapy, in which a person discusses various psychological and emotional issues with a trained therapist, can be effective for treating mild to moderate depression. Cognitive-behavioral therapy (CBT) helps a person examine their negative thought patterns and to practice responding to negative thoughts in a new way.[26]

In interpersonal therapy (IPT), the therapist attempts to understand a patient's relationships, in order to link relationship changes and problems to the onset of depression. By addressing these issues, which can either be the cause or the consequence of depression, depressive symptoms can be reduced.[27] Although the thought of shock treatments or electro-convulsive therapy (ECT) may be unpleasant and frightening, it can actually be a fast and effective treatment for severe depression. When medication and/or psychotherapy are ineffective or are too slow to relieve severe symptoms, ECT may be useful.

Timed exposure to daytime-intensity light is the treatment of choice for SAD, the seasonal winter blues.

Light Therapy. Timed exposure to daytime-intensity light is the treatment of choice for SAD, the seasonal winter blues. This consists of sitting before an appropriate lighting device that simulates outdoor lighting. Morning light therapy is better than evening light exposure, and the wavelength or type of light (incandescent or fluorescent) is not as important as the intensity. But white light may work better than light with narrow-band wavelengths.

Response to light therapy generally begins within two to four days, and measurable improvement is often seen in one week. But therapy should last at least two to four weeks. Otherwise, depressive symptoms may recur soon after light therapy is discontinued. It is still not known exactly how the mechanism of bright light works, but it has been suggested that light exposure may reinforce the normal settings of our biological clock, and/or restore normal levels of the "feel-good" neurotransmitter serotonin.[28]

A Chinese Medicine Perspective

Chinese medicine has a very different outlook on depression. According to traditional Chinese medical philosophy, emotions and internal organs are so closely linked that they affect each other constantly. All classical Chinese medical texts also place great emphasis on how our moods and emotions affect our physical health. Because our feelings are such an important part of our everyday life, they say, we should consciously guard them all the time, from as early in life as possible. According to this tradition, the best strategy is to check emotional extremes whenever they arise. Harmony and balance are considered to be the best preventive health measures, especially for depression.[29]

Any one emotion can be harmful if it is experienced in excess. The *Yellow Emperor's Manual of Corporeal Medicine*,[30] a famous medical text that dates back to 1000 B.C., lists seven emotions to watch out for—joy, anger, worry, contemplation, sorrow, fear, and shock—and defines how such emotions may be harmful to the five basic internal organs:

➜ Too much joy is harmful to the heart.
➜ Too much anger is harmful to the liver.
➜ Too much contemplation or thinking is harmful to the spleen.
➜ Too much worry is harmful to the lung.
➜ Too much fear is harmful to the kidney.

Each emotion also has a particular effect on the movement of the life energy, qi, which is believed to be circulating within the body:

➜ Anger causes energy to flare upward in sudden, intense explosiveness.
➜ Joy causes energy to relax and slow down. But being overwhelmed with joy can make a person feel high and giddy, then weakened and drained.
➜ Contemplation causes energy to knot up, creating stagnation and making a person feel tired and lethargic.
➜ Sorrow causes energy to disperse, making a person feel like withering away.
➜ Fear causes energy to sink downward, making people feel frozen and causing them to break out in a cold sweat.
➜ Shock causes energy to scatter and become disorderly, making a person feel chaotic and panicky.

According to traditional Chinese medical philosophy, emotions and internal organs are so closely linked that they affect each other constantly.

Acupuncture and herbal medications can be used to release energy blocks resulting from repeated improper movements of the life energy, qi.

Treatments for depression are developed from these principles. Acupuncture and herbal medications, for instance, can be used to release energy blocks resulting from repeated improper movements of qi (caused by having too much of any emotion). They also correct any imbalances in the functions of internal organs triggered by excess emotions.[31]

As to everyday lifestyle, traditional Chinese medicine offers the following advice:

→ Eat a simple diet of fresh foods in moderate quantities, with lots of variety and including brown rice, cucumbers, apples, cabbage, fresh wheat germ, kuzu root, blue-green microalgae, leafy dark green vegetables, seaweed, and bitter-tasting foods.
→ Discontinue any harmful habits such as staying up late.
→ Drink alcohol and have sex in moderation. Do daily physical exercise that includes plenty of stretching, for better energy and blood circulation.
→ Do spiritual exercises to calm the mind.
→ Do deep breathing to relieve tension and stress.[32]

Addicted to Feeling Good

All forms of addiction are based on a desire for the feel-good system to be activated. And all addictive substances lead to increased availability of dopamine in the gaps between neurons, which increases the "feel-good" stimulation of the brain. In people who become addicted, the natural process of dopamine release becomes an overwhelming, artificially induced priority in their lives. The intensity of feel-good responses they seek pales in comparison to anything and everything else. According to San Franciscan David Smith, the world expert on addiction, addiction is defined as the persistent pattern of dysfunctional use of a substance that involves any or all of the Three Cs: Compulsive Use, Loss of Control, and Continued Use despite harmful consequences. More than a third of people suffering from depression are also suffering from addiction.[33]

With repeated use of an addictive substance, specific alterations in the proteins and enzymes within the neuro-pathways for dopamine and other neurotransmitters are repeatedly induced. As the body becomes accustomed to the intensity of feel-good sensations, greater and greater amounts of the addictive substance are needed to produce the same effects (a process called *neuroadaptation*). Attempts to stop bring on more craving as withdrawal symptoms take place because the body has now adapted to needing the addictive substance.

While dopamine is the key neurotransmitter in addiction, glutamate, which is associated with thinking and memory, also plays an important role. When high dopamine levels lead to feel-good responses, glutamate affects memory and thinking, producing the conditioned response of craving. The whole affair is like giving the brain a repeated wrong memory, and that's why relapse is a lifelong risk.[34]

Humans are not alone in being susceptible to addiction. Most animals will gladly take any drug that humans use, with the exception of marijuana and certain psychedelics such as LSD. Researchers at the New England Regional Primate Research Center reported that pigeons, rats, and monkeys will all press levers to access cocaine or opiates, suggesting that the potential of addiction is common to many species.[35]

However, people differ in their susceptibility to substance abuse, and they differ in their ability to stay away from an abused substance without relapsing. Having one addiction also seems to lower the threshold for another.[36] The reasons for this are not entirely clear, but researchers are suggesting that substance abuse leads to changes in gene expression at the molecular level. American pharmacologist Ken Blum, for example, first linked alcoholism to the specific gene A 1 allele, one of four forms of a gene that is programmed for a particular dopamine receptor.[37] Even though his work is controversial, researchers in France, Japan, and Finland have since confirmed associations of this gene to other substance abuse and compulsive disorders.[38]

Nevertheless, there is hope that the biochemical aspects of addiction may be treated with medications. In fact, new drugs that will aim to attack addiction at the level of specific brain targets and neurotransmitters are on the horizon. One experimental drug, for instance—MK-801—has been shown to prevent mice from becoming sensitized to cocaine and amphetamines.[39]

The brain "is so immersed in pleasure that it happily eats away at the bases of its own existence."
—Japanese philosopher Daisaku Ikeda

Post-Vietnam Lessons in Addiction

The root of addiction seems to lie in both brain chemistry and behavior. American researcher Lee Robins studied Vietnam War veterans when they returned home in 1971 and found that 45 percent admitted to having tried addictive opioids (specifically opium or heroin) while on duty. Of these men, 20 percent had developed dependency.[40]

When the same group was re-examined three years later, half of them had tried opioids again, but had not become regular users. Only 12 percent of those who had a dependency history relapsed into addiction. This suggests that exposure alone does not necessarily lead to addiction. Social and cultural contexts, availability of the substance, genetic susceptibility, and individual psychological or personality traits also contribute to the development of or relapse into an addiction.

A recent study has shown that substance abusers may have unknowingly trained themselves to respond to environmental and social triggers associated with the pleasure and experience of the high. The Brookhaven National Laboratory study published in the *European Journal of Pharmacology* in March 2001 revealed that when lab rats trained to associate cocaine with a given environment were later exposed to such an environment, they showed an approximately 25-percent increase in dopamine levels compared to the non-addicted control group, even in the absence of additional cocaine.[41]

During this study, the researchers also investigated the efficacy of the therapeutic agent GVG (gamma-vinyl GABA), which can indirectly deplete dopamine and the resulting pleasurable feelings by inhibiting an enzyme that breaks down a dopamine-modulating neurotransmitter. A new drug with this agent, brand-named Sabril or Vigabatrin, is awaiting clinical trials in North America for use in the treatment of addiction.

However, even with the help of a therapeutic agent, social situations that may lead to the triggering of environmental cues should be avoided. It is also important to be prepared, since avoidance may not always be possible. Knowing that cravings are temporary can help; when attention is diverted away from the addictive substance, life purpose can be reasserted.[42]

"All addiction feeds the ego, the self," says U.S. psychiatrist Stephen Bergman. "The ego is insatiable; if you're into ego, you'll never get enough of sex, money, drugs, relationships, not enough of anything. Getting beyond the ego helps. Redirecting attention away from the self-reinforcing, addictive activity interrupts the addictive cycle. Love someone, love yourself. Love not only competes with ... addiction; it replaces addiction in a non-addictive way."

Recovery has to start, however, with self-awareness and acknowledgement of the problem. Information on how to get out of addiction is also empowering. And it is important to accept the reality of relapse and deal with it.

The mind capable of understanding the workings of the brain must be more complex than the brain itself. The mind can either short-circuit the brain and decide that ready access to the temporary rewards of an addictive substance is the ultimate priority, or it can re-establish life priorities and choose to learn how to stay away from the addictive substance. In the end, the mind has to make a decision to break free from the addiction and then act on it.

> Having one addiction seems to lower the threshold for another.

From Depression to Addiction ... and Back Home Again

The following interview with Sydney, a 25-year-old ex-cocaine addict living in Toronto, demonstrates how depression can lead to addiction "by default." Cocaine is a particularly insidious drug because its abuse is hidden and permeates all walks of life. This drug ensnares its victims—be they supermodels or down-and-out crack users—with the allure of living in the fast lane of "sex, drugs, and rock 'n' roll." And in a society that almost reveres the increased alertness, confidence, and endurance brought on by cocaine, it's all too possible for this drug addiction to go unnoticed and unchallenged.

WellnessOptions (WO): How long was it from your first time, to becoming addicted to cocaine?

Sydney: It was really gradual for me, about three years. I'd just gotten out of a really abusive relationship, and I was sitting there feeling depressed one day when I thought, "Screw it, I'll just get high." That's when I started doing it a lot. Coke just takes over your mind. You start to rationalize yourself into thinking it's okay. You become really good at making excuses for yourself, like "I could get a lot more done today if I just had a tiny little rail to get me going." Sounds ridiculous but you start to think that way. All of a sudden you wake up one morning and you realize you've been making excuses for two years.

"There is no such thing as a life of passion, any more than a continuous earthquake, or an eternal fever."
—Lord Byron

WO: Is that why you quit, you woke up one morning?

Sydney: I got woken up by a motor vehicle accident that almost killed me. I wasn't driving, but I got seriously injured and I thought about it in the hospital—"I don't want to die a cokehead." If you're lucky, you find out one day that you're worth more than 60 bucks a gram. I was also lucky that the hospital had me on all sorts of painkillers and I slept through the worst of any withdrawal syndrome I might have had.

WO: Are you worried you're going to get addicted again?

Sydney: Well, again, I'm lucky. I have two things, a loving relationship and a creative career that I love. I'd lose them both if I got addicted again. When I was doing it every day, I didn't realize it, but everything that was important to me slowly took a back seat to getting high. I could do stuff, but there was no heart in it. And for a creative person, or anyone for that matter, it can feel like slow death, or "soul death."

WO: What can you do to quit cocaine then? Any advice?

Sydney: Stop for a minute and find something that you love. Stop thinking so fast, stop looking for the next "thing"—whatever that is for you. Just stop for a second and realize there's something special and great about you, and as much as you think it does, coke does not make it better. Get away from everyone and everything—go someplace that your dealer won't and just enjoy being you for a while. The only way I know to stop doing coke is to love yourself.

Perpetual High?

In today's fast-track society of excess, we expect increasing and instant rewards all the time. We are expected to be perfect and perfectly happy, from now to eternity. Every problem has a built-in help manual; every blue mood has a cure in a glass of red. If only we knew which button to press, which magic pill to reach for ...

But even the great poet and master of excess Lord Byron said this about the eternal quest for lasting excitement: "There is no such thing as a life of continuous passion, any more than the continuous earthquake, or an eternal fever." Coming from the creator of *Don Juan*, this remark rings particularly true. Life cannot sustain a perpetual high. Neither our brains nor our bodies are wired for it.

When being high becomes the norm, more and more is needed to get less and less. And there's a price to pay when we pursue an unreal, fireworks-beautiful, kaleidoscopic biochemical quick-fix: it's the crushing slide into a black hole. Depression is more common than most of us realize, and major depression, if left untreated, can easily lead to the tormenting hell of addiction, or even suicide, which ruins many more lives in its wake.

Why are happy moods so elusive? Why is contentment so difficult to maintain?

As science unravels the mystery of the brain, we are beginning to learn about the physiological reasons for good moods, depressions, cravings, and gratification. And there are other contributing factors: psychological, social, cultural, interpersonal, environmental, what we eat, how we sleep ... There are also things that we can do to improve mood, lessen depression, or recover from addiction.

There may even be magic pills available in the near future to get us out of a particular addiction just as quickly as we got hooked. But in the end, neither the satisfied body nor the gratified brain alone seems to fulfill the mind or pacify the soul. Perhaps fluctuation is necessary after all, with the momentum of the fall propelling us on to the next rising. Perhaps it is the tension and transition, the discipline and calm between changing moods, and the lessons and wisdom drawn from the continuum of the flux of feelings that expand our capacity for happiness.

True contentment of the mind requires more than an instantly gratified brain. It probably requires time and effort to nurture and grow. Instead of feeding on highs, it probably feeds on knowledge and appreciation of the inner self, of the outer world, of others, and of the interrelatedness of all there is.

It is the tension and transition, the discipline and calm between changing moods, and the lessons and wisdom drawn from the continuum of the flux of feelings that expand our capacity for happiness.

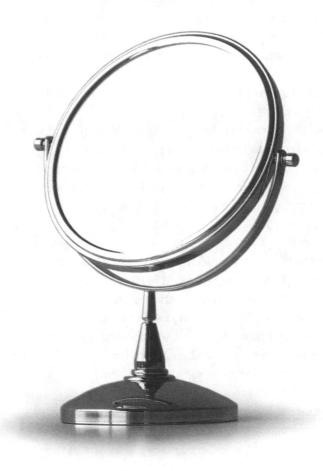

5 How Are You Doing as the Years Go By?

As for me, I could leave the world with today in my eyes.
—Truman Capote, *A Christmas Memory*

What do you see?

In Greek mythology, Eos is the goddess with the rosy fingers, the goddess of dawn who brought the first glimmer of day to earth. She was a lovely young goddess who evoked desire in men, earning the enmity of Aphrodite, the goddess of love and beauty. As revenge, Aphrodite inspired Eos to fall in love with the mortal Tithonus, the handsome son of the King of Troy. Wishing to be bound to Tithonus for eternity, Eos pleaded with Zeus to allow Tithonus to live forever. The wish was granted, but unfortunately Eos had forgotten to ask for perpetual youth as well.

As the years went by, Tithonus became an old man with a wrinkled brow. Eos fed him with celestial ambrosia, which made flesh incorruptible, but her efforts were to no avail. As old age led to decrepitude and impotence, Eos confined Tithonus to his chamber. Finally, she relieved him of his suffering by changing him into a grasshopper.

Is It Growing or Aging?

The issue is not one of aging but of quality. Adding life to years is even more important than adding years to life.

We are all being propelled up a magnificent mountain called life by something called time. It is a non-stop journey, which some people call aging and others call growing. Under any name, the phases of transformation in our lives are like the seasons or the tides, each with its own characteristics and beauty. Our appearance may change as we grow older, and we may express ourselves differently, but our essence remains unaltered—that of a living, walking wonder.

The word *aging* certainly conveys a sense of decline. But it can also refer to a process of change that leads to a desirable quality—as in wine, which matures until it becomes perfectly mellow. Nevertheless, some wines do not age well. The issue is not one of aging but of quality. Adding life to years is even more important than adding years to life. And it all begins with today.

Society's perceptions about aging also need radical updating. As American obstetrician/gynecologist Christiane Northrup points out, the decline that many people experience as the years go by "is not a natural consequence of aging—it is a consequence of our collective beliefs about aging. In our ageist culture, many aging individuals, instead of believing in their capacity to remain strong, attractive, and vital throughout their lives … come to expect their bodies and minds to deteriorate with age. Chronological age and biological age are two different things and we must decide to age with power, strength, and beauty."[1]

Adding Life to Years

"To add life to years, not just years to life" was the slogan chosen for the debut issue of the Gerontological Society of America's *Journal of Gerontology* in 1946 and it marked the beginning of a worldwide trend to combat the effects of aging. [2]

The basic philosophy of this revolution is to integrate the "forever young" part with the "well" part of growing and aging. It seeks to promote a state of well-being regardless of age so that life may be enjoyed and lived to the fullest until its end. The purpose of this mentality is to ensure that all of us stay well and can enjoy being productive for as long as possible.

Why and How Do We Age?

Although the specific biological basis of aging is unknown, there is general agreement that the answer lies at the cellular or molecular level. This has given rise to numerous theories about why we grow old. The neuroendocrine theory suggests aging is programmed into the brain's hypothalamus-pituitary system.[3] The free radical theory postulates that oxygen-derived free radical cells cause progressive random damage.[4] The functional capacity of the immune system may also decline with increasing age.[5] And some researchers have discovered telling information about the tiny, stabilizing knots at the ends of our chromosomes called *telemeres*, which maintain the integrity of the cell. Every time a cell divides, these telemeres become shorter. This has led to the theory that there may be a timepiece of aging that shortens every time the cell divides.[6]

Aging is characterized by progressive declines in many areas of our body's functioning:

→ muscle mass and strength;
→ aerobic capacity and stamina;
→ hormone function;
→ sleep quality;
→ bone density;
→ lifestyle quality;
→ mental capabilities (impaired memory, inability to concentrate);
→ sexual function.

Common disorders such as cardiovascular disease, hypertension, cancer, stroke, dementia, and diabetes have also been equated with aging because of their increasing prevalence in later life. But this

Longest Recorded Lifespans

MAMMALS	YEARS
Virginia opossum	3
Little brown bat	3
House mouse	4
Black rat	5
German shepherd, Great Dane (dogs)	11
Pekinese, terrier (dog)	15
Wolf, arctic	16
Sheep	20
African fruit bat	22
Tiger, Bengal	24
Pig	27
Domestic cat	28
Lion, African	30
Bottlenosed dolphin	35
Rhesus monkey	35
Brown bear	37
Horse	46
Beaver, Canadian	50
Chimpanzee	50
Elephant, Indian	70
Blue whale	110
Human	122

BIRDS	
European robin	11
Starling	20
Feral pigeon	30
Herring gull	49
Andean condor	75
Parrot	90

REPTILES	
Chinese alligator	52
Galapagos tortoise	175

AMPHIBIANS	
Common European frog	12
Common toad	36

FISH	
Guppy	5
Perch	25
Carp	50
Halibut	60
Pacific rockfish	120

INVERTEBRATES	
Fruit fly	0.3
House fly	0.3
Quahog (clam)	200

PLANTS	
Bamboo	120
Bristlecone pine	5000

Longest Recorded Lifespan data from
R. Gosden, "Cheating Time" (New York:
W.H. Freeman, 1966); J. George et al.,
Canadian Journal of Zoology 77 (1999)
751; R.M. Nowak, "Mammals of the
World," 5th Edition (Baltimore: Johns
Hopkins University Press, 1991).

World Aging Trends data from
World Health Reports, World Health
Organization, United Nations.

World Aging Trends

WORLD MEDIAN AGES (YEARS)

	1950	2000	2050
World total	23.6	26.5	36.2
Africa	19.0	18.4	27.4
Asia	22.0	26.2	38.3
Europe	29.2	37.7	49.5
North America	29.8	35.6	41.0
Latin America Caribbean	20.1	24.4	37.8
Oceania	27.9	30.9	38.1

PERCENTAGE OF DIFFERENT AGE GROUPS IN SELECTED COUNTRIES

MORE DEVELOPED COUNTRIES	2000 Age 0-14	2000 Age 15-59	2000 Age 60+	2050 Age 0-14	2050 Age 15-59	2050 Age 60+
Canada	19.1	64.2	16.7	16.3	53.2	30.5
Italy	14.3	61.7	24.1	11.5	46.2	42.3
Japan	14.7	62.1	23.2	12.5	45.2	42.3
U.K.	19.0	60.4	20.6	15.0	51.1	34.0
U.S.	21.7	62.1	16.1	18.5	54.6	26.9

LESS DEVELOPED COUNTRIES	2000 Age 0-14	2000 Age 15-59	2000 Age 60+	2050 Age 0-14	2050 Age 15-59	2050 Age 60+
Angola	48.2	47.3	4.5	36.7	58.1	5.2
China	24.8	65.0	10.1	16.3	53.8	29.9
Jamaica	31.5	58.9	9.6	19.3	56.7	24.0
Nigeria	45.5	50.2	4.8	25.1	64.6	10.3
Republic of Korea	20.8	68.2	11.0	16.5	50.4	33.2

FIVE COUNTRIES WITH THE OLDEST/YOUNGEST POPULATIONS IN 2000 & 2050 (BASED ON PROJECTED WORLD POPULATION OF 9.3 BILLION)

A. Oldest population

2000 Country	Median age	2050 Country	Median age
Japan	41.2	Spain	55.2
Italy	40.2	Slovenia	54.1
Switzerland	40.2	Italy	54.1
Germany	40.1	Austria	53.7
Sweden	39.7	Armenia	53.4

B. Youngest population

2000 Country	Median age	2050 Country	Median age
Yemen	15.0	Niger	20.4
Niger	15.1	Yemen	21.1
Uganda	15.4	Angola	21.2
Burkina Faso	15.6	Somalia	21.5
Congo	15.6	Uganda	22.1

Prevalence of Common Age-Related Chronic Diseases

DISEASE	Prevalence at age (cases/1,000 patients on general practice list)		
	75+	65-74	45-65
Osteoarthritis of hip/knee	326	163	35
Deafness	254	127	30
Obesity	218	204	150
Hypertension	207	233	114
Cataract	196	60	6
Heart failure	149	44	5
Chronic ischemic heart disease	148	110	27
Chronic obstructive pulmonary disease	111	150	36
Diabetes mellitus	109	84	27
Stroke	100	44	9

association varies greatly among people in different circumstances and cultures, challenging the idea that these are necessary conditions of growing older.[7]

Determining factors for the likelihood of having aging disorders seem to be more environmental than genetic. Members of one Kenyan tribe, for instance, have low blood pressure when they live in a rural environment, but their blood pressure increases with age when they move to the city.[8] Japanese people living in Japan have much lower blood-cholesterol levels and lower rates of coronary heart disease than white Americans, but this difference disappears when Japanese people migrate to the United States.[9] And Dutch women living in the Antilles have a higher level of bone mass and lower rates of fracture than Dutch women of the same age living in the Netherlands.[10] In fact, genes account for only about one-third of the health problems associated with aging, with lifestyle and environmental factors accounting for the rest.[11]

To a large extent, we as individuals can determine how long and how well we live.

How Our Hormones Change as We Age

Evidence suggests that many aging processes in our body are related to declines in various hormonal systems and the development of hormone deficiencies.[12]

These hormonal changes include: decline in the release of growth hormone from the pituitary gland; reduction in the luteinizing and

Members of one Kenyan tribe have low blood pressure when they live in a rural environment, but their blood pressure increases with age when they move to the city.

To a large extent, we as individuals can determine how long and how well we live.

follicle-stimulating hormones, leading to lower levels of testosterone in males and causing andropause (the same hormonal reductions in females lead to lower levels of estrogen/estradiol, causing menopause); decrease in adrenal activity resulting in lower levels of dehydroepiandrosterone (DHEA) in both sexes; reduction in the release of melatonin, a sleep-promoting hormone, leading to sleep problems; and increased insulin resistance as well as decreased glucose tolerance.[13]

How We Age (besides too quickly)

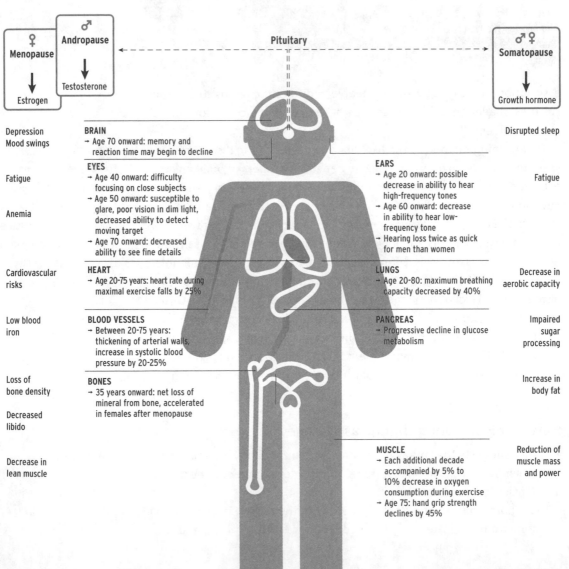

♀ **Menopause** ↓ Estrogen

♂ **Andropause** ↓ Testosterone

Pituitary

♂♀ **Somatopause** ↓ Growth hormone

Depression
Mood swings

BRAIN
→ Age 70 onward: memory and reaction time may begin to decline

Disrupted sleep

Fatigue

EYES
→ Age 40 onward: difficulty focusing on close subjects
→ Age 50 onward: susceptible to glare, poor vision in dim light, decreased ability to detect moving target
→ Age 70 onward: decreased ability to see fine details

EARS
→ Age 20 onward: possible decrease in ability to hear high-frequency tones
→ Age 60 onward: decrease in ability to hear low-frequency tone
→ Hearing loss twice as quick for men than women

Fatigue

Anemia

Cardiovascular risks

HEART
→ Age 20-75 years: heart rate during maximal exercise falls by 25%

LUNGS
→ Age 20-80: maximum breathing capacity decreased by 40%

Decrease in aerobic capacity

Low blood iron

BLOOD VESSELS
→ Between 20-75 years: thickening of arterial walls, increase in systolic blood pressure by 20-25%

PANCREAS
→ Progressive decline in glucose metabolism

Impaired sugar processing

Loss of bone density

Decreased libido

BONES
→ 35 years onward: net loss of mineral from bone, accelerated in females after menopause

Increase in body fat

Decrease in lean muscle

MUSCLE
→ Each additional decade accompanied by 5% to 10% decrease in oxygen consumption during exercise
→ Age 75: hand grip strength declines by 45%

Reduction of muscle mass and power

"I Need All the Preservatives I Can Get!"

Sometimes age is a frame of mind.

When, in fact, does growing stop and aging start? They both start when life begins, and measurable signs of decline actually begin at a much earlier age than previously expected. For instance, growth hormone secretion peaks at age 20; cardiorespiratory fitness decreases at a rate of 1 percent each year after age 20; muscle strength and endurance decrease at a rate of 10 to 15 percent per decade. By age 60, the size of our thymus, headquarters of the immune system, will have shrunk to less than 5 percent of that of a newborn, weakening our immune responses.[14]

As George Burns, the American comedian, joked when he was 95: "At my age, I stay away from health foods. I need all the preservatives I can get."

Happiness, much like age, is also often a frame of mind, and a matter of perspective. A half-filled glass can be half-full or half-spilled. It can also be totally full-filled or completely spilled. On any day, at any age.

The ongoing search for the fountain of youth has resulted in new techniques to combat the aging process. In fact, anti-aging is now such a hot topic that it is becoming its own subspecialty in medicine. It is also evolving into an extremely lucrative commercial industry. Some interventions, such as regular exercise programs and lifestyle changes, are non-pharmacological, but there is strong interest in a variety of hormone replacement therapies (HRT) that might stabilize or reverse age-related declines. These strategies for increasing blood-hormone levels remain controversial. However, since they are gaining so much attention, it is important to look at the risks and benefits of these therapies, which include replacement of growth hormones, sex hormones, androgen, and estrogen.[15]

> When, in fact, does growing stop and aging start?

Growth Hormone Replacement

After we reach the age of 40, the amount of muscle in our bodies decreases progressively. Our muscle power goes down by 3 to 5 percent each year, and the total amount of fat in our bodies increases, particularly in the intra-abdominal regions.[16] We also experience decreasing bone mass and an increased incidence of osteoporosis and fractures.[17] This set of aging symptoms is called *somatopause*.

Many symptoms of somatopause are the same as those that mark a syndrome called adult-onset growth hormone deficiency. The growth hormone (GH) is secreted by the pituitary gland in a pulsating fashion, the greatest levels of secretion occurring during the first three to four hours of sleep. Daily secretion of GH is highest in early adulthood, peaking before age 20 and then declining to a minimal level by age 60.[18] In 1990, ground-breaking evidence was published indicating that GH replacement therapy in the elderly could reverse some of the symptoms of somatopause.[19] And there are now many studies examining the benefits and risks of growth hormone replacement therapy in humans.[20]

Because of these new revelations, some have proposed that GH treatment may be a panacea for fading youthfulness.[21] But this therapy is not without its side effects—including joint pain (arthralgia), water retention (edema), and carpal tunnel syndrome. Though many of these problems may be dose-related and may disappear when treatment stops, studies of the long-term effects of prolonged use of GH are required before it can be promoted as an everyday medical treatment.[22]

Male Menopause

Many setbacks created by andropause can be overcome through a continuous exercise regime.

The average healthy aging male experiences gradual declines in the principal male sex hormone, testosterone. About 7 percent of men between 40 and 60, 21 percent of those between the ages of 60 and 80, and 3 percent of men older than 80 have subnormal levels of testosterone, a condition known as *hypogonadism*.[23] This decline will continue until the end of life. And though few men experience the dramatic level of symptoms that women go through during menopause, about 40 percent of men in their 40s experience symptoms to some degree as they start to go through andropause.[24]

Symptoms of Male Andropause

PSYCHOSOCIAL	PHYSIOLOGICAL
Increased irritability	Loss of bone density
Depression	Decrease in lean muscle mass
Mood swings	Increase in fat
Decreased libido	Decrease in strength
Lethargy, or fatigue	Decrease in aerobic capacity
Decreased sense of well-being	Erectile dysfunction

These difficulties can be aggravated by smoking, drinking too much alcohol, high blood pressure or hypertension, certain drug use, poor diet, psychological problems at work or at home, and most importantly, the lack of a continuous exercise regime.[25]

For many andropause conditions, androgen replacement seems to be a helpful treatment, but more large-scale, long-term studies are needed to confirm benefits.[26] Some of the effects of androgen on different body systems are shown in the following table.

Different men age differently, so if you are considering therapy, make sure that you are first evaluated for levels of what is called "free testosterone" in the blood—not "protein-bound" testosterone. Testosterone supplementation can bring benefits such as increased bone density, increased muscle mass and strength, decreased body fat, return of libido and sexual function, feelings of greater well-being, and less fatigue.[27] But there are risks as well: worsening of existing cardiovascular problems, prostate enlargement and cancer, hypertension, and sleep apnea (a serious disorder in which a sleeping person repeatedly stops breathing).[28] Before you even consider supplementation, have a checkup to find out whether you have these conditions or are at risk for them, and obtain advice from a physician.

Risks and Benefits of Testosterone Supplementation

BODY SYSTEM	EFFECTS
Cardiovascular	Declining free testosterone levels and increasing atherosclerosis with age in men suggests that low blood levels of free testosterone increase risk of coronary atherosclerosis. Others claim that high testosterone increases risk of coronary heart disease. Additional large-scale, long-term studies needed.
Body composition	Supplementation in adult men increases lean body mass and strength and decreases body fat. Evidence is consistent that androgen therapy is beneficial.
Bone metabolism	Bone density decreases in hypogonadism. Androgen supplements increase bone mineral density.
Respiration	Testosterone can exacerbate sleep-related breathing disorders and pulmonary problems. Risk in patients with sleep apnea and pulmonary problems.
Fluid balance	Androgens cause fluid retention. Could aggravate hypertension, peripheral edema, and congestive heart failure.
Sugar metabolism	Low testosterone is associated with increased development of diabetes. Testosterone treatment has a positive effect on decreasing insulin resistance and fasting blood glucose levels.
Behavior/mood	Deficiencies adversely affect behavior and mood. Supplements improve mood, energy, and sense of well-being; decrease nervousness and irritability.
Sexual function	Addition of androgens to hypogonadal men significantly increases sexual and erectile function.

Adapted from Y.C. Kim, International Journal of Impotence Research 11 (1999): 343–352.

Menopause and Estrogen

Women in their 50s undergo a near-total decline in their female sex hormones, usually over a period of one to three years.[1] In this phase of aging, production of hormones—primarily estrogen and progesterone—declines dramatically to levels that can change both inner feelings and outward appearance. Reduction in estrogen and progesterone production in women can cause a loss of skin tone, thinning of tissues along the reproductive tract, loss of libido, abdominal weight gain, and mood changes. It can also result in loss of bone mass or osteoporosis, hair thinning, urinary incontinence, increased risk of cardiovascular disease, sleep disturbances, fatigue, and a general sense of malaise.

Researcher J.C. Prior and colleagues point out in *The New England Journal of Medicine* that our culture has defined menopause as a "point in time rather than a process, and ... [has labeled] it an estrogen deficiency disease ... all reflections of nonscientific, prejudicial thinking by the medical profession."[29] But this negative view of menopause is not unique to our lives and times. The "change of life" has been surrounded by a culture of negativity for centuries. Today, however, more than 40 million postmenopausal American women can expect to live one-third of their lives after menopause.[30] And average life expectancy for women has increased to approximately 84 years, up from 48 years for a woman born in 1900.

This means that in North America, a woman is now likely to live 35 to 40 years after menopause, which in effect is the springtime of the second half of her life. As Christiane Northrup states, a woman can "make the most of the menopausal transition" and "think of it as a process for creating the healthy body she needs to last her until the end of life."[31]

From the perspective of prevention, bone mass, for one, should be evaluated much earlier in life than during or after menopause. By then, hormone replacements and medications may be the only option. The risk of cardiovascular disease, stroke, and maturity-onset diabetes in postmenopausal women is also significant. Even though 75 percent of women have menopausal symptoms, most of these can be treated immediately with hormone replacement therapy, physical activity, homeopathy, meditation, acupuncture, or herbal remedies.[32]

Today, more than 40 million postmenopausal American women can expect to live one-third of their lives after menopause—which in effect is the springtime of the second half of a woman's life.

Hormone Replacement Therapy Risks

If you are thinking about hormone replacement therapy, you do need to take into account some of the risks. Conventional treatment of menopause tends to rely on estrogen, along with progesterone in women with a uterus, but generally no progesterone for a woman who has had a hysterectomy. A 2002 Women's Health Initiative study funded by the U.S. National Institute of Health assessed risks and benefits of hormone replacement therapy for menopausal symptoms and came up with some important findings.[33]

Be sure to check with your doctor whether one type of estrogen—estradiol, which is considered most potent—is enough for you. (Women produce at least three estrogens: estrone [E1], estradiol [E2], and estriol [E3]).[34]

Hormone Replacement Risk (Common Prescriptions)

DRUGS	BENEFITS	POSSIBLE SIDE EFFECTS
Estrogens → oral tablets → skin patches → vaginal preparations → injections → gels	→ reduce hot flushes → improve mood and concentration → relieve vaginal symptoms → prevent osteoporosis → prevent dementia	→ breast tenderness → nausea → headache → bloating → increased risk of breast cancer → increased risk of endometrial cancer
Progestins → oral tablets → injections	→ reduce risk of endometrial cancer (from estrogen)	→ edema → bloating → mood alteration
Testosterone → oral tablet → injections	→ improve sexual desire → increase sense of well-being → increase muscle tone	→ voice changes → acne
Selective estrogen receptor modulators (raloxifene) → oral tablets	→ reduce risk of bone fractures	→ flushing → leg cramps → flu syndromes
Bisphosphonates → oral tablets	→ prevent and treat osteoporosis	→ abdominal pain → nausea → diarrhea
Calcitonin → nose spray	→ reduce bone fractures	→ nose dryness → nose bleeding

If There's Life after Sex, Is There Sex after Mid-Life?

How we see ourselves and take care of ourselves as sexual beings will have a great impact on all aspects of our well-being. The effect is often far-reaching, extending to people around us and to future generations.

A man's sexual desire wanes in mid-life, and some women also experience a decline, but for a significant proportion, libido may go into overdrive. This can change a well-matched relationship that has matured over many years into a difficult case of sexual desire discrepancy. To cope with these potential changes, partners need to be understanding of each other as they may go through mid-life and its physical transitions at different times and rates. A variety of other factors such as career changes, self-esteem problems related to aging, and financial issues surrounding retirement may also account for or aggravate an imbalance in partners' desire.

When desire discrepancy causes problems in your sex life, there are strategies you can use to make things better. It is very important not to blame each other. Sex can be redefined as a continuum, from cuddling to kissing to caressing to masturbation to various types of intercourse—and this eliminates the need to "go all out" every time you are intimate with your partner.

D.H. Lawrence wrote in *Lady Chatterley's Lover* "I thought I'd done with it all. Now I have begun again," (said the Lover). "Begun what?" (asked Lady Chatterley). "Life."

Sex and love are part of life. At some point in our lives, we may begin to make love twice a month instead of twice a day, and eventually we may be very happy if we can have sex twice a year. Our love may come to be expressed as gentle companionship rather than mad passion, but our capacity for affection, joy, and love will not diminish as we age. Weathering seasons side by side and going through life transformations together can bring special rewards in a relationship. Few images are more peaceful, touching, and spiritually uplifting than that of an old couple holding hands and looking into each other's eyes.

Hormone Replacement Risk (Natural Approaches)

APPROACH	BENEFITS	POSSIBLE SIDE EFFECTS
Calcium and vitamin D	→ reduce bone loss and fractures → prevent and treat osteoporosis	→ constipation → nausea → vomiting
Isoflavone in soy products	→ reduce vaginal dryness → reduce hot flashes	→ interaction with estrogen → increased breast cancer risk
Black cohosh	→ regulate periods	→ stomach upset → nausea → vomiting → decreased blood pressure
Ginkgo biloba	→ improve memory	→ stomach upset → headache → skin reaction → prolonged bleeding time
Dong Quai	→ effectiveness is still being evaluated	→ increased skin cancer risk → can be toxic → prolonged bleeding time
Yam and Evening primrose oil	→ effectiveness is still being evaluated	→ side effects not known
Exercise	→ reduce osteoporosis and bone fractures → decrease risk of heart problems → increase muscle tone → increase sense of well-being → reduce hot flushes	→ should be preceded by cardiovascular health analysis → safe if appropriate for one's age and fitness level

Data from **Hormone Therapy** (January 2003), The National Women's Health Information Center, U.S. Department of Health and Human Services.

Together and Beyond

It is so easy to withhold and to withdraw from living fully, and to look for something or someone else to complete the living for us. This can happen at any age, to anybody. But as we age, there is a greater tendency to seek perfection and glory in the past or in others. Especially when it comes to matters of sex and sexuality.

Sexuality did not evolve for completion. It evolved to advance *life*, to make *life* better and last longer, whether it occurs in an organism or a person, or as an event between mates.

When I was younger, I thought love and sex was about the right time, the right place, and the right person. Now, I think it is much more than that. It is the right chemistry, the right food, the right job(s), the right in-laws, the right words, the right temperature, the right pressure, the right timing, the right move, and the right ... *everything*. It is also probably continuously evolving, as we change on the inside and on the outside. Environment, history, inheritance, traditions, potential, all that was, that is, and that will be are woven together.

Our sexuality is a reflection of us and the totality of who we are. And a sexual experience, at any age, is about expressing, absorbing, projecting, and embracing the totality of the moment, the being(s), and the experience.

Adrenopause and Sex Hormones

The hormone steroid dehydroepiandrosterone (DHEA) and its sulfate ester (DHEAS) are secreted by adrenal glands, and when these secretions decrease with age, the condition is called *adrenopause*.

Decline in DHEA may contribute to a shift from anabolism (the building-up phase of metabolism) to catabolism (the destructive phase of metabolism) associated with aging. And this shift results in a series of age-related symptoms such as loss of muscle mass, osteoporosis, and heart conditions. Because DHEA and DHEAS are converted into both the female hormone estrogen and the male hormone androgen in the peripheral tissues, they are also sometimes called sex hormones.[35]

Much publicity that makes radical claims for DHEA is not based on scientific clinical data. And the DHEA that is available outside the conventional medical network in North America poses a real public health concern. The quality—and even the very presence—of DHEA in products on sale in the marketplace is unregulated and not governed by official quality-control standards. There are also concerns about the abuse of DHEA and about some of its side effects. By increasing sex steroids, DHEA can promote the development of ovarian, prostate, or other types of cancer. Other side effects include acne, unwanted hair growth, hair loss from the scalp, irritability, aggression, and menstrual irregularity, sometimes even in postmenopausal women.[36]

Some Lifestyle Factors and Aging

Free radicals are the highly reactive by-products of cell metabolism. Some of them are essential to many intracellular metabolic reactions, but others are potentially harmful, causing damage to cell proteins, DNA, fat lipids, and membranes through oxidation.

Antioxidants. Oxygen-derived radicals (ROs)—the highly reactive by-products of cell metabolism—are produced in abundance in all animal cells and tissues as part of our normal metabolic processes. It has been estimated that each human cell undergoes ten thousand "hits" by free radicals each day. Some free radicals are essential to many intracellular metabolic reactions, but others are potentially harmful, causing damage to cell proteins, DNA, fat lipids, and membranes through oxidation. This results in the generation of dysfunctional molecules responsible for conditions as diverse as cancers, lung disease, dementia, cardiovascular disease, and eye diseases.[37] The number of damaging free radicals can also be increased by smoking, ultraviolet rays, air pollution, or a diet of high saturated fats.[38]

Fortunately, the body has numerous mechanisms that either prevent the formation of ROs or neutralize ROs once they are formed—and this has led to the theory that the lifespan of an organism can be increased by slowing the rate of random free radical reactions.[39] Many studies have shown that the addition of a number of well-known antioxidants—such as bioflavonoids and vitamins A, C, and E—to a rodent's diet can increase its lifespan by an average of 20 to 30 percent.[40] Some of the dietary sources of antioxidants for humans include vegetables, fruits, and tea.

The Immune System. The aging of the immune system, referred to as *immunosenescence*, brings on a dramatic reduction in the ability of the body to respond to foreign invaders (or antigens). And functional decline has been observed at many levels, including chemical changes within disease-fighting immune cells, called lymphocytes. Although the overall number of lymphocytes does not change greatly in old age, the composition of lymphocytes in the blood and their reaction to infectious agents are altered considerably. As the body ages, the lymphocytes it produces are less vigorous and less effective in combating challenges. They are like a weakened army of aging soldiers guarding the border and an aging police force patrolling the body.[41]

The body also loses its ability to distinguish what is self and what is foreign—a problem that can lead to autoimmune diseases and prevent the immune system from identifying and fighting cancerous or malignant cells effectively. This is one of the reasons why the risk of many cancers increases with age.[42]

The body's ability to create a fever response to infection is not always automatic in elderly people. In fact, more than 20 percent of adults over age 65 who have serious bacterial infections do not have fevers. At this age, the central nervous system is simply less sensitive to immune signals and no longer reacts as quickly or efficiently to infection.[43]

Unfortunately, there is no magic anti-aging drug or anti-aging pill, so the healthiest way to slow the age-associated decline in immune function may be to adopt a regimen of proper nutrition and regular physical activity. A good immune-system-building diet includes plenty of fresh fruits and vegetables and low intake of saturated fat. Vitamin and dietary supplements are also effective—especially vitamin E and zinc.[44]

As for exercise, regular moderate activities may increase resistance to infections such as the common cold, but hard training is not a good idea, because it is often associated with increased respiratory tract infections.

The healthiest way to slow the age-associated decline in immune function may be to adopt a regimen of proper nutrition and regular physical activity.

For more on diet and supplements for improving the immune system, see Chapter 8, "Gourmet Wellness."

Napping is associated with decreased mortality and lowers diastolic blood pressure; it improves mood; and it decreases fatigue.

Obtaining preventive vaccinations is one way to help the aging immune system work. But, in general, older adults do not respond to vaccines as well as younger people do—and that pattern also applies to streptococcal pneumonia. This is a particular problem in the case of influenza because the elderly account for more than 80 percent of deaths during flu epidemics. Tetanus is another problem, since more than 70 percent of people over the age of 70 worldwide did not receive the necessary tetanus vaccinations in their younger days and so are more susceptible to the illness. On the other hand, some people are allergic to vaccines. It is best to check with your doctor regarding vaccinations.[45]

Sleep Patterns and Coping Options. As we grow older, we sleep more restlessly and wake up more often. And when we wake up in the middle of the night, we have more trouble getting back to sleep. With aging, we also tend to shift from being "owls" (evening types) to acting like "larks"(morning types). Over a 24-hour period, however, older adults seem to need the same amount of sleep as younger adults.[46]

As we grow older, we are also more likely to take afternoon naps. Healthy seniors have a napping rate of 24.3 percent compared to 7.9 percent for younger adults—and these power naps pay great dividends. A short afternoon nap (less than 30 minutes) improves older people's psychological, behavioral, and physiological arousal in the afternoon to adequate levels.[47]

Growth Hormones and Sleep

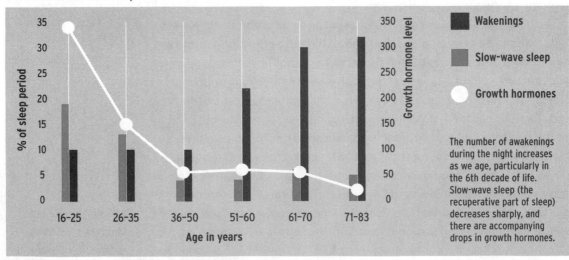

The number of awakenings during the night increases as we age, particularly in the 6th decade of life. Slow-wave sleep (the recuperative part of sleep) decreases sharply, and there are accompanying drops in growth hormones.

Data adapted from Vancauter et al., **Journal of the American Medical Association** 16 (2000): 861.

Sleeping and the Social Whirl

As we age, our nightly sleeping pattern may get worse because our social lives are more restricted, with reduced mobility, limited social interactions, fewer professional activities, and reduced exposure to light.

Scheduled exposure to bright light can help improve the situation. And planned activities can also make a difference. Here is one sequence that can improve sleep, as well as cognitive performance:[48] 10 minutes of stretching and 20 minutes of light physical activity (walking, stationary light exercises), then 30 minutes of seated social interactions (board or card games), followed by about 30 minutes of activities such as croquet or dancing.

In fact, as Barbara Phillips, professor at the University of Kentucky Medical Center, points out, napping has a number of useful results: it is associated with decreased mortality and lowers diastolic blood pressure; it improves mood; and it decreases fatigue.

Lifestyles of the Forever Young and Well?

It's never too late to adopt a wellness lifestyle. Research with heart-attack survivors, for example, has shown that those who exercise regularly can reduce their risk of a second fatal heart attack by up to 25 percent.[49] Other studies have demonstrated that people with healthier habits experience half as much chronic disability.

Here are a few lifestyle tips that, if followed regularly, could add years to your life and delay the onset of diseases related to aging.

Exercise. Regular, moderate exercise is the best antidote to many of the effects of aging. In fact, it is likely the most important part of an anti-aging lifestyle, as it helps prevent or ease a whole list of age-related ailments: coronary artery disease, high blood pressure, stroke, diabetes, obesity, osteoporosis, arthritic pain, stress, depression, insomnia, and senility.

Research shows that resistance exercise training programs can improve muscle size, strength, and endurance even in very old and frail men and women. Data compiled from 29 studies showed that exercise programs increase cardiorespiratory fitness in adults over 60 years of age by 22 percent on average.[50] It is never too late to start.

A short afternoon nap (less than 30 minutes) improves older people's psychological, behavioral, and physiological arousal in the afternoon to adequate levels.

See Chapter 8, "Gourmet Wellness," for a table listing indoor/outdoor chores and their calorie-burning values.

Simply put, exercise is the closest you can come to an effective anti-aging therapy. At least 30 minutes a day of moderately rigorous physical activity will help you stay younger—and daily chores count if they are rigorous enough!

Whatever routine you choose, you should make sure it includes these three components:

→ An aerobic activity to gradually raise your heart rate and improve your heart's health.
→ Weightlifting every other day to build muscle and bone and to improve balance.
→ Stretching for as little as 10 minutes every other day, to help prevent stiffness.[51]

See Chapter 9, "Our Bodies in Motion," for more on exercise and fitness.

Food Tips. As we grow older, we may not think a healthy diet is as necessary as it was when we were younger, had heavier workloads, and were more active. But a balanced diet can decrease your risk of cancer, high blood pressure, coronary artery disease, diabetes, osteoporosis, and memory loss.[52]

Other Lifestyle Tips:
→ If you use tobacco, stop. Stopping offers immediate and long-term health rewards.
→ Prevent obesity by keeping your weight between 5 percent below and no more than
20 percent above normal for your size.
→ Drink alcohol in moderation. Chronic abuse of alcohol is an age accelerator.
→ Protect your skin from the sun. Too much sun ages skin and raises your risk of getting
skin cancer.
→ Sleep seven to eight hours a night. Too little or too much sleep can shorten your years.
→ Talk to your doctor. Find out which screening tests you should have and how often. Regular checkups will help identify and manage risk factors for various medical problems.[53]

Optimal Mindset

A number of negative emotions tend to creep up on us as we grow older, and they can become major obstacles to wellness. As the years go by, we may become saddled with feelings of disappointment/regret, anger/frustration, loneliness/abandonment, and fear/insecurity. We'll take a look here at the first two obstacles, which tend to become more pronounced with age, and discuss other overall emotional fitness issues in Chapter 10, "From Daily Hassles to Spiritual Fitness."

Disappointment/Regret. Disappointment is most often caused by expectations, especially those we impose on ourselves, on those close to us, and perhaps on life in general. As we age, unmet expectations and the realization that some of these may never come to fruition can cause an overwhelming sense of disappointment. As our personal history becomes longer and longer, we could very easily become victims of the past: not only because of things left undone or unsaid, but also because we realize we cannot repeat yesterday's glories.

We need to keep in mind every day, especially when we are growing old, that yesterday does not exist anymore. It doesn't matter how tragic or glorious that past was. Today is the moment. You can always treasure a moment that you lived fully in the past. And when that moment is already fully lived or completely relived, how can there be any room left for regret? or for frustrated yearnings?

Of course, not all moments are so rich. But the value of any point in time can be maximized—changed from negative to positive—so that perspectives and wisdom from that moment are gained and shared. You can live today, embracing yesterday and tomorrow, actively engaging the past and future for the benefit of the present.

Anger/Frustration. According to the conventional wisdom of many cultures, "letting off steam" is good for health—and as we grow older, we often feel that we are more entitled to "get things off our chest." As the list of life's limitations grows with age, we may feel more and more frustrated and irritated with ourselves, with our situations, or with people around us. Before we know it, we can become much angrier people.

But anger is bad for your health—especially for your heart's health. Recent research studies show that the risk of heart attack is two times greater within two hours after an angry episode.[54] Cultivating an

See Chapter 8, "Gourmet Wellness," for more information on diet to reduce age-related physical problems.

You can live today, embracing yesterday and tomorrow, actively engaging the past and future for the benefit of the present.

Recent research studies show that the risk of heart attack is two times greater within two hours after an angry episode.

See Chapter 10,
"From Daily Hassles
to Spiritual Fitness,"
for more detailed
information on
these issues.

increased awareness of the irritations and frustrations that set off anger, and learning specific techniques to reframe anger when it occurs, are two ways of effectively reducing the intensity and duration of anger.

Some negative emotions often associated with anger are guilt and blame. Consciously countering these emotions with forgiveness of yourself and others may also be therapeutic.

An Oriental Perspective

Chinese medicine and meditation philosophy have a totally different perspective on growing and aging. According to this approach, all living beings are endowed at birth with the three elements of life: essence (*jing*), energy (*qi*), and spirit (*shen*).

The degree to which we protect and preserve these life elements determines the state of our health and well-being. This excerpt from the *Yellow Emperor's Manual of Corporeal Medicine* (Huang Di Nei Jing, 1000 B.C.), the earliest medical classic in China, describes the lives of ancient centenarians who benefited from following a life-protecting

Yin—Yang

According to traditional Chinese medicine, health is a simple state of equilibrium. It is not a composite of quantifiable entities such as chemical levels in the blood. So the practice of Chinese medicine is based on precise perception of disharmony, as indicated in the manifested signs and symptoms of a disorder. And practitioners begin by studying disharmony and disorder before proceeding to an understanding of harmony and health.

That is why *yin* and *yang* make up one of the most fundamental concepts of Chinese medicine. This philosophy sees two inseparable extremes in all energy and entities—a dual nature, positive and negative, male and female. These two energies are constantly interacting, with one advancing while the other is retreating, until one peaks and the direction of advance is reversed. Yin and yang and their interactions with each other are what account for all changes in the universe and in human bodies.

In anatomy, yin is the internal region—including tendons and bones—while yang is the external region, including the skin. In clinical diagnosis, yin and yang describe the nature of a disease. Classifying all symptoms of a disorder into yin and yang categories is the first step of any diagnosis. And treatments always aim to maintain or restore the balance of yin and yang, sedating any excess, for instance, and toning up any deficiency.

regime: "These people ... followed the principles of yin and yang, practiced body-building exercises best suited to their environment, were moderate in food and drink, maintained strict regimen in daily life and did not overexert themselves. That is why they remained in a good physical and mental state, enjoyed naturally endowed life spans."[55]

Jing: The Essence. Natural immunity factors and resistance to disease are found primarily in the body's vital jing, in three essential fluids:

→ Blood fluid includes all elements carried in the bloodstream.
→ Hormonal fluid includes all regulators for growth, immunity, sexuality, metabolism, and aging.
→ The third form of fluid includes regulators of waste products, digestive enzymes, perspiration, tears, and urine.[56]

Qi: The Energy. Qi is the vital force that activates every function and drives every process in the human body, voluntary and involuntary. It is a form of bioelectric energy that connects and travels throughout the body along complex channels called meridians. When this energy is balanced, the entire organism flourishes, and conversely, when it is disrupted or runs empty, the organism's vital functions fail.

Pre-natal qi is the primal power of the universe manifested in such things as light, heat, motion, and sound. *Post-natal qi* manifests itself in humans as the energy of the major organ systems, including body heat, breath, pulse, muscle activity, and other forms of bioenergetics. This post-natal energy comes from food, water, herbs, nutrients, and air. Through digestion and breathing, the body extracts vital nutrients and elements from external sources and transforms them into internal energy circulation.[57]

Shen. The spirit *shen* refers to the multiple facets and functions of our mental faculties, including consciousness, rational thought, intuition, psyche, personality, will, ego, and sensory awareness.

Balance and Harmony. *Shen* is the flowering blossom, *jing* is the root, and *qi* is the connecting stem. Only well-nourished roots planted in fertile soil generate strong stems and beautiful blossoms.[58]

Chinese medicine and meditation propose regulating the senses, dissipating negativity, and balancing energies so we can look inward with tranquility, beyond the mind. This tradition maintains that we are born with the full potential for life, but during the ordinary course of

Shen is the flowering blossom, **jing** is the root, and **qi** is the connecting stem. Only well-nourished roots planted in fertile soil generate strong stems and beautiful blossoms.

Adding Life and Years with "Emptiness"

An ancient Taoist maxim sums up the virtues of restraint and moderation as keys to health and well-being in Chinese medicine:

Empty mind: Keep the mind free from confusion and worry.
Empty stomach: Eat when you are hungry and stop before you are full.
Empty kitchen: Keep only enough food for a few days to ensure freshness.
Empty room: Avoid clutter and noise in living quarters to enhance serenity.[59]

> Good health and well-being depend on optimal balance and harmony among the energies of the vital organs and between the human body and its natural environment.

living, the demands of the world gradually pollute essence, dissipate energy, and exhaust spirit. This state leads to poor health and sickness.[60]

Good health and well-being, on the other hand, depend on optimal balance and harmony among the energies of the vital organs and between the human body and its natural environment. Toxins, germs, and pernicious elements that cause disease can invade only if the body's resistance is impaired. According to Chinese medicine, a loss of vital energy as we age results in a disruption of the body's inherent ability to maintain its structures and functions and to repair itself.[61]

4,600 Years Old ... and Going Strong

The will to survive and the spirit of life are truly astounding. Take, for example, the oldest living things in the world: the venerable bristlecone pines. Their average age is 4,000 years, and the longest-living of them all is more than 4,600 years old. These trees average about 9 meters (30 feet) in height, and they live on steep, barren slopes of shattered stone about 2,700 meters (9,000 feet) up the flanks of White Mountain, about 350 kilometers (215 miles) from San Francisco. On hard ground where even weeds find it difficult to survive, we find these longest-living organisms in the world.[62]

The world's oldest, tallest trees and those with the greatest girth belong to the same species, and they are all found in California. The *Sequoia sempervirens* grow about 600 kilometers (370 miles) northwest of White Mountain, and the tallest among them soars to 110.4 meters (368 feet). About 100 kilometers (60 miles) to the south are stands of trees that have the greatest girth in the world, the Giant Sequoia. The diameter at the base of the largest Giant Sequoia currently in existence is more than 9 meters (30 feet). This tree is 81.6 meters (272 feet) tall, and at 36 meters (120 feet) from the ground its diameter is 5.1 meters (17 feet). The first branch alone is 2.1 meters (7 feet) in diameter and projects 37.5 meters (125 feet) through the air, tall enough to tower over a 12-story building.[63]

Surprisingly, these trees have truly humble beginnings: their seeds are so tiny that it takes more than 91,000 of them to make up a pound, or close to half a kilogram. And they come from cones produced only by trees more than 200 years old. Why do they live and remain standing tall for so long?

These trees have roots that extend more than 150 meters (500 feet) around in the ground. As they reach out, they expand their sphere of nourishment, enriching themselves in every possible way. But this expansion is not aggressive, exclusive, or competitive. In fact, the roots of these trees all merge and grow together with those of neighboring trees, creating a common network.[64]

It is because of this unbreakable mutual support that they are able to withstand the rigors of an environment that would be almost impossible to bear if they were alone.

Perhaps, after all, if we look long and hard enough, our world can actually be seen in a single seed, and the secret of "forever young and well" can be found in the ancient Sequoia. Maybe some do grow older *and* wiser!

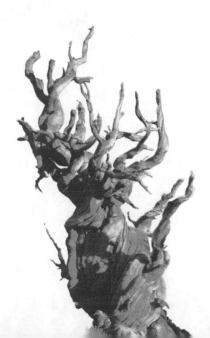

On barren slopes of shattered stone, a four-thousand-year-old tree.

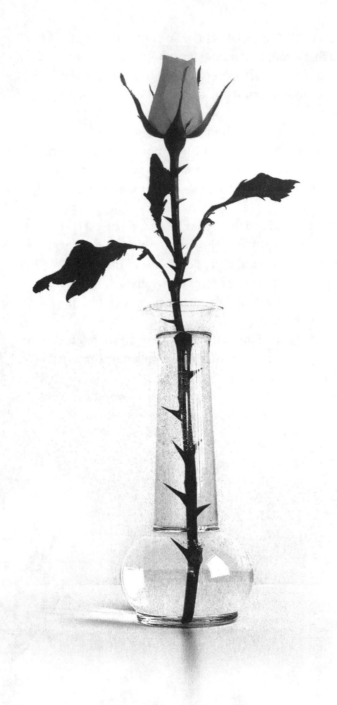

6 What Is Your Body Telling You?
Understanding Pain

*Our brain allows us to agonize over future pain, past pain,
and the pain of loved ones ... Suffering, like love, requires
a human dimension in addition to the raw biology.*
—Frank T. Vertosick Jr., *Why We Hurt*

Pain question: Is there a rose without thorns?

Awareness and intelligence are double-edged swords. They allow us to perceive pain and suffering but also give us the tools to understand the process, making wellness choices possible. "When it comes to the treatment of pain," says American neurosurgeon Frank T. Vertosick Jr., "knowledge is the best weapon."[1]

Why is knowledge so important? Because it helps us create strategies, a necessity when dealing with an enemy as formidable as pain. When facing foes, the best strategy is certainly to eliminate them. But pain is felt differently for different reasons by different people, so the more knowledgeable you are about your pain, the more effectively you will be able to eliminate it with proper devices.

If elimination is not possible and you have to live with the enemy, it is even more essential to develop strategies. For example, since pain is perceived and felt because there is awareness, you may be able to change the focus of your awareness. And it is true that pain is greatly reduced by distraction. The capacity of your awareness may be modified and the pain threshold expanded. Numerous treatments also exist that may help us manage or reduce the intensity of pain.

Where there's knowledge, there's hope for wisdom. Where there's wisdom, there's always hope for a sense of well-being and optimal living.

Historical Views of Pain[2]

Pain is a complex, subjective, multidimensional phenomenon that is perceived through human consciousness. It is influenced by genetic predisposition, psycho-sociological expectations and conditioning, and cultural and family dynamics. Pain can also be intensified or reduced depending on general health and mental condition; the nature and severity of the pain; environmental factors; and the personal meaning attributed to the experience. The list of influences goes on and on. As in any other experience filtered through human consciousness, pain is both something that we can change and something that is constantly changing by itself, improving or worsening, appearing or disappearing, amplified or forgotten. And any of these shifting perceptions can happen at a moment's notice.

The ancient Egyptians believed pain was the spirit of the dead entering the body through the ears or nose, but the ancient Indians thought it arose from a frustration of desires, an ailment of the heart. Plato believed it was an emotional experience of the soul, and Hippocrates thought pain was caused by an imbalance among the four humors (the physical elements that were considered to be part of every body). Similarly, the ancient Chinese attributed pain to an energy and nutrient imbalance or insufficiency.

Galen, the 2nd-century court physician to Emperor Marcus Aurelius in Rome, prescribed opium for pain and blamed the phenomenon on "hard nerves"—peripheral nerves in the brain and spinal cord system. The 17th-century philosopher Descartes described pain as being transported by tube-like nerves connecting the skin to the brain.

By the late 1800s, Scottish neurosurgeon Charles Bell, French physiologist François Magendie, German physiologist Johannes Mueller, and British physiologist Charles S. Sherrington had formulated the dedicated neural pain pathway principle. They established that the function of pain is not to heal, but to provide warnings about cell and tissue damage in the body. Pain, they theorized, is transmitted in the form of nerve impulses by connecting peripheral receptors to spinal neurons and then to brain receptors. This pathway was thought to be like a telephone line.

In 1965, Canadian psychologist Ronald Melzack and British physiologist Patrick Wall developed the gate control theory, which suggested that the brain controls the amount of pain information it receives. The central nervous system contains a mechanism, they said, that is closed to normal stimulation but open to pain sensations.

> Pain is both something that we can change and something that is constantly changing by itself.

Today's Pain Concepts

According to the International Association for the Study of Pain, pain is the most common reason why people seek medical attention, accounting for more than 70 million health/medical visits each year in the United States alone. The association defines pain as "An unpleasant sensory and emotional experience associated with actual or potential tissue damage or described in terms of such damage." Pain is a perceived threat or damage to a person's biological integrity.

The skin and other sensitive parts of the body, such as the tongue and eyes, have large numbers of pain receptors. Internal organs, on the other hand, have fewer pain receptors and are insensitive to most types of injury. Pain caused by tissue damage (skin, muscle, internal organs) is known as *nociceptive pain*, but pain caused by nerve damage or abnormal nerve function is called *neuropathic pain*, or neuropathy. This is the usual cause of chronic pain, and it may involve any part of the nervous system, from a small nerve in a toe to a nerve in the spinal cord.[3]

Damage to a tissue by perforation, fracture, sprain, contusion, infection, or lack of blood supply (as in angina) stimulates specialized nerve cell endings, known as nociceptors or pain receptors. These receptors send signals through the spinal cord to the brain, where they are interpreted as pain. At the same time, the damaged tissues release chemicals called prostaglandins, which cause inflammation and swelling at the injury site. This further stimulates the pain receptors.[4]

A Pain in the Brain?

Pain: Can't live with it; can't live without it.

The pain experience involves simultaneous activities in various regions of the brain and in multiple neural pathways. The feeling of pain is probably produced by a neuromatrix (a pattern-generating mechanism of the brain) as sensory inputs mix with information already stored in the brain such as memory and expectations. For instance, pain signals from our skin, muscle, bone, or other tissues travel to the brain through two neural pathways that run in the spinal cord. One relays information to the brain regions that analyze the precise location and nature of the pain (e.g., burning, crushing, sharp). The second pathway communicates with brain regions that produce arousal, and process emotion to ensure that pain sends an intense, unpleasant signal. In this way, our nervous system protects us from repeated damage. Unfortunately, this emotional hardwiring also means that pain can be accompanied by emotional suffering, compounded by past experience. With chronic pain, this shows up in many people as depression.[5]

In chronic pain, it's either as though an initial assault has altered the transmission of the pain signals, keeping the pain "knob" set on "high," or else as if pain has somehow become the default mode. Genetic researcher Jeffrey Mogil of the University of Illinois is trying to localize genes that might explain this phenomenon. He claims genetic differences may explain why some people's pain signals cannot be turned off.[6]

Injury not only produces pain; it also results in stress as the body tries to return to a stable state. This process takes place in different parts of the body, not just at the injury site, and it is affected by many genetic factors that exist at the injury site, in the adrenal medulla (which secretes stress hormones), throughout the immune system, and in many areas of the brain.

Pain and Suffering in the Mind and Heart

Conditioning and memory play key roles, and neuroscientists are just beginning to unravel the mystery of what exactly these roles are and how they are executed. However, it is now clear that pain behavior can be generated or perpetuated by learned cues in the environment or by the expectation of pain.

McGill University neuropsychologist Catherine Bushnell applies functional magnetic resonance imaging to visualize the activation of neural pathways while the patient is actually experiencing pain. She finds that the brains of people experiencing severe, chronic pain show different patterns of neural activation than normal subjects. Pain-related areas in the cortex are overactivated in pain patients.

Pain and suffering are two different things, but not all pain causes suffering. And not all suffering is expressed as pain or stems from pain, even when the two are happening at the same time. Pain is a perceived threat or damage to a person's biological integrity and survival, but suffering is the perception of a serious threat or damage to the self. Suffering occurs when there is a discrepancy between what the person expected of the self and what the person actually is or does.

When we are in pain, discomfort and functional limitations foster negative thinking and create a vicious cycle of stress and disability. The idea that the pain is uncontrollable leads to stressful fear, and the feeling that the pain is undeserved creates anger. The sustained longing to get back to a pain-free state then results in more fatigue, and the inability to participate fully in life, play, and work brings frustration and regrets.

The pain experience is about plugged-up knees and shooting needles. It's about the lump in the throat, the sinking feeling in the stomach, and the heartache when a person is served with divorce papers. Suffering is the consequence of perceived, impending destruction of some essential part of the person, either in the body or in the heart. Suffering emerges because the pain changes who we are—for instance, from a happy spouse to a lonely divorcée.

> Pain and suffering are two different things, but not all pain causes suffering. And not all suffering is expressed as pain or stems from pain, even when the two are happening at the same time. Suffering emerges because the pain changes who we are.

Types of Pain[7]

Transient Pain. Transient pain occurs in the absence of any tissue damage. It warns the body of physical damage by the environment or by overstressed body tissues.

Somatic Pain. When stimulated, certain nerve cells (sensory pain neurons) throughout the body send signals to the brain, where pain perception is thought to begin. Throbbing somatic pain is caused by increased blood flow to the damaged tissue or by vasodilation (an increase in the diameter of blood vessels), as in the case of migraines. Severe shooting pains, resulting from such problems as sciatica, are caused by pressure on, or irritation of, nerves at the point where they emerge from the spinal cord. Burns or stimulations from stepping on a nail, which happen at the body surface, are perceived by the brain and projected back to the site of the injury so that one feels the pain there. This kind of pain provokes an immediate reaction to move away from the stimulant.

Referred pain: Hip problems may be felt as knee pain, while problems with a tooth may be felt as an earache.

Referred Pain. Referred pain originates at internal (visceral) structures and is often felt at a superficial area that may be some distance away from the point of origin. The area to which the pain is referred generally receives its nerve supply from the same level of the spinal cord as the visceral organ involved. For example, an arthritic hip joint may cause referred pain in the groin, buttock, or knee, and the pain worsens as the day wears on.

Similarly, problems with a tooth may be felt as an earache. A person with angina who feels cardiac pain in his left arm is also experiencing referred pain. The pain that begins in his heart due to a lack of blood supply (ischemia) is felt in his arm most likely because the neurons from both the heart and the arm converge upon the same neurons in the central nervous system.

Since somatic pain is far more common than visceral pain, the brain interprets the pain as being from the arm's surface instead of from the heart. However, when visceral pain is felt both at the site of the distress and as referred pain, it means that the sensation is radiating from the organ to the superficial area.

Phantom Pain. Phantom pain is pain in a part of the body that no longer has any sensation at all or is even missing. This kind of pain is experienced by up to 80 percent of all amputees. They have the distinct feeling that the missing limb is still attached and is held in a distorted and intensely painful position. Other phantom pain sensations, such as cramping, burning, and squeezing, may also be present.

For amputees who report burning, throbbing, or tingling phantom pain, the pain intensity seems to change readily with blood flow changes in residual limbs. And since the temperatures of residual limbs in amputees are also cooler when compared to intact limbs of healthy subjects, heat treatment and exercises that reduce muscle tension in residual limbs have been proposed as ways to reduce phantom pain. It seems that these approaches are helpful in diminishing cramping phantom pain. "Pain memory" also plays a role in generating phantom pain. In fact, pain memories established before an amputation may be a powerful factor in determining the level of pain.

A similarly phantom-like phenomenon is causalgia. Patients suffering from this disorder experience burning pain and sensitivity after their injuries have healed at sites some distance away from the original wound site, usually in the hands or feet.

Tormenting Sensory Ghosts

Causalgia was first described in 1872 by American neurologist Silas Weir Mitchell (1829–1914), based on his work with soldiers injured in the Civil War. According to Mitchell, after an injury had healed, a causalgia patient would experience intense, burning pain, usually in the hand or foot, but at a site some distance removed from the original wound. Many more injured soldiers have since been afflicted by causalgia and by phantom pain, baffling doctors such as French surgeon René Leriche (1879–1955) in World War I and Harvard-trained physician William K. Livingston (1892–1966) in World War II.

In his book *Injuries of Nerves and Their Consequences*, Mitchell described phantom pain as "*Sensory hallucination* ... the sensorial delusions to which persons are subject in connection with their lost limbs ... a phantom of the missing member, a sensory ghost ... faintly felt at times, but ready to be called up to his perception by a blow, a touch, or a change of wind."[8]

In 1937 Leriche published *La Chirurgie de la Douleur* (*The Surgery of Pain*), about his work on causalgia and phantom limbs. In it, he gave this description of a World War I amputee he'd helped in 1916: "I saw the patient on the 20th June: the upper (residual) limb was completely paralyzed ... arm, forearm, hand and fingers ... dominating everything, was an intense burning pain, concentrated particularly in the palm of the hand and on the pulp of the finger-tips."[9] He operated on the patient in August, and this patient had less pain after the operation. But in other cases, the relief was only temporary, and the ghost pain returned.

Acute and Chronic Pain

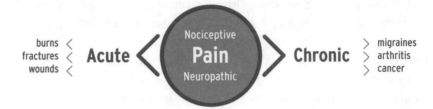

For more information on treatment options available to those who are suffering from **acute pain**, see the "Treatment Spectrum" later in this chapter.

Acute Pain. Acute pain occurs almost immediately after tissue damage or injury has occurred and lasts a limited time (seconds, minutes, hours, days, weeks, or months). When the body tissue is damaged, nociceptors at the site of the injury are activated. Since the healing process usually takes a few days or weeks, pain that persists for months or years is not classified as acute. However, in malignant diseases, the invasion of body tissues can produce continuous acute pain.[10]

Acute pain plays a protective role by warning us of imminent or actual tissue damage and by coordinating reflexes and behavioral responses—thus keeping such damage to a minimum. If tissue damage is unavoidable, changes in the peripheral and central nervous systems establish profound but reversible hypersensitivity to pain in the inflamed and surrounding tissue. This process makes wound repair possible by protecting the damaged area from contact until healing has finished.

Although acute pain is a normal physiological response to an adverse stimulus, social and psychological factors also greatly affect the

Painful Predictions

As we age, we will encounter a greater and greater likelihood of suffering from chronic pain. And since the entire world's population is aging rapidly, the prevalence of chronic pain conditions such as arthritis, lower back pain, and cancer will increase around the globe. People in every country would benefit from better pain management methods and programs. Fortunately, new methods are being actively sought. In fact, in the last few years, there has been an explosion of research in the field of chronic pain mechanisms and management.

The World Health Organization (WHO) has projected that the number of people diagnosed with cancer over the next 20 years will double to 20 million cases per year. And they have published guidelines, including *Achieving Balance in Opioids Control Policy 2000*, as a way of helping governments develop less restrictive drug laws governing the prescription of opioid painkillers for medical purposes.

immediate experience of acute pain—among them, a person's attitude, expectations, and beliefs, as well as the individual's personality, family background, and culture.

Chronic Pain. Chronic pain is usually the result of an initial injury or disease, but we have very little knowledge of how or why it takes hold. Some people have terrible injuries with disabilities and never suffer chronic pain; others do well through several car accidents until the "final straw," after which even a relatively minor injury somehow triggers a cascade of increasing pain. It is possible that chronic pain sets in when the original injury causes damage to the nervous system, interfering with the healing process, and the intensity of the pain may be out of proportion to the original injury or tissue damage.[11]

Is genetic makeup a determining factor in the development of chronic pain? Is it a function of aging? Sleep? Nutrition? Attitude? Neuronal chemistry changes? It is probably a combination of factors, but the exact causes are not yet entirely clear.

Chronic pain takes a toll in all areas of life—emotional, financial, familial, and functional. In North America, for example, the cost of back injuries in 1986 was about US$20 billion (about Cdn$31 billion at today's exchange rate). Painful arthritis and recurrent headaches cost US$17 billion and $16 billion, respectively, and other chronic painful musculoskeletal disorders cost $11 billion. In the United States, 50 million people suffer from recurrent headaches, and 70 percent of migraine sufferers spend at least one day a month in bed trying to recover from these severe headaches.

Chronic pain patients often experience depression, sleep disturbance, fatigue, and decreased overall physical and mental functioning. The depression accompanying chronic pain often responds to conventional anti-depressant treatments, even if the pain cannot be fully eradicated. But due to the misplaced idea that it's normal for the pain sufferer to feel down and out, depression is often left untreated. If depressive symptoms persist, the victim of chronic pain needs to be evaluated and vigorously treated.

Chronic pain ... often imposes severe emotional, physical, economic, and social stresses on the patients and their families. It is one of the most costly health problems for society.
—Anesthesiologist John J. Bonica (1917–94), founder of the International Association for the Study of Pain

Managing the Mechanisms of Chronic Pain

Because chronic pain is caused by such a wide variety of conditions, it is important to diagnose the mechanisms producing the problem in each individual, in order to review as broad a range of treatments as possible. According to one expert on the issue, physician Harriet Wittink of the New England Medical Center, therapies that decrease the intensity of chronic pain don't automatically lead to increased functioning or decreased disability. "A person's beliefs, appraisals, and expectations play a substantial role in determining functional limitations," Wittink notes.[12]

"Avoidance behaviors stemming from fear of pain and/or fear of re-injury can limit a person as much as the pain itself. Successful treatment of chronic pain must therefore entail a cognitive shift from helplessness to being able to function despite pain. To achieve this, an active partnership must be established between the patient and the pain management team. The essence of successful chronic pain management is that patients regain control over their lives."

It is essential for both patient and physician to understand that the treatment of chronic pain extends beyond the limits of biological medicine. Total pain must be addressed, not just physical pain.

Early Pain Control

Early control of pain can shape its subsequent evolution. Research shows that stimulation of pain receptors due to tissue damage can lead to important physiological responses even in unconscious, anesthetized patients. Even brief intervals of acute pain can induce chronic pain with changes and sensitization to the pain perception system combined with lasting psychological distress. Methods to control acute pain have greatly progressed since this discovery.[13]

Treatment Spectrum

How Do Painkillers Work? Analgesics, drugs that alleviate pain, can be separated into those that can be used externally and those that can be taken internally.[14]

External Analgesics. External analgesics include ointments and lotions that can be applied to the skin. Many of the products on the market may contain more than one agent and most work as sensory depressants or counter-irritants. Sensory depressants suppress the sensory response and decrease the sensitivity of the area to pain. Counter-irritants are designed to provide pain relief by stimulating the nerve endings—based on the Pain Paradox Theory. According to this theory, our brains can process only a certain amount of information at a time. When people apply counter-irritants to their skin, they create new stimuli in that area. This causes their brains to pay more attention to the new stimuli and to focus less on the existing pain.

External analgesics can be irritating, however, and should not be used on an open lesion or damaged skin. Unless a health-care professional says otherwise, they should not be used more often than indicated on the product or longer than a week. After applying these agents, it's also important not to put on any airtight dressing or tight bandages. Many external analgesics are toxic when ingested, and should never be used on young children.

Internal Analgesics. Internal analgesics are usually more effective in providing pain relief than external ones. Their effect can cover more than one area of the body and last much longer. For mild to moderate pain, acetaminophen, acetylsalicylic acid (ASA), and non-steroidal anti-inflammatory drugs (NSAIDS—including ibuprofen, naproxen, and indomethacin) can usually give enough relief. In more severe cases, opioids (including codeine, morphine, and oxycodone) can provide better painkilling effects. They may be taken in various ways—as oral tablets, injections, or suppositories, for example.[15]

Internal analgesics have a number of side effects, which must be taken into account. Opioids, for example, can cause drowsiness and affect a person's ability to drive or operate machinery, and NSAIDS and ASA have the potential to cause stomach ulcers. Since these analgesics work throughout our bodies and not just locally, they could also interact negatively with other medications. That's one reason why you need to consult a doctor or a pharmacist before taking any internal analgesics. Anti-depressants, anti-convulsants, tranquilizers, and anesthetics have been used in combination with analgesics to provide additional pain relief, but again, these combinations should be made only on a physician's orders.

> Analgesics work throughout our bodies and not just locally. They could also interact negatively with other medications. Consult a doctor or pharmacist before taking any internal analgesics.

Opioids: Helpers and Destroyers[16]

Opioids have been known for thousands of years for their painkilling, euphoric, and addictive effects. The term *opiate* was once used to designate drugs derived from opium: morphine, codeine, and many

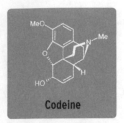

Codeine

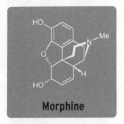

Morphine

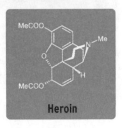

Heroin

derivatives of morphine. But soon after the development of totally synthetic compounds with morphine-like actions (such as methadone, propoxyphene, and fentanyl), the word *opioid* was adopted to refer to all drugs, natural and synthetic, with morphine-like actions.

Opioid activities can cause suppression of the cough reflex, respiratory depression, mood alteration, mental clouding, and brain-wave pattern changes. Nausea, vomiting, orthostatic hypotension (a sudden fall in blood pressure when a person stands up), and fainting can also occur. Inhibition of intestine mobility can lead to constipation, while an increase in sphincter tone may cause urinary retention. Large doses can cause excitation or seizures. Morphine and its derivatives also cause miosis (contraction of pupils).

The discovery of opioid receptors in the central nervous system during the early 1970s led to the discovery of several types of natural opioids found in our bodies. These natural painkillers produced in our central nervous system such as endorphins, dynorphins, and enkephalins are found in the brain and are also released from our pituitary, along with several stress hormones. They cause behavioral effects similar to those induced by morphine, which can be reversed with the morphine antagonist naloxone.[17]

History of Opioids

Raw opium contains about 25 different alkaloids, including morphine and codeine. Special chemical procedures are needed to isolate morphine and codeine from opium, and another chemical process is used to convert morphine to heroin. The opium poppy was cultivated by Sumerians around 3400 B.C., making it most likely the first drug used by humans, preceding even alcohol. Egyptian medical texts mentioned opium use for different conditions as early as around 2000 B.C. In addition to its use as a painkiller, the Romans used it to commit suicide or kill others at around 150 A.D. Swiss physician Paracelsus started to popularize the use of opium as "laudanum" in the 1500s. Morphine was isolated in 1800 by German pharmacist Friedrich Serturner, and was medically accepted and commercially available by 1820. It became even more popular by 1853 when the hypodermic syringe was perfected and it was thought that injection (as opposed to ingestion) would not cause addiction. Heroin, five times more effective than morphine as a painkiller, was produced in 1874. It was soon made commercially by Bayer. It was prescribed for respiratory illness, and as a cough suppressant.

In 1914, the *Harrison Act* in the United States reclassified opioid abuse as a criminal activity, rather than a medical sickness. [18]

Marijuana

Marijuana is the most widely used psychedelic drug known to humans, and varied uses of the hemp plant are literally woven into the fabric of human history. Archeological evidence from an ancient village in Taiwan suggests that humans were already using part of the marijuana plant as early as ten thousand years ago, during the Stone Age.

Public opinion and legislation concerning the use of marijuana have fluctuated throughout history from the lenient to the harshly intolerant. But one of the most important issues facing us today relates to the wise development, use, and legislation of marijuana for medicinal purposes.

In July 2001, Canada implemented regulations allowing for the possession, production, and use of marijuana for certain medical purposes under specifically defined conditions. The Marijuana Medical Access Regulations established a compassionate framework to allow the use of marijuana by people who are suffering from serious illnesses and where the use of marijuana is expected to have some medical benefit that outweighs the risk of its use.

Under the regulations, those who fall into one of three categories can apply for an "Authorization to Possess" marijuana for medical purposes. Holders of this authorization may possess a maximum 30-day treatment supply of marijuana at any given time.

Category 1 is for applicants who have terminal illness with a prognosis of a lifespan of less than 12 months. Category 2 is for applicants who suffer from specific symptoms associated with certain serious medical conditions, namely: multiple sclerosis (MS), spinal cord injury and diseases, cancer, AIDS/HIV infection, severe forms of arthritis, and epilepsy. Category 3 is for applicants who have symptoms associated with a serious medical condition other than those described in Categories 1 and 2, where conventional treatments have failed to relieve symptoms.

Marijuana remains an illegal drug in Canada except when authorized legally by the application and approval process. More information about these regulations and the application procedure is available at the Health Canada Web site.

Increase Your Body's Own Painkillers. Today, accumulated evidence has shown that responses to both acupuncture and prolonged exercise activate the central opioid systems. For instance, endogenous opioids (naturally produced in our bodies) are as potent as morphine at the same molecular concentration. Many studies show that exercise and training programs can also elevate endorphin concentrations in the body, and these have been linked to increases in pain threshold and

There is potential in using exercise to treat pain conditions.

decreases in pain perception. Acupuncture is also effective in controlling pain, even during some surgical procedures. These discoveries have led to a new theory of pain perception mechanisms, in which "non-pain" is perceived as an equilibrium between pain signals and "anti-pain" signals generated by the workings of naturally produced opioids in our bodies. There is potential in using exercise to treat pain conditions, as well as addiction, eating disorders, hypertension, depression, and anxiety.[19]

The Other Side of the Coin. Opioids are currently the most powerful painkillers, and most clinicians and scientists agree that the proper medical use of opioids does not create drug addiction. This is because a person in pain has a different physiological reaction to opioids than someone who is not in pain. The mechanism behind this pharmacological difference is not entirely clear, but research has shown that dosages given when there is no pain or doses beyond the amounts needed to relieve pain caused respiratory depression. There is apparently no respiratory depression when dosage levels are correct.

This difference also applies to addiction. Drug addiction does not occur in patients after pain relief with opioids in childbirth or operations, or after a myocardial infarction.

As University of Oxford pain researcher Henry McQuay says, the "clinical message is that opioids need to be titrated against pain" and the "political message is that medical use of opioids does not create drug addicts, and restriction hurts patients." However, support for use of opioids in non-cancer pain is not unanimous. There are concerns that opioids are harmful, and that increased availability of opioids would have adverse social repercussions.

Opioid analgesics definitely have the potential for abuse. Psychological or physical dependence and tolerance can follow repeated administration. In addition to "street abuse," medical abuses of opioids sometimes occur in individuals at high risk, including those in the medical profession. People with chronic pain syndromes may also misuse prescribed drugs.

Natural Remedies and Vitamins

PABA (para-aminobenzoic acid) is an over-the-counter natural remedy that can relieve pain. In low doses, it has the ability to slow the breakdown of cortisol (a natural pain-relieving hormone) in the liver. This action can

Warning Signs of Inappropriate Opioid Abuse

→ Preoccupation with drugs
→ Refusal to participate in a medication taper
→ Reports that nothing but a specific opioid works
→ Strong preference for short-action over long-term effect
→ Use of multiple prescribers and pharmacies
→ Use of street drugs or other patients' drugs
→ Not taking medications as prescribed
→ Loss of medications more than once
→ Decreased function

reduce pain or enhance the benefits of painkillers. D-phenylalanine can reduce pain by enhancing the action of our own natural painkillers. It also promotes the effects of acupuncture and of Aspirin and other non-steroidal anti-inflammatory drugs, thus reducing the amount of medication required. Known side effects of D-phenylalanine include anxiety, headaches, and high blood pressure.[20]

Vitamin B1 may suppress neural stimuli that produce pain, and vitamin B6 may increase the conversion of tryptophan, a precursor to the synthesis of the neurotransmitter serotonin. Serotonin is involved in pain perception and is often deficient in chronic pain patients. Vitamin B12 can also have pain-reducing effects.[21]

Botanical Medicines

White willow trees provide pain relievers, too. Extract from their bark contains salicin, which is metabolized to salicylic acid and has known anti-inflammatory and antioxidant properties. One natural compound found in willow-tree bark is acetylsalicylic acid (ASA). A more stable form of ASA has been the best-selling medication in the world since 1897—Aspirin. Devil's claw can have similar pain-reducing and anti-inflammatory properties.[22]

Hot cayenne pepper brings us a different kind of pain reliever. Known also as Capsicum, this plant contains capsaicin, and capsaicin depletes a chemical called substance P when applied on a person's skin. Substance P is an integral part of central nervous system pathways involved in psychological stress and pain, and when it is depleted, nerve transmissions from peripheral nerves to the spinal cord are blunted.[23]

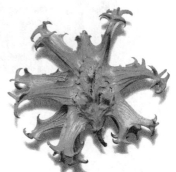

Devil's claw can have pain-reducing and anti-inflammatory properties.

How Do Painkillers Work?[24]

EXTERNAL ANALGESICS	HOW DO THEY WORK?	PRECAUTION
Camphor	It has weak local anesthetic and analgesic properties. In low concentration, it is a sensory depressant; but it becomes a counter-irritant when used in high concentration.	Too much rubbing can cause flushing of the skin. Ingestion of even a small amount of camphor could be life-threatening, especially for children. It should be kept out of reach of children.
Capsicum/Capsaicin	Capsicum is extracted from cayenne pepper. It works as a counter-irritant and causes redness and warmth on the areas where it is applied. It is one of the most studied external analgesics. Capsicum is believed to provide relief by depleting a substance that is responsible for pain transmission in our nerves.	Capsicum causes pain and burning sensations when first applied. With repeated applications, these sensations will disappear. Patience is needed when using capsicum. You may need to apply at least three to four times each day on the area and it may take up to two to four weeks of continuous usage before pain relief occurs. It can irritate your eyes just like pepper. Wash hands after applying.
Salicylates: Triethanolamine salicylate, Methyl salicylate	Salicylates are commonly used as counter-irritants in various topical preparations. Although they are related to ASA and are absorbed through skin into the body, they are very unlikely to have any systemic anti-inflammatory or analgesic effect.	They can be absorbed into our bodies. Heat should not be applied together with salicylates, since it could increase absorption and may damage the skin. People who are using anticoagulants/blood thinner should avoid using salicylates because of increased risk of bleeding. Salicylates should be applied only on intact skin and should not be used by children.
Menthol	Similar to camphor, it can be both a sensory depressant and a counter-irritant. In low concentration, menthol provides a cooling sensation where it is applied. In higher concentration, it creates a burning or warm feeling.	Adverse effects are unlikely to occur with menthol.
Eucalyptus oil	Eucalyptus oil is present in many external analgesic products. It is not recognized as a counter-irritant and its role is not totally clear. It produces a cooling sensation similar to menthol and camphor.	Ingestion of eucalyptus oil can cause gastrointestinal symptoms.
INTERNAL ANALGESICS	HOW DO THEY WORK?	PRECAUTION
Acetaminophen	Even though acetaminophen is one of the most commonly used internal analgesics, we still do not completely understand how it helps to relieve pain. It has only weak anti-inflammatory activity but it may interfere with signal generation and transmission in our nervous systems.	Acetaminophen is usually well tolerated, but alcoholics and patients with liver conditions should consult a doctor before taking it. It is important to follow recommended dosage because an excessive amount could lead to serious toxicity.
Acetylsalicylic acid (ASA) and NSAIDs	ASA and NSAIDs provide pain relief through similar mechanism. They suppress the production of the chemicals that trigger inflammation and pain response.	Compared to acetaminophen, ASA and NSAIDs have more side effects. Common ones include gastrointestinal upset, water retention, and prolonged bleeding time. They can also provoke asthmatic attacks in sensitive individuals. Patients with gastrointestinal, heart, or liver conditions should consult their doctors before taking ASA or NSAIDs. Pregnant women in their third trimester should avoid using these agents unless directed by their doctors. Aspirin is usually not recommended for children.
Opioids	Among the different types of analgesics, opioids are the strongest. They act on both the peripheral and central nervous systems to decrease sensitivity and increase tolerance to pain.	Opioids are the strongest analgesics and have many side effects such as mood changes, sedation, gastro-intestinal upset, and constipation. With prolonged use, opioids lead to tolerance and dependence.
Willow bark	This is a herb that is traditionally used to treat fever and pain. It is believed that constituents in willow are converted in our bodies to salicylic acid and provide pain relief.	The same precaution should be used for willow as for ASA and NSAIDs. With limited clinical information available, it should not be used during pregnancy, lactation, or for children.

Healing Therapies

Physiotherapy, chiropractic treatment, different types of massages, and many other therapies are useful in treating or reducing pain. Anything that relaxes you and gives you a sense of well-being— such as aroma-therapy, music, art, and theater therapies—may also be helpful.

Pain by its very nature defines limits and makes us not want to move joints, structures, or tissues. This is a reaction that must be respected, since it's through guarding that the body protects its own structures. However, any treatment plan that deals with pain must also include strengthening of supporting tissues and structures. And a combination of treatments marrying nutritional and physical fitness will lead to a much stronger resolution of pain.

Anything that relaxes you and gives you a sense of well-being—aromatherapy, music, art—may be helpful in treating pain.

Acupuncture

Most patients who undergo acupuncture treatments do so because of pain conditions, and this originally Oriental practice is becoming more widespread around the world. A conference organized in 1997 by the Office of Alternative Medicine and the Office of Medical Applications of Research (attached to the U.S. National Institutes of Health, NIH) came to this conclusion about acupuncture after hearing from a panel of 25 experts who presented 2,302 scientific studies: "Promising results have emerged for the use of acupuncture in treating the nausea and vomiting related to chemotherapy and postoperative dental pain," they said, and they went on to present a long list of other situations where acupuncture could be useful: "addiction, stroke rehabilitation, headache, menstrual cramps, tennis elbow, fibromyalgia, myofascial pain, osteoarthritis, low back pain, carpal tunnel syndrome, and asthma."[25] They also concluded that further research would likely lead to knowledge of more areas where acupuncture could be beneficial.[26]

One of the advantages of acupuncture is that it has a much lower incidence of adverse effects than do many drugs or other accepted medical procedures. Since acupuncture treatment does not require drugs that might lead to side effects or even addiction, it is gaining acceptance in Western countries. The World Health Organization now lists more than 40 conditions in which acupuncture can be helpful, and many of these conditions are associated with pain.[27]

The Five Elements

The five elements in Chinese medicine actually refer to five processes that lead to different conditions of the internal body landscape. These are: fire, wood, earth, metal, and water, which correspond to five organs: heart, liver, spleen, lung, and kidney. The heart function, for instance, generates heat and warmth, which is essential for maintaining body temperature. But when the process is overactive, the rate of metabolism speeds up and may result in fever. Chinese medicine aims at keeping a balanced amount of "fire" in the body.[29]

The theory behind acupuncture is based on the concepts of yin and yang, the five elements, and the meridians, which are central to Chinese medicine. Optimal health is achieved when these systems are in harmony.[28]

Since acupuncture treatment does not require drugs that might lead to side effects or even addiction, it is gaining acceptance in Western countries.

Acupuncture is described in the *Yellow Emperor's Manual of Corporeal Medicine* (1000 B.C.). in terms of the interrelationship between "meridians" and the use of acupuncture in diseases. Meridians are the channels, or pathways, that carry qi and blood throughout the body. *Qi* refers to life energy and its circulation. "Blood" is not meant in a literal sense, but rather in terms of its function as an invisible lattice that links together all fundamental textures and organs, and the circulation of nutrients within this network. To maintain good health, it is essential that blood, qi, and the meridian system maintain their harmonious balance and are properly nurtured.

The classical meridian system consists of a regular meridian subsystem and an extra meridian subsystem. (The regular one is known as *jing* — a different jing from the one mentioned in Chapter 5, on aging. Though the two words are pronounced in the same way, they are different Chinese characters.) Acupuncture treatment is based on the theory that the insertion of very fine needles into points along the meridians can remove blockage or stimulate better flow of qi and blood. Then the system is rebalanced and harmony restored.[30]

Another method to work on the points without puncturing the skin is acupressure. With this treatment, stimulation of the acupuncture points is performed, with fingers or a small ball or round instrument that does not puncture the skin, to remove blockages and encourage smooth flow of qi and blood.[31]

Acupuncture meridians

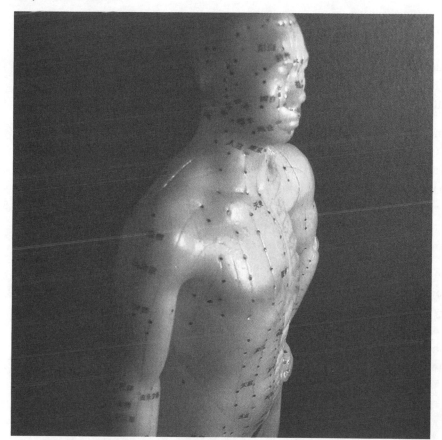

For more about yin and yang, see Chapter 5, "How Are You Doing as the Years Go By?"

There are 12 pairs of meridians in the main meridian subsystem, and they are distributed symmetrically on each side of the body. Each pair has its own definite pathway. There are 6 pairs within the upper extremities. Three of these pairs are located on the ventral side and they run from the chest to the hand. The other 3 pairs are on the dorsal side and run from the hand to the face. Similarly, there are 6 pairs for the body's lower extremities. There are 3 pairs on the lateral side, and they run from the face to the foot; the 3 pairs on the medial side run from the foot to the chest.

365 Acupuncture Points[32]

Meridians may be compared to a railway network and acupuncture points to stations. Classical texts on acupuncture recognize about 365 acupuncture points on the surface meridians of the body. In recent literature, this has increased to more than 2,000 possible points. In practice, however, a typical doctor's repertoire might be only about 150 points. Each acupuncture point has a defined therapeutic action, and a typical treatment requires the insertion of 5 to 15 needles.

The depth to which a needle penetrates depends on the particular point. Immediately following insertion, based on the ailment, an acupuncturist may manipulate the needle in several ways. These include raising and thrusting; twirling or rotation; a combination of raising/thrusting and rotation; plucking; scraping (with a vibration sent through the needle); and trembling (another vibration technique). Electro-acupuncture uses very small electrical impulses through the acupuncture needles. Other methods use laser and sound waves (sonopuncture). All variations apply vibration through the points.

A related technique, moxibustion, involves the application of heat from burning substances at the acupuncture point. Acupuncture needles were originally made of bronze, copper, tin, gold, or silver, but they are now made of hair-thin stainless steel. The U.S. Food and Drug Administration regulates acupuncture needles in the same category as surgical scalpels and hypodermic syringes, and they are manufactured under single-use standards of sterility. It is important to check the safety and sterility standard of the needles.

A number of theories have been developed to try to explain the mechanisms of pain relief by acupuncture:[33]

→ The gate theory put forward by Ronald Melzack, of the Department of Psychology at McGill University, and British physiologist Patrick Wall suggests that stimulation from the needle jams the nerve signal, so that other pain signals (from an incision, for instance) cannot reach the brain.

→ The insertion of acupuncture needles may stimulate the release of endorphins, a class of opioids naturally produced within the brain. Bruce Pomeranz of the Department of Zoology at the University of Toronto has contributed much to the understanding of endorphins and acupuncture with his studies on animals.

→ Stimulation by acupuncture may also activate the hypothalamus and pituitary gland in the brain, resulting in a broad spectrum of effects that have an impact on entire systems within the body.

Recent Discoveries about the Meridian

Amazing scientific studies, including some conducted by French researcher Pierre de Vernejoul and Korean researcher Kim Bong Han, have shown that the meridian system is a separate network, entirely independent of the vascular, nervous, and lymphatic systems. It seems to consist of several duct systems interlinking within itself, as well as interconnected with many tissue cell nuclei. They carry ductal fluids with high concentrations of deoxyribonucleic acid (DNA), ribonucleic acid (RNA), amino acids, and hormones such as adrenaline, estrogen, and corticosteroids.

➙ Documentation also exists to show a relationship between acupuncture and alternation in the secretion of neurotransmitters and neurohormones; changes in the regulation of blood flow both centrally and peripherally; and immune functions.

It has been reported that more than one million Americans receive acupuncture each year, an indication of its degree of acceptance in North America in general. Since many patients seek health-care treatment from both physicians and acupuncturists, communication between these providers should be encouraged and improved. If you are investigating acupuncture or are already receiving treatments for one problem, inform all the practitioners helping you in case any pain you are experiencing is masking other health problems.[34]

Working in Pain

Canadian workers suffering pain during some (in ligher shade) or most (in darker shade) of the time in a working week:

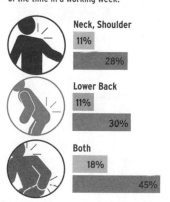

Neck, Shoulder
11%
28%

Lower Back
11%
30%

Both
18%
45%

Proportion of 1,541 workers suffering from lower back and shoulder pain during a working week:

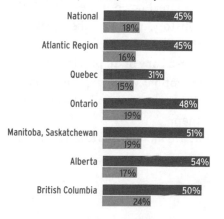

National 45% 18%
Atlantic Region 45% 16%
Quebec 31% 15%
Ontario 48% 19%
Manitoba, Saskatchewan 51% 19%
Alberta 54% 17%
British Columbia 50% 24%

■ pain a bit of the time last week
■ pain most of the time last week

Data from Earl Berger, **Berger Health Survey**, October 1999.

The Posture Problem

How does posture lead to pain? Posture is a collection of characteristics that encompasses the way you sit, stand, walk, talk on the phone, watch TV, surf the Internet—in other words, it is the position your body takes whenever you do anything. The more mundane the task, the more important it is to note your posture when you are performing it, since mundane, everyday tasks make up most of our daily activities. The effects of repeating certain postures, keeping the body in a certain posture for too long, or assuming an improper posture can accumulate and lead to chronic pain.[35]

Pain Checklist

To help understand your pain, and to provide doctors with clues for causes and treatment options, list these items:

1. When and how did the pain start?
2. List and classify each type of pain you experience.
3. Rank them in order of importance, in terms of how they affect you negatively.
4. Describe the pain:

   a. Feelings: burning, knife cutting, aching, squeezing, throbbing, pounding, etc.
   b. Duration
   c. Severity
   d. What brings it on? What makes it worse?
   e. What can you do to release it? Or reduce it?
   f. Symptoms: numbness; nausea; weakness; tingling; sensitivity to light, sound, and noise, etc.

5. How is this pain affecting your life? Any disability?
6. List treatment history, including therapies, medications, and the response you've had to each treatment.
7. Test history: keep a copy of all previous tests.
8. Describe your emotions when experiencing pain.
9. Make a list of how you dealt with the emotions, and other ways that you can imagine dealing with them.
10. List things that are more important to you than the pain.[36]

Expanding the Pain Threshold[37]

Excerpt from a Diary of Pain. This pain in the knees makes me feel like something inside is plugged up, and there is a pressure expanding from the inside out. It starts as a very dull and blunt pain, increasing as the pressure increases. When it becomes unbearable, the thing to do is to get up and walk along the edge of the room, walking around furniture that stands in the way, counting all the time. By about a hundred, the piercing needles have come. Tiny and everywhere at first, the tingling grows sharper with fewer needles at work. Another hundred counts or so, the last needles that are the sharpest are gone. Everything is fine until next time.

I always find that so unfair. If someone has pinched me, I can pinch back. If I have pinched myself, I deserve the pain. But something inside starts it at will, and it isn't me. There is nothing that I can do, except to get up and walk and count. There is no control, and there is nobody else and nothing else to get mad at. And it has nothing to do with whether I have been good or bad. What's the point?

Three levels of pain are at work here: physical pain, "total pain," and spiritual or "existential pain," each compounding and amplifying the others. We have already addressed many issues related to physical pain. Heartache, emotional stress, and mental anguish increase physical pain. Other worries, including work and money concerns, family dynamics, and relationship problems, as well as negative emotions such as anxiety, stress, depression, anger, resentment, conflict, and feelings of injustice, all amplify physical pain. These are referred to as "total pain."

Expanding the Total Pain Threshold[38]

The best strategy for mastering an enemy is probably by elimination. But what if that is impossible? How can we live with pain?

For one thing, it is very important that everyone involved in the pain treatment process, including family, health-care givers, doctors, friends, and public health policy makers, all work to help you reduce and overcome negative emotions and stress. However, it is ultimately you who has to make the effort to transform this experience. Here are some things you can do:

Many pain patients get stuck in the recovery process because of the "Why me?" mentality. Their symptoms become more severe whenever they think of the problem and become angrier.

→ *Take good wellness measures.* The ability to withstand any stress, including pain, has to do with the overall ability of the body to function. Improving the general state of your health will help you cope better with pain. It is important to stop harmful habits and take good wellness measures such as eating properly and sleeping regularly.

→ *Research and investigate the pain condition.* Understanding the condition brings back a certain sense of control. If you have to live with an enemy, knowing the enemy is winning half the battle. Knowledge leads to realistic expectations and better adjustment to limitations. It will also help you locate better care for the pain condition.

> Knowledge leads to realistic expectations and better adjustment to limitations.

→ *Take responsibility for recovering.* Many pain patients get stuck in the recovery process because of the "Why me?" mentality. Their symptoms become more severe whenever they think of the problem and become angrier. It is as though they cannot let go of the injustice and are therefore unable to let go of the pain. Ultimately, whether we are responsible for the cause of our pain or not, we are responsible for our present-day well-being and happiness. The value, meaning, and purpose of our lives belong to us and no one else.

→ *Find a distraction.* Researchers have discovered that pain can be reduced if the sufferer is somehow distracted—engaging in an unrelated activity or one that serves as a partial antidote to the pain.

→ *Reduce pain through relaxation.* Many things contribute to aggravating or dampening pain: music, lighting, temperature, environment, our senses, clothing, posture, and position, among others. Learn relaxation techniques and make the effort to relax.

→ *Appropriate, gradual, and progressive exercises and activities* help increase pain tolerance. Weak muscles and inactivity lower one's pain threshold and increase the likelihood of further damage due to poor circulation.

→ *Find something meaningful in life.* Instead of focusing on the pain, the incentive to reach goals in life will distract you from and dampen the pain. When we are involved deeply in something useful and meaningful, we forget the pain or it becomes much more tolerable. In contrast to negative emotions, positive feelings such as love, a sense of security, appreciation of beauty, compassion, and hope have calming effects and reduce physical pain.

Pleasant Distractions for Pain Relief

McGill University neuropsychologist Catherine Bushnell has discovered that a person's emotional state affects the perception of pain. For example, someone with intestinal cancer will find stomach pain more alarming than someone who attributes the pain to indigestion. Bushnell has also shown that if a person is distracted, pain feels less severe. Distraction reduces pain-related activation in both sensory and limbic regions of the cerebral cortex. Distraction may also activate the brain's pain-inhibition circuits, causing them to send less powerful signals to the cortex. Distraction can be achieved by many methods, including hypnosis.

A form of distraction (Immersive Treatments) was developed at the University of Washington Burn Center for burn victims, who regularly experience agonizing pain especially when bandages are changed and wounds are cleaned. Even morphine is insufficient to curb the excruciating pain. Researchers at the burn center reported that patients experienced significantly less pain during wound care when engaged in virtual activities.

One virtual game allows patients to fly through an icy canyon with a river and a frozen waterfall, and to throw snowballs. Since patients often report that they re-experience the original burn pain during wound care, *SnowWorld* was designed to help cool things down.

Burn Pain during Physical Therapy

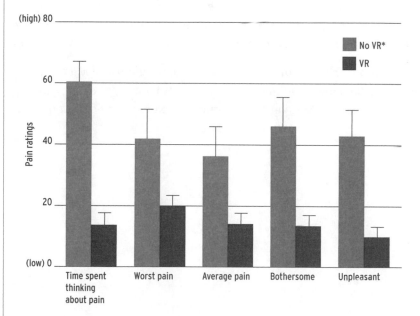

Immersive Treatments were developed by David Patterson from the Harbourview Burn Center, and Hunter Hoffman from the Human Interface Technology Lab at the University of Washington. This table shows the significant reductions in patients' pain levels during physical therapy when distracted (in virtual game reality) compared to when having conventional treatment only.

Data from H.G. Hoffman, D.R. Patterson and G.J. Carrougher, "Use of virtual reality for treatment of adolescent burn pain during woundcare." **Pain** 85 (2000): 305–309.

Spiritual Pain Management

The spiritual or existential aspect of pain also needs to be addressed. Pain—especially intense sustained pain or pain related to terminal illness—usually leads to questions about our existence, the meaning of life itself, and fear of loss: losing awareness, the self, and sanity, losing loved ones or possessions, fear of more suffering, and mental anguish about an uncertain future.

To deal with spiritual pain, we need to confront the reality of our own mortality and limitations and try to understand the essence of our own being. This is where spirituality or religion comes in. The role of spirituality and religion is to enable people to deal with existential anxiety and suffering, to reach an understanding of the process of life and death, and to find comfort and reassurance.

To expand the spiritual pain threshold:

→ Establish a sense of fulfilling your life and of living fully.
→ Establish a sense of appreciation. Keep a record of your positive experiences and also record the things you have learned from negative experiences.
→ Recognize the overwhelming value of love.
→ Realize that the life and death process is a continuum of learning and evolving, so each moment is valuable. Yesterday is history, tomorrow is mystery, and today is a gift for us to appreciate, enjoy, and make use of.

I remember these words from Percy Bysshe in *Julian and Maddalo*: "Most wretched men/ Are cradled into poetry by wrong; / They learn in suffering what they teach in song." I touch my pain and sing a song.

I can feel well in comfort and in pain.

> To deal with spiritual or existential pain, we need to confront the reality of our own mortality and limitations, and understand the essence of our own being.

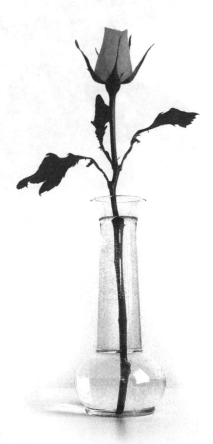

Pain question: Is there a life without pain?

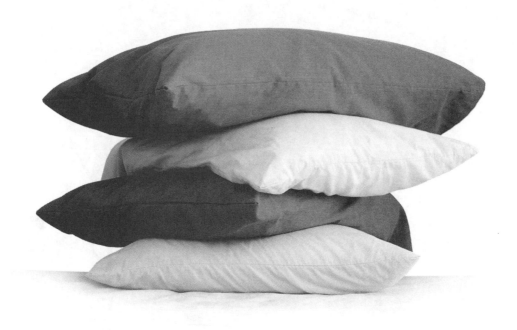

7 How Are You This Morning?
Sleeping Well

An immobilized dance.
A silenced sonata.

Nowhere …
yet here,
in the landscape of my sleep.

… In the landscape of my sleep …

In ancient cultures, sleep was associated with a metamorphosis into an inactive state or a crossing over into a new land. In more recent times, scientists have clarified differences between the "sleep" and "awake" modes of the brain by recording brain-wave patterns, and we know that our "journeys to the Land of Nod" are different from other sleep-like states such as hibernation or a coma. But the precise purpose sleep serves still remains a mystery.

The total amount of time that different species spend sleeping every day differs greatly, ranging from a mere 4 hours to a lengthy 18 hours.

Most people sleep between 4.5 and 10.5 hours each night, and if we live to be 80 years old, we will have slept up to 35 years! Since nature has intended us to spend so much time engaging in this activity—or inactivity—it must be profoundly important for our survival. And this nightly loss of consciousness of our environment obviously fulfills some restorative function, because we need adequate sleep in order to feel refreshed and effective.[1]

Mammals and birds are the only living things that are known for certain to sleep; it is unclear whether reptiles, fish, insects, and other life forms do the same. But the total amount of time that different species spend sleeping every day differs greatly, ranging from a mere 4 hours to a lengthy 18 hours. Interestingly, larger animals tend to sleep less than smaller ones.[2]

Sleep is not a passive process of simple withdrawal from wakefulness. Rather, the current notion is that sleep is composed of distinct states, each actively generated by specific brain regions. It is also thought that each of these states has distinct effects on a variety of physiological processes. Our sleep is also a highly organized and active process, regulated by specific neurotransmitters. There are actually more chemical and electrical activities going on in the brain when we're sleeping than when we're awake.[3]

Average Hours of Sleep Each Day for Different Species

	AVERAGE TOTAL HOURS OF SLEEP	% OF 24 HOURS		AVERAGE TOTAL HOURS OF SLEEP	% OF 24 HOURS
Brown Bat	20	83	Dog	11	44
Human (infant)	16	67	Human (adult)	8	33
Squirrel	15	62	Human (Elderly)	5.5	23
Mouse	12	50	African Elephant	3.3	14
Cat	12	50	Horse	3	12

Data from Tobler et al., "Is Sleep Fundamentally Different Between Mammalian Species?" **Behavioural Brain Research** 69 (July, 1995): 35; Rattenborg et al., "Half Awake to the Risk of Predation." **Nature** (Feburary, 1999): 397.

Half-Asleep and Half-Awake?

Most mammals are *bihemispheric* sleepers—that is, both hemispheres (or halves) of their brains are in "sleep" mode while they are slumbering. However, studies of brain-wave patterns among a number of dolphin species, as well as the pilot whale and the porpoise, show that only one hemisphere of their brains is in "sleep" pattern while the other half is "awake." This is called unihemispheric sleep.[4]

Birds appear to sleep both kinds of sleep. In unihemispheric sleep, the bird actually has one eye closed and one eye open, and the open eye is associated with the "awake" hemisphere. (Resist the temptation to ask yourself whether the bird is half-awake or half-asleep!)

Why are birds so ambiguous about their sleep behavior? When do they exhibit "half-awake" sleep? A team of biologists at Indiana State University sought answers to these questions by arranging mallard ducks in rows of four and continuously videorecording their sleep behavior. The tapes were then analyzed to determine how often each bird engaged in unihemispheric sleep (with one eye open).

They found that the sleeping birds at either end of a row engaged in unihemispheric sleep 32 percent of the time—almost three times as often as the birds in the middle. The birds at the ends of the row also oriented their open eye away from the center of the group 86 percent of the time, while the interior birds showed no preference for direction in their gaze.[5]

This behavior suggests that the birds at the ends were alert to possible danger. And it is true that sleep can be a dangerous activity for animals because it makes them easy prey for their enemies. Further studies have shown that the "awake" hemisphere is functioning even when the other half of the brain is asleep.

Do We Have to Sleep?

When we sleep, our metabolic rate is reduced by only 15 percent from a quiet, restful state. And by increasing food intake by only a small amount, we can compensate for the energy loss of a sleepless night. So do we really have to sleep? This idea was tested by Randy Gardner, who at the age of 17 tried to refrain from sleeping for as long as he could. He achieved a record 264 hours of sleeplessness but finally fell asleep when nature simply took over.

We have to sleep to survive, but scientists still don't know exactly why. Research has shown that all laboratory rats chronically deprived of sleep die after about two to three weeks. They develop septicemia, a condition in which large amounts of different bacteria and their toxic products are

We have to sleep to survive, but scientists still don't know exactly why.

present in the bloodstream. Normally, these bacteria are confined to the intestine and are harmless. But in the research rats, when these bacteria migrated through the bloodstream from the intestine to the lymph nodes, the liver, and other organs, the rats' immune systems collapsed and they died. The cause of death seemed to be the loss of the protective functions of the immune system. It's not clear how their systems collapsed; the only certain conclusion was that sleep deprivation suppresses the immune system.

Several theories have been suggested to explain why sleep occurs. According to the repair theory, sleep serves a biological need, replenishing key areas of the brain or body that have been depleted during the day. Studies have shown that even people who show little or no physiological impairment after several days of sleep deprivation inevitably do show impaired intellectual performance.[6]

The adaptive theory suggests that sleep prevents us from wasting energy and exposing ourselves to predators, thus aiding survival.[7]

Since the regulation of body temperature (thermoregulation) became a part of the physio-genetic makeup at the same time as sleep, it's also suggested that sleep may have a cooling and heat-retention function.

What Goes On When We're Asleep?

Behaviorally, four characteristics are associated with sleep:

→ reduced motor activity (a ball will drop out of a person's hand during sleep);
→ decreased response to external stimulation (the sleeping person is disengaged from the environment and is not communicating);
→ stereotypic sleeping postures (such as lying down with eyes closed, although some people can sleep standing up);

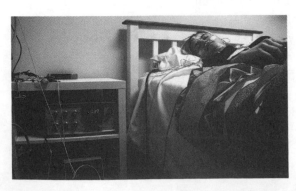

Measuring Sleep in a Sleep Clinic
Scientists are able to study sleep using three basic electro-physiological signals recorded from surface electrodes: 1) An electroencephalogram (EEG) is used to measure brain activity and is recorded from electrodes placed on the head overlying the cortex. 2) Separate electrodes placed beside each eye are used to record eye movements in an electrooculogram (EOG). 3) An electromyogram (EMG) is used to monitor postural muscle tone by surface electrodes placed under the chin.

➜ a loss of consciousness that can be reversed with relative ease, compared with other sleep-like states such as a coma.[8]

Canadian sleep researcher Harvey Moldofsky described these physiological aspects of sleep: "Changes in the whole body occurred during sleep," he said. "A person can pretend to be asleep, but no one can fake the brain-wave patterns associated with sleep in a laboratory. During sleep, the characteristic pattern of wakefulness disappeared and different brain-wave patterns appeared."[9]

Through the monitoring of brain waves during sleep, five stages of sleep (known as stages 1, 2, 3, 4, and the rapid eye movement or REM stage) have been identified. Each stage is characterized by distinctive brain-wave frequencies. Stages 1 through 4 are grouped together in the category NREM (non-rapid eye movement) sleep and are further identified as follows: stages 1 and 2 are light sleep, and stages 3 and 4 are deep, or slow-brain-wave, sleep (SWS).[10]

Sleep begins with about 80 minutes of NREM sleep followed by REM sleep of about 10 minutes, so an entire cycle of NREM and REM sleep lasts about 90 to 110 minutes. This cycle is then repeated about four to six times during the night. But sleep does not progress uniformly starting with stages 1 through 4, then entering REM sleep, and finally repeating the cycles before waking up. Instead, repeated episodes of NREM and REM sleep of various durations alternate throughout the night.[11]

In Stage 1, our eyes begin to roll, and rhythmic brain waves give way to slower-frequency irregular waves as we become less responsive to stimuli and experience fleeting thoughts and images. In Stage 2, our electroencephalogram (EEG) tracings show fast-frequency bursts of brain

> "A person can pretend to be asleep, but no one can fake the brain-wave patterns associated with sleep in a laboratory."
> —Canadian sleep researcher Harvey Moldofsky

Sleep Pattern Changes with Age
Percentage of total sleep time spent in each phase

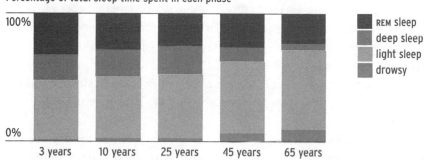

Legend: REM sleep, deep sleep, light sleep, drowsy

Ages: 3 years, 10 years, 25 years, 45 years, 65 years

activity called sleep spindles, marked by muscle tension and accompanied by a gradual decline in heart rate, respiration, and body temperature. Stages 3 and 4 normally occur 30 to 45 minutes after a person falls asleep. In this slow-brain-wave sleep (sws), low-frequency brain waves mark the deepest levels of sleep, when our heart rate, respiration, body temperature, and blood flow to the brain are further reduced.

If roused from Stage 4 sleep, we will be groggy and confused. The body appears to be at its most obviously quiescent during this stage of sleep and shows little postural muscle tone. sws (slow-brain-wave sleep) is the most difficult sleep stage to be awakened from, and it is considered to be the most restorative. It is important to mental and physical recovery.[12]

Changes in hormonal and immune functions also occur during the sws stages. Growth hormone production increases during Stage 4, while adrenaline and cortisol production declines, and about 80 percent of the daily release of growth hormones occurs during the first two sws cycles. Certain immune functions are activated while others decline during both sws stages. For example, there is increased production of T-cells, natural killer cells that fight off virus infections.

The neurons most critical to earlier stages of NREM sleep control are in the basal forebrain. Some of these neurons become most active before and during sleep, and it has been shown that people with injury to these parts of the brain have difficulty falling or staying asleep. Many of these neurons are activated by heat, which explains why a hot bath or a hot day causes sleepiness.[13]

Rapid eye movement, or REM, sleep is an active form of sleep in which the discharge patterns of most neurons resemble those that characterize active wakefulness. Our brain waves, heart rate, breathing, and blood pressure increase to the same levels or to levels greater than those observed in the alert, wakeful state. In men, penile erections occur regularly; and in women, the vagina often becomes engorged.

Despite the internal state of heightened brain arousal in REM sleep, responsiveness to external arousing stimuli such as noise is markedly reduced compared to responsiveness observed in non-REM sleep. It's as if we are so "active" in our sleep landscape that we have to shut off the physical world.

Some neurons are active only in REM sleep, while others are entirely inactive. The combined effect of sleep-active and sleep-inactive neuronal

In rapid eye movement (REM) sleep, our brain waves, heart rate, breathing, and blood pressure increase to the same levels or to levels greater than those observed in the alert, wakeful state.

balance explains the tranquil appearance a person has at a time when brain activities increase with vivid dreaming.

REM sleep appears critical to mental stability and memory, and lack of REM sleep causes irritability, disorientation, and attention deficits. Sleep researcher J. Allan Hobson notes in his book *The Dreaming Brain* that REM sleep is the time when recently acquired information is consolidated in the memory. We spend more time in REM sleep when we are learning new things, and if REM sleep is disrupted, we remember less the next day.[14]

Rats and Their A-maze-ing Dreams

A study of rats and their REM sleep has shed some light on how REM sleep is associated with learning and memory. Experimental studies conducted by neuroscientist Matthew Wilson of the Massachusetts Institute of Technology show that after a hard day's running in a maze, laboratory rats dream in their REM sleep about ... running the maze![15]

By implanting electrodes in the brain, it was possible to record activities of 13 different nerve cells simultaneously, and the pattern of nerve cell activities changed as the rats ran through the maze. Research results showed that after maze-running, rats in REM sleep demonstrated a pattern almost identical to the one shown while they were running the maze. It's not clear exactly why and how the rats replayed the maze-running experience during their REM sleep, but the study lends support to the link between REM sleep and learning and memory.

Dozing Off Again: How Much Sleep Do We Need?

In a sleep study, researcher Daniel F. Kripke and colleagues at the University of California, San Diego, gathered sleep habits and health information on more than a million Americans, and followed those individuals for 6 years. The age of participants ranged from 30 to 102 years, with an average age of 57 for women and 58 for men.

As a result of comparing participants' sleep patterns and their death rates, the researchers concluded that a good night's sleep lasts 7 hours. They also found that participants who slept for 8 hours or more tend to have died sooner. The statistically calculated risk of death over 6 years for those who slept 8 hours increased by 12 percent. For those who slept 9 hours, it increased 17 percent, and for those who slept 10 hours, the risk increased 34 percent. The risk of death for those who slept 10 hours or more was equivalent to the risk for people who are moderately obese. But the risk of death for those who slept *less* than 8 hours did not seem as

Some neurons are active only in REM sleep, while others are entirely inactive. The combined effect explains our tranquil appearance at a time when brain activities increase.

Do Intelligent People Sleep More? Or Less?

A number of famous people of superior intelligence, such as Thomas Edison, Napoleon Bonaparte, and Leonardo da Vinci, needed little sleep at night, but they napped often. Albert Einstein, on the other hand, slept a lot.

The amount or length of sleep we require does not seem to correlate with intelligence or personality. It's as individual as the amount of food we need.

Researchers concluded that a good night's sleep lasts 7 hours.

great as for those who slept more. While these findings are statistically significant, they do not translate into much of a real-life risk.[16]

The point is that sleeping more is not always better for your health. On the other hand, it is almost impossible for a healthy person to oversleep. So if you sleep more, it may be because your body needs the extra hours. Also, according to Kripke, those who complain of insomnia are not necessarily in bad health, but those who often take sleeping pills have a 25-percent increase in death risk—equivalent to the risk incurred by sleeping only 3 hours a night.

Sliding into Sleep Debt

If we go without enough sleep for some time, the sleep debt we accumulate must be paid back. In the past century, since Thomas Edison invented the light bulb, we have reduced our average sleep time by about 20 percent. Specifically, our average sleep duration in general has decreased from more than 9 hours per night in 1910, to between 8 and 9 hours in 1959, to between 7 and 7.5 hours in the mid-1990s. Today, 27 percent of us have only an average of 6 to 6.9 hours of sleep every night.[17]

By some accounts, each hour of lost sleep translates into a temporary loss of one IQ point.

One or two fewer hours per night may not sound like a huge difference, but cumulative sleep debts have serious consequences. According to international sleep authority William C. Dement and his colleagues, our brains keep an accounting of how much sleep is owed. Sleep deprivation also leads to deterioration in our mood and behavior, reduced mental cognition and concentration, and lower levels of alertness and energy. Lack of sleep makes us clumsy and less able to think creatively, quickly, or clearly, and it reduces short-term memory. By some accounts, each hour of lost sleep translates into a temporary loss of one IQ point.[18]

Seriously sleep-deprived people may experience "microsleeps" lasting about 10 to 60 seconds, when the brain enters a sleep state regardless of what the person is doing. Microsleep can be deadly. If a driver is traveling at 48 kilometers (30 miles) an hour and falls into a microsleep for 10 seconds, the vehicle will have traveled more than the length of a football field before he awakens from the momentary blackout.[19]

In his book *Sleep Thieves*, Canadian sleep researcher Stanley Coren points out that the day after North Americans move their clocks one hour ahead (losing an hour of sleep), traffic accidents increase by 7 percent.[20] However, in the fall, when we turn the clocks back and gain an hour of sleep, there is a *reduction* in traffic accidents by approximately 7 percent. It's frightening to learn that we are such a sleep-deprived society that one hour of sleep gained or lost in a single night can cause a 7-percent change in the accident rate!

How do we repay our sleep debts? Researchers have found that the brain keeps some kind of sleep account. People lacking REM sleep will recoup REM sleep first when they catch up. The same applies to NREM sleep. This would seem to indicate that we need an adequate amount of both kinds of sleep. How the brain keeps the sleep balance is a mystery; the accounting seems to take place, and at some point, we have to repay the debts. But it appears that we do not have to repay our sleep debts hour for hour.[21]

Sleep Rhythms

Our bodies house a precise biological clock that regulates and synchronizes a vast array of physiological functions, from our sleep-awake cycle to hunger, body temperature, heart rate, hormone levels, and sensitivity to pain. For example, Swiss researcher Kurt Krauchi has also shown that the body readies itself for sleep by dilating blood vessels in the feet and hands. The greater the extent of the dilation, the shorter the time needed for sleep onset—so warming your hands and feet is a simple and effective way to get to sleep more quickly.[22]

The timing of this dilation of blood vessels is governed by an internal pacemaker that regulates our rhythms according to a cycle lasting about 24 hours. This rhythmic cycle is known as a circadian rhythm, from *circa* meaning about and *dies* referring to day. Some of these rhythmic changes may occur while we are sleeping, but they are not all related to sleep: even if we stay awake during our normal sleeping hours, certain physiological functions in our bodies will continue to be activated and/or slow down according to our circadian rhythms.

If a driver is traveling at 48 kilometers (30 miles) an hour and falls into a microsleep for 10 seconds, the vehicle will have traveled more than the length of a football field before he awakens from the momentary blackout.

For many, the "sleepiest" hours are between 2 and 5 a.m. and from 2 to 5 p.m.

How Large Is Your Sleep Debt? (Questionnaire)

To determine whether you have a sleep debt, answer each question checking the box for "YES." Each "YES" counts as one score.

- ☐ Do you usually need a loud alarm clock to wake you up in the morning?
- ☐ Do you usually hit the snooze control to get a few minutes more of sleep when the alarm goes off (or simply turn off the alarm and try to catch a bit more sleep)?
- ☐ Do you find getting out of bed in the morning usually a struggle?
- ☐ Do you sometimes sleep through the alarm?
- ☐ Do you usually find that a single beer, glass of wine, or other alcoholic drink seems to have a noticeable effect on you?
- ☐ Do you sleep longer on weekends than you normally do during the week?
- ☐ On vacations and holidays, do you sleep longer than you normally do on regular workweeks?
- ☐ Do you often feel that your "get-up-and-go" has gotten up and gone?
- ☐ Do you find it more difficult to attend to details or routine chores than it used to be?
- ☐ Do you sometimes fall asleep when you had not intended to?
- ☐ Do you sometimes find yourself getting very sleepy while you are sitting and reading?
- ☐ Do you sometimes find yourself getting very sleepy or dozing off when you are watching TV?
- ☐ When you are a passenger in an airplane, car, bus, or train and the trip lasts over an hour without a break, do you commonly find yourself getting very sleepy or dozing off?
- ☐ Do you usually feel extremely sleepy or doze off when you are sitting quietly at a public meeting, lecture, or in a theater?
- ☐ Do you usually feel extremely sleepy or doze off when you are sitting quietly after a large lunch without alcohol?
- ☐ Have you sometimes found yourself getting extremely sleepy with the urge to doze when you drive and are stopped for a few minutes in traffic?
- ☐ Do you drink more than four cups of coffee or tea (containing caffeine) during the day? (Remember to count refills; also count extra large take-out cups as two cups.)

Scores:

4 or less: You are obtaining an adequate amount of sleep and are not showing significant signs of any sleep debt.

5 or 6: You are probably getting an adequate amount of sleep on most days, although on some days your sleep account is a bit short, which may cause you to be less than 100% alert on some activities.

7 or 8: You are showing evidence of sleep debt that may cause a noticeable reduction in your efficiency at work and your ability to finish all your required activities on time. Things to watch for are little errors and short episodes of inattention. You will occasionally just "slip up," act clumsy, reach a wrong conclusion, or miss an important detail. Usually at this level, you will catch the errors if you have a chance to recheck your work.

9 to 11: You definitely have a large sleep debt. You may commit large, random errors or omissions in your work, miss small errors even when you go over your work a second time, miss appoint-ments, and not remember instructions or information. Other symptoms may include: episodes of minor clumsiness, mood changes, feelings of reduced motivation (a "why bother" attitude), brief bouts of depression or annoyance, and feelings of being swamped or overworked.

12 to 14: Sleep debt may be taking a major toll on your life. In addition to the symptoms outlined above, your general quality of life may be suffering; you may have inexplicable instances where you make a major mistake or leave out an important item and don't notice it, with loss of patience for detailed work, loss of interest in many of the things that were previously interesting, less inclination to socialize, tendency to be a bit more accident prone, occasional crises in loss of confidence, and temporary memory loss.

15 and above: Sleep debt is a major problem. Your level of sleepiness is in the range of those people with clinical levels of sleep disturbances. You almost certainly need a marked change in sleep behavior to ensure your physical and psychological safety. Sleep more.

Adapted from Stanley Coren, **Sleep Thieves** (Free Press, 1996). Reprinted with permission.

Control of Melatonin Secretion by Light and Darkness

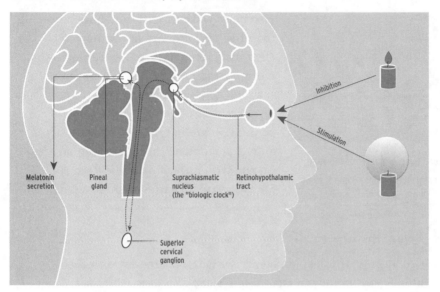

Sleep is affected by signals such as light and darkness, and the internal clock that maintains the sleep pattern is a section of the brain called the suprachiasmatic nucleus (SCN) (which consists of two pin-sized clusters of cells). When light strikes our retina, neural input is transmitted to the SCN and to the pineal gland, stimulating the secretion of the hormone melatonin. The melatonin regulates circadian rhythms, sleep, mood, and body temperature.[1,5,10]

Most of us have two windows within a 24-hour cycle when we are sleepiest or most alert. For many, the "sleepiest" hours are between 2 and 5 a.m. and from 2 to 5 p.m. The most alert times are generally from 8 to 10 in the morning and 8 to 10 in the evening. Variations in body temperature can serve as an easy indication of mental alertness and performance. Mental performance, mood, and willingness to work are poorest when our body temperature is at its lowest level.[23]

> Mental performance, mood, and willingness to work are poorest when our body temperature is at its lowest level.

Are You an MT Lark or an ET Owl?

One way to keep track of your own alert-sleepy windows is to monitor your body temperature throughout the day. This information will also help you determine scientifically what circadian type you are: a morning person (MT), an evening person (ET), or neither.[24]

Body Temperature and MT, ET

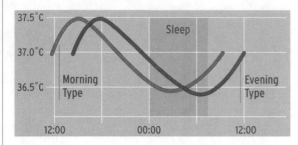

Variations in body temperature over 24 hours for morning and evening types. Mental performance mirrors changes in body temperature.

MT types wake up early and have better cognitive performance in the morning. Their body temperatures rise earlier in the morning and drop earlier in the evening. ET people follow the opposite pattern. An estimated 12 percent of the general population are MT types; 27 percent, ET; and 61 percent, neither. More women are MT, and with increasing age, everyone tends toward an earlier sleep schedule.

Desynchronization

Two categories of sleep problems exist: desynchronization, caused by external environmental factors; and sleep disorders, which are physiological health conditions.

Desynchronization may occur when our circadian rhythms are upset by shift work or by long-distance travel, especially across time zones. A mismatch takes place between the internal physiological cycles, including the sleep-wake rhythm and the external environment. The end result is a variety of symptoms such as sleep loss, fatigue, digestive problems, and constipation, as well as psychological symptoms including confusion, irritability, general loss of mental efficiency, mood impairment, headaches, and anxiety.[25]

Jet Lag. Jet lag is an artificial and temporary condition resulting mainly from air travel across time zones. The severity of the condition increases with the number of time zones crossed and the frequency of time-zone changes. A recent study has provided evidence that repeated exposures to jet lag occur in airline cabin crew when there are only short intervals between out-of-zone flights. This elevates levels of the stress hormone cortisol, resulting in cognitive and memory impairment.[26]

A number of strategies can be used to reduce the impact of jet lag, including programmed exposure to bright light and to social activities, diet adjustment (meals higher in protein when you want to be more energetic, and complex carbohydrate foods when you want to relax), melatonin medication, and acupressure.[27] It also helps to follow the

For more general information on how to fall asleep or how to sleep better, see the "Sleep Strategies" section later in this chapter.

bedtime and meal schedules of the new time zone after you arrive at your destination.

Shift Work. Sleep problems associated with shift work, or "shift lag," affect more than eight million North Americans who must work permanent or rotating shifts. This is because a changed schedule of bright light and darkness can reset the biological clock by up to 12 hours within two to three days, causing sleep problems and conditions similar to jet lag. Studies have shown that workers may not be able to adapt well to a shift change even after six nights if they work under ordinary room lighting (150 lux).[28]

Some shift workers may also suffer from "night shift paralysis." This condition is a temporary but incapacitating paralysis that occurs in about 12 percent of night nurses and 6 percent of air traffic controllers. During a night shift, most frequently at about 5 a.m., the sufferer is suddenly unable to move, even though he or she is still fully conscious. Attacks may last from a few seconds to a few minutes. This is a very frightening experience, and may easily lead to accidents. Males appear to be more prone to the condition than females, and it is most likely an indication of the amount of sleep deprivation the worker has accumulated.

Shift rotation adaptation problems can be treated effectively by a schedule of exposures to different levels of bright light at night and darkness during the day. Workers' "sleep type" also affects their ability to adapt to shift work, and this should be taken into consideration when a shift system is established. Evening type (ET) people are better able to adjust to rotating shifts than morning type (MT) people.[29]

> "Night shift paralysis" is a temporary but incapacitating paralysis that occurs in about 12 percent of night nurses and 6 percent of air traffic controllers.

> For more information on light therapy, see Chapter 4, "How Are You? Feeling Bad, Feeling Good."

Sleep Disorders

Everyone knows how it feels to experience the occasional sleepless night: tossing and turning, dreading the exhaustion that will dampen the next day, worrying about not being able to function at work with a sharp mind or steady hands. We try counting sheep, drinking hot milk, reading a boring document ... but unfortunately, for the millions of people who suffer from a sleep disorder, these tricks don't always work.

Insomnia. Insomnia can be defined as having difficulty falling asleep or staying asleep, waking up too early in the morning, or having non-refreshing sleep at night.[30] The *Diagnostic and Statistical Manual of Mental Disorders* (DSM-IV), a handbook of psychological and psychiatric

> Insomnia is the most common sleep disorder, affecting an estimated one in four adults.

diagnoses, uses the "insomnia" label when sleep problems continue for one month, cause significant daytime fatigue, and lead to impaired functioning in various realms of daily life.[31]

Insomnia is the most common sleep disorder, affecting an estimated one in four adults. Epidemiological studies show that up to 38 percent of the population in North America suffers from insomnia. The percentage of insomniacs also increases with age, and more than 50 percent of people over the age of 65 complain of the disorder. But fewer than half of those affected seek medical advice. Furthermore, many people who are exhausted during the day may not even be aware that they are waking up repeatedly during the night. Consequently, too many people continue to experience long nights and endure exhausting days.[32]

You don't really have to count sheep to put yourself to sleep.

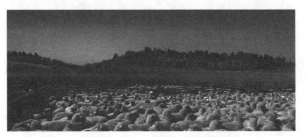

Most sleep experts agree that insomnia and other sleep disorders are usually symptoms of underlying psychological or medical issues. So to develop an effective healing plan and sleep strategies, these root causes need to be investigated. A survey of American physicians revealed that 30 percent of patients who came for help with insomnia were also diagnosed with depression. Twenty percent of these patients had other mental disorders (anxiety disorder, obsessive-compulsive disorder, schizophrenia), 19 percent had other underlying medical disorders, and 31 percent were diagnosed with primary insomnia (i.e., insomnia was the only complaint).[33]

Primary insomnia is a preoccupation with not being able to sleep, when there is no other medical or psychiatric condition present. Those who suffer from primary insomnia may be experiencing anxiety on a subconscious level while they are awake, but do not express those feelings except through their sleeping habits. The condition becomes worse if they begin to associate their bedroom and bedtime with sleeplessness.[34]

Traditional Chinese medicine maintains that health is a simple state of equilibrium and either too much or too little sleep is an indication of disharmony. In classical Chinese medical texts, insomnia is described as "yang unable to return to yin"—that is, the active does not become passive when it should. Yin and yang energy are constantly interacting, with one advancing while the other retreats, until one peaks and the direction of advance is reversed. This interplay continues during sleep. We fall asleep and wake up when a certain threshold of this energy interplay is crossed. When the process continues smoothly during sleep, we have restful, undisturbed sleep. But when the active yang energy cannot quiet down as it should, it causes insomnia. When the yin energy is overpowering, however, internal energy circulation becomes stagnant, and sleep is also compromised.[35]

Chinese medical texts also point out another fundamental cause of insomnia: "the heart failing to contain the spirit." In this case, *heart* is defined not as the physical organ itself but by its activities and functions. *Spirit* refers to the summation of our emotions, thoughts, memories, judgments, and so on. When the *heart* stores the *spirit,* it means that the heart and its activities are affecting and being affected by the summation of our emotions and thoughts. If the heart is not calm and fails to contain the spirit, palpitations occur, body energy is in chaos, and other internal processes are upset, leading to insomnia or restless sleep.

Insomnia Caused by Medical Conditions. Sleep disturbances can be caused by a whole compendium of medical problems: Parkinson's disease; cardiac failure; kidney disease; Alzheimer's disease; hypo- and hyperthyroidism; gastroesophageal reflux disease; asthma;

> In classical Chinese medical texts, insomnia is described as "yang unable to return to yin"—that is, the active does not become passive when it should.

Insomnia and Mood Disorders

Insomniacs with anxiety disorders generally have more trouble falling asleep, while those with depression, post-traumatic stress disorder, and schizophrenia are more likely to have difficulty *staying* asleep. Depressed people also often experience early morning awakening, and depression is the most common psychiatric cause of insomnia.[36]

In fact, sleep is an extremely sensitive indicator of mood disorders. Up to 90 percent of patients with major depression experience difficulty sleeping. Those who have a personal or family history of mood disorders and experience a disruption in their normal sleep pattern should seek medical advice immediately. Conversely, among patients who have experienced insomnia for more than one year, there is a higher risk of developing a new major depression, anxiety disorder, or alcohol problem.

For more information on principles of Chinese medicine, see Chapters 4, 5, and 6. For more on traditional Chinese treatments of insomnia, see the "Sleep Strategies" section later in this chapter.

A person with sleep apnea is more likely to complain of severe fatigue during the day than someone who is suffering from insomnia.

allergies; chronic obstructive pulmonary diseases (bronchitis and emphysema); chronic pain from fibromyalgia, arthritis, and cancer; and prostate problems requiring frequent nighttime urination.[37]

Sleep Apnea. People who have sleep apnea suffer from repetitive pauses in breathing and gasping for air while they are sleeping. These episodes disrupt their sleep so much that they become extremely tired during the day. In fact, a person with sleep apnea is more likely to complain of severe fatigue during the day than someone who is suffering from insomnia. Other symptoms of sleep apnea include loud snoring, morning headaches, and morning dry mouth.

Sleep apnea may be treated with continuous positive airway pressure (CPAP). A small, comfortable mask is fitted over the nose, leaving the mouth uncovered. Patients must sleep with their mouth closed, aided by a chin strap, while a machine gently blows air into the nose at a pressure slightly higher than the surrounding air pressure.[38] Avoiding sedatives and alcohol may also reduce the severity of the problem.

Restless Legs Syndrome (RLS). This syndrome, characterized by unpleasant sensations in the legs or feet, is another disorder that causes insomnia. Moving the lower limbs may temporarily relieve the discomfort, but symptoms worsen in the evening and may make it difficult for a person to fall asleep. RLS is usually caused by an underlying medical condition such as iron-deficiency anemia, kidney failure, or pregnancy. Anti-depressant drugs, such as Prozac, may also cause RLS.

Hormone fluctuations may cause insomnia.

Hormonal Fluctuations in Women. Low levels of progesterone, during or immediately before menstruation, or progesterone fluctuations during pregnancy may cause insomnia. During menopause, many women also experience frequent waking episodes associated with hot flashes, which are caused by low levels of estrogen.[39]

Insomnia Caused by Medications or Other Substances. Many medications affect the body's nervous system, the brain, and neurotransmitters, and this affects the onset or quality of sleep. Commonly prescribed drugs that may cause insomnia include steroids, some anti-depressants, and beta blockers. Insomnia may also be brought on by alcohol, nicotine, caffeine, and some over-the-counter medications such as cough and cold remedies, decongestants, and antihistamines. Some sedatives that are used to treat insomnia actually lead to sleeplessness when they are discontinued.[40]

Adjustment Sleep Problems. When we experience sudden emotional stress brought about by a job change, personal loss, an examination, or hospitalization, we may have trouble sleeping. But once the situation is resolved or time has passed, the insomnia disappears and no specific treatment is required.

Sleep Strategies

Fortunately, there are ways to help us fall and stay asleep. Simple things like warming your hands or feet and eating the right foods can make a big difference.

Sleep Smart Practices. Here are a few simple but effective sleep tips:

→ Warm your hands and feet, or take a warm bath before bedtime.
→ Stick to a regular sleep and wake-up schedule.
→ Use the bed for sleep and sex only. Try not to work or watch TV in bed.
→ Keep your bedroom dark, and avoid bright lights before bedtime.
→ Keep your bedroom comfortably cool but not cold.
→ Decorate your bedroom in soft, peaceful colors, such as light green or pink.
→ Avoid any mental or emotional overstimulation, such as watching a thriller on TV, reading a murder story, or debating an issue before bedtime. Doing exercises less than three or four hours before bedtime may also overstimulate.
→ Do exercises during the day! Studies have shown that physical activities and exercise during the day improve sleep patterns and general well-being. It's best to do exercises of moderate intensity (preferably aerobic) 3 to 6 times a week for 30 to 45 minutes at 50 to 70 percent of maximum heart rate and appropriate to your age and physical condition.
→ Keep your bedroom quiet or listen to continuous low noise that is nondescript, soothing, and soft. Sounds of waves, soft music, or humming noises from fans may relax you and induce sleep.
→ Unplug the telephone and use earplugs to shut off possible sudden loud noises.
→ Hide the clock if you have a habit of checking the time when you're still awake.
→ Drink a glass of warm milk or eat a light snack before bed.
→ Avoid heavy meals, caffeine, or alcohol close to bedtime.[41]

> Keep your bedroom dark and avoid bright lights before bedtime—and hide the clock if you have a habit of checking the time when you're still awake.

Sleeping the Right Way Round

According to Michael Tetley, a British physiotherapist who has studied native peoples at sleep all over the world, most people adopt similar sleeping positions, and very few positions lead to musculoskeletal problems.[42] In Kenya, for example, indigenous people lie on one side with their knees slightly bent and one arm folded under their head instead of using a pillow. In Tibet, caravanners sleep in the open in cold, wet conditions, so they lie down with their shins flat on the ground, bending their bodies forward, with their heads resting on animal skins. In this position, they have minimal body contact with the ground, and by folding their bodies, they conserve heat.

According to Chinese traditional medicine, the best sleeping position is on the right side, with the legs slightly bent and the right arm bent and resting in front of the pillow. The left arm should rest on the left thigh. Sleeping on the back, according to this thinking, indicates that excess active energy is at work. Sleeping on the stomach indicates weakness of the stomach, and constantly sleeping on one side indicates a weakness on that side, or excess on the other side.[43]

Most sleep experts agree that the best way to sleep is in the fetal position because it minimizes back stress and abdominal pressure. Putting a pillow under the head lessens the weight on the shoulder nearest the mattress and avoids stressing neck muscles. If you are pregnant, you should sleep on your left side so that blood from the lower half of your body can return to your heart. The uterus may press on the large inferior vena cava vein and diminish blood flow back to your heart if you lie on your back.[44]

Sleeping on the stomach puts excessive pressure on the diaphragm and prevents full lung expansion, which leads to reduced oxygen intake. Lying flat on your back may place more stress on your back. This position may also exacerbate a hiatus hernia or gastroesophageal reflux disease. Placing a small pillow under your knees may reduce stress on your back.

Sleep positions

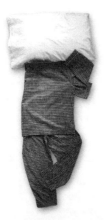 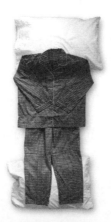 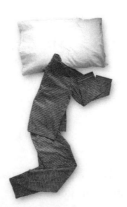 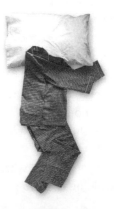

Eating and Drinking for Better Sleep. What we eat and drink can determine whether we have a good night's rest. Diets high in complex carbohydrates, for instance, can increase levels of the amino acid tryptophan, and this increases levels of the brain chemical serotonin, which regulates sleep, relaxes the body, and may promote sleepiness. Eating foods rich in complex carbohydrates (pasta, potatoes, vegetables) in the evening may promote sleep. On the other hand, high-protein foods such as meats, dairy products, and eggs may promote wakefulness, so they should be eaten earlier in the day. According to traditional Chinese medicine, red dates, lotus seeds, asparagus, bananas, bamboo shoots, rice, yams, ginger, and cinnamon promote and improve sleep.[45]

Throughout history and in many parts of the world, alcohol has been widely recognized as a medicine, especially because of its hypnotic and anesthetic effects. But it is not always helpful in promoting or maintaining sleep. For people without sleep problems, moderate drinking can improve sleep, but heavy drinking can have adverse consequences. Alcohol is a fairly strong diuretic, which stimulates the kidney to produce more urine. This means more getting up in the middle of the night for trips to the bathroom.[46]

The diuretic action of alcohol on the kidney also results in body dehydration and a drop in blood pressure. This falling blood pressure then warns the brain and nervous system of impending danger, and a flood of adrenaline hormones and neurotransmitters is unleashed. The resulting arousal responses include sweating, fast pulse, headache, excitability, fear, and nausea. These symptoms cause wakefulness and may begin less than two hours after a person falls asleep.

If heavy alcohol consumption occurs before a person falls asleep and the drinking is stopped abruptly, the body has no opportunity to adjust to a gradual decline in blood alcohol concentration. This sharp drop stimulates the adrenaline system even more and causes worse symptoms. A small glass of alcohol upon awakening in these cases will actually help the person resume sleep because it stops the adrenergic response in its tracks.

The metabolic characteristics of an individual, the amount of alcohol, and the time over which the alcohol is consumed are factors that determine whether the symptoms will develop and how severe they will

Most sleep experts agree that the best way to sleep is in the fetal position because it minimizes back stress and abdominal pressure.

be. If you are not accustomed to drinking, you may be ill prepared to handle large amounts of alcohol quickly, especially before bedtime.

For people with sleep disorders, it is best to avoid alcohol completely, or at least during the four to six hours before bedtime. A number of sleep disorders can be aggravated by alcohol. Alcohol depresses the respiratory system, for instance, reducing oxygen intake, creating excess carbon dioxide, and increasing nasal stiffness. Drinking also makes sleeping more difficult for people with sleep apnea.

Hypnotics and Herbal Remedies. Prescription and over-the-counter medications and herbal remedies known as hypnotics can help a person sleep, but as with any medication, they must be used with caution.[47] For a listing of common hypnotics and their risks and benefits, see the following table, "Risks and Benefits of Common Hypnotics." Consult your doctor before taking any drugs or remedies, especially if there's any danger of cross-medication with something else that you're taking.

Acupuncture Points. Sleep research shows that acupressure applied to the wrists at acupuncture point 7C can induce sleep. Hard plastic beads (these are available commercially) held in place by adhesive tape may be applied to the points.

Pills and Booze: Why They Don't Mix

If you are taking sleeping aids you must exercise extreme caution with alcohol consumption. When sedatives or tranquilizers and alcohol are consumed a reasonable amount of time apart, the effects of one may degrade or inactivate the effects of the other. In other words, drinking makes the sedatives less effective, and taking sedatives can lead to greater tolerance of alcohol. This is because the body can naturally expand the supply of enzymes and other chemical components in order to break down and metabolize the full amount of alcohol and sedatives presented to it—if they are presented one after the other, so that the body has the time to process it.

If sedatives are taken with alcohol, however, the two compete for enzymes and chemicals when they metabolize, so each will block the other and the effects of both will be prolonged. Sleeping pills will have more powerful action, and the alcohol will add to the total sedative effects. Serious and dangerous conditions may develop as a result and may lead to an unintended overdose.

Risks and Benefits of Common Hypnotics

Sleep disorders may be symptoms of other health concerns. It is important to consult your doctor before you consider taking any of the following sleeping aids, especially if you are already taking other medications or have other health issues besides sleep problems. Taking any of the following with alcohol or other drugs, including over-the-counter products for common cold and cough, may pose serious health problems. Consult your doctor about potential risks.

HYPNOTICS	BENEFITS	RISKS
Melatonin A natural occurring sleep hormone released by the pineal gland in the brain. Melatonin is stimulated by darkness and inhibited by light.	Promotes sleep, affects sleep duration and quality. Used to lessen effects of jet lag. Classified as a prescription medicine in the United Kingdom, some European countries, and Canada, but available over-the-counter in the U.S.	No long-term safety data available, especially for larger doses over prolonged periods of time. Some common side effects are excessive sedation, headache, and irritability.
Over-the-counter sleeping aids Often contain antihistamine as an active ingredient.	Antihistamines are designed to treat cold symptoms or allergy response, not to promote sleep, but many antihistamines have sedating effects.	Development of tolerance and dependence with prolonged use. Should not be used consecutively for more than 7 days. May cause daytime confusion, dizziness, blurred vision, dry mouth, constipation, and urinary retention.
Benzodiazepines These include the most prescribed classes of drugs in the world and in history.	Widely used to provide temporary relief for insomnia and other chronic sleep problems.	Sedative residual effects such as cognitive impairment, loss of motor skill, mood swings, confusion, and withdrawal symptoms. Estimated 60% of sleeping pill users become accidentally addicted. About 43% of emergency-room suicide attempts or overdoses involve sedative-hypnotic drugs. Cross-addiction to other drugs or alcohol is common.
Non-benzodiazepine drugs such as zolpidem and zaleplon	May have less sedative residual effects and a shorter circulatory time in the body.	Allergic reactions such as difficulty breathing; swelling of lips, face, or tongue; hives; hallucinations; abnormal behavior; or severe confusion.
Herbal remedies Include **Valeriana officinals, Passiflora incarnata, Avena sativa,** and **Melissa officinalis.** Commercially available as a tea, tincture, capsule, or tablet. Chinese herbs with sedative effects include ginseng, astragalus, and royal jelly.	Some clinical studies have demonstrated that valerian may be useful for initiating or improving the quality of sleep.	Hangover, headaches, excitability, and heart disturbances have been reported. Not for people with liver dysfunction or who are pregnant. Herbal products are not required to undergo the same rigorous testings as drugs do. More research is needed.

Data from W.C. Dement, **The Promise of Sleep** (New York: Living planet Press, 1999); J. Horne, **Why We Sleep** (New York: Oxford University Press, 1988); M.W. Radomski, "Sleep Strategies and Military Effectiveness," **WellnessOptions** (February/March 2001): 25–27; I.V. Zhdanova, R.J. Wurtman, H.J. Lynch et al., "Sleep-Inducing Effects of Low Doses of Melatonin Ingested in the Evening," **Clinical Pharmacology & Therapeutics** (1995) 57: 552–558.

Cognitive and Behavioral Therapies. Recent evidence suggests that combined cognitive and behavioral therapy is the best way to help a person stay insomnia-free in the long term. Cognitive techniques can change insomnia-inducing misperceptions about how much sleep is required and about the impact of sleep deprivation—as well as dealing with deep-rooted stress that causes sleeping problems. Behavioral techniques include controlling stimuli (helping the sufferer associate the bed and bedroom with sleep instead of wakefulness); temporal control (sleeping and waking up at regular times and eliminating frequent naps); and sleep restriction (limiting the amounts of time spent lying awake in bed before sleeping).[48]

One recent study shows that people with primary insomnia have improved sleep after reading cognitive-behavioral self-help books, even without seeking professional help.

Cognitive-behavioral therapy treats insomnia effectively and helps maintain recovery, especially in older adults. One recent study has shown that people with primary insomnia (i.e., those whose only complaint is insomnia) have improved sleep after reading cognitive-behavioral self-help books, even without seeking professional help.[49]

Relaxation. Progressive muscle relaxation, aromatherapy, massage therapy, yoga, tai chi, meditation, other relaxation techniques, and biofeedback may also be beneficial.

Strategic Naps. In some cases, such as shift work, long-haul flying or driving, and special continuous military operations, cumulative sleep deprivation may be impossible to avoid. But there is a coping method: strategic napping. Nap timing, length, and placement in the sleep cycle can be optimized, and sleep inertia that occurs upon awakening from a nap can be minimized. Studies have shown that after a person has been deprived of sleep for 24 hours, a nap of 15, 30, 60, or 120 minutes can increase alertness. The highest improvement is recorded after a 60-minute nap, but no greater improvement was recorded after the 120-minute nap.[50]

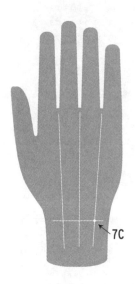

Sleep research shows that acupressure applied to the wrists at acupuncture point 7C can induce sleep.

When we first wake up, we enter a transitory period of decreased alertness called sleep inertia, which lasts from 30 to 120 minutes.[51] It poses a real problem for people such as pilots, truck drivers, and radar operators, who are required to perform highly skilled tasks shortly after abrupt awakenings. It is also a difficulty for military commanders who must make critical decisions after sudden awakenings. The magnitude and duration of after-nap sleep inertia are affected by the sleep stage the person was in when their sleep was interrupted, and awakenings from deep Stage 3 and 4 sleep are the worst. Sleep inertia has a greater effect on cognitive tasks than on motor tasks.

Naps should be scheduled in the early morning when there are fewer occurrences of sws (slow-brain-wave sleep).[52] Post-nap grogginess can persist for about 2 hours after a 2-hour nap taken late at night (e.g., at 11 p.m), but naps of about 80 to 90 minutes can minimize the probability of awakening from sws. The worst sleep inertia often occurs upon awakening from a 50-minute nap.

From Sleep Onward ...

The days when most sleep problems were treated with sleeping pills are gone forever. Sleep is now recognized as an integrated behavior that requires an integrated clinical, medical, and healthy lifestyle approach for treatment.

But science is just beginning to explore the landscape of sleep, and many territories are still uncharted. What happens in the brain to move us over the thresholds of falling asleep and waking up? Is "sleep learning" a good idea? Or would it interfere with the consolidation of memory and learning from the day before? Is it important to go to bed feeling happy in order to wake up happy? Why, after a lifetime of knowing the difference between reality and dreams, are we still usually unable to tell that dreams are dreams until we wake up? Why do we never see our own faces in our dreams? Why are about 20 to 30 percent of dreams in black and white and the rest in multiple colors?

One thing is certain: maze-running lab rats have shown us that daytime experience is carried over into sleep. As we dream on, we relive those events, file memories, and consolidate lessons. And the way we venture through the landscape of sleep at night affects our well-being the next day.

What we eat and drink can determine whether we have a good night's rest.

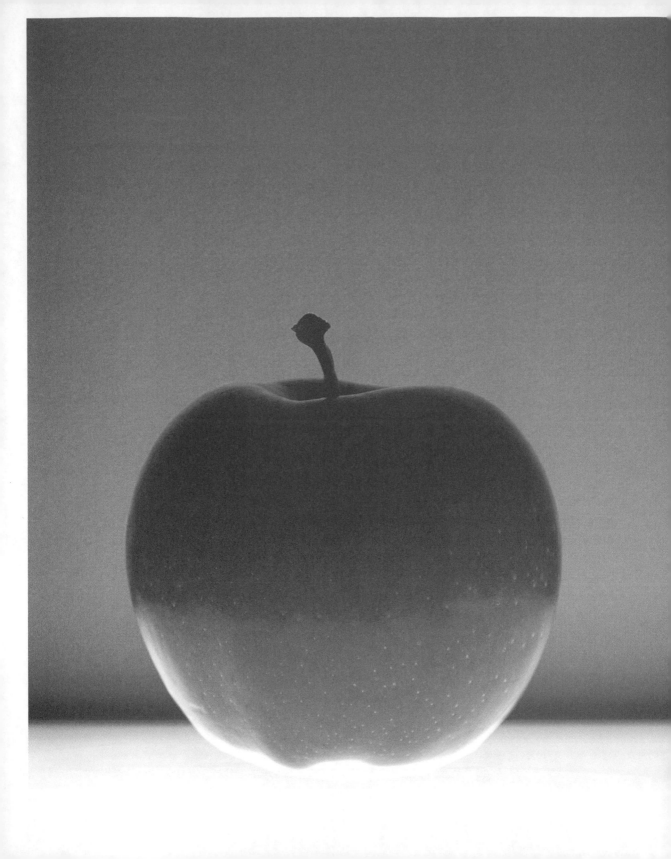

Part III

Forging Your Own Path to Wellness: Healthy Lifestyle Practices

Intellectuals solve problems; geniuses prevent them.
—Albert Einstein

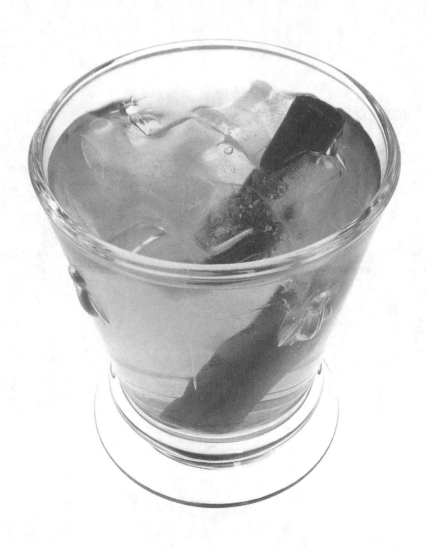

8 Gourmet Wellness:
The Tao of Food and Nutrition

The winning general won before engaging in warfare;
the losing general engaged in warfare trying to win.
—Sun Tzu, *The Art of War*

Cinnamon Water

The word *Tao*, which is often translated as "the Way," is actually derived from the Chinese character (道). It is made up of two parts: the head with hair (首) and the act of walking with one's head bent forward, looking up and down (辶). So Tao means moving forward with your head looking up at times, to see where you're going, and looking down at other times, to see how you're getting there. It's not just "the Way." It's a very involved activity of consciously thinking while physically advancing. Different Taos serve different purposes. They are not completed sets of rules and they are developing all the time.

Everyone engages the body when they eat, but we are not all conscious of exactly what and how we are eating. To develop a Tao of nourishment is to do more than engage the body while we eat and drink. It is to eat consciously, knowing what, why, and how we are eating and enjoying the process all the while.

Like viewpoints on scenic routes that give us a sense of the entire landscape, many landmark experiences in my life have shaped my Tao of nourishment. For example, I had a tricolored toy boat that I used as a meal box when I was very young. The white cabin contained soup and rice in two compartments, the blue deckhouse was for the main course, and the pink tower was actually a small cup for dessert. I would carry the boat with me, absent-mindedly and infrequently picking at the food while focusing on whatever game I was playing. Over the years the containers changed, but my inattention to food did not. This only began to change after that motorcycle accident I described at the beginning of this book. When I found myself still alive in the hospital, I enjoyed the first drink offered to me so much that I have since learned to savor, not just gobble up.

Two incidents in 1973 were food-thought provoking for me, too.

The first occurred toward the end of the Chinese Cultural Revolution, when I traveled to China to cover a story. It was my first visit, and I went to a very poor coastal village. The children had to collect cockroaches for chicken feed, and they traded the feed for their dinners. As a privileged visitor, I could eat whatever I could buy. But the foods available were limited to grayish rice, pickled vegetables, and tea. I have since learned to respect the freedom to choose and to treasure our access to an abundance of food and drink choices.

The second incident happened in November of the same year. That's when Bobby Fischer, the eccentric, publicity-shy international chess champion, came to Hong Kong for a four-day visit. He secretly checked into a hotel but was soon discovered by the press. To avoid further exposure, he moved out to stay with the vice-president of the Hong Kong Chess Club, who happened to be a friend of mine. Even though I was a reporter working in Hong Kong at the time, I was given the opportunity to meet with Bobby Fischer for breakfast. I will never forget what he ate at that meal: 11 extra-large, sunny-side-up eggs! "The eggs help me think," he said. And that was my introduction to conscious eating!

What's in an Egg?

Many of the essential nutrients required for proper functioning of the body are found in eggs. They contain nine essential amino acids, for example, and they're rated at 93.7 percent—higher than any other food—in terms of how efficiently the human body uses the protein for building new tissue.

Other nutrients and health benefits provided by eggs include:

→ Vitamins A, D, and K.

→ Choline: essential for brain development and memory.

→ Lutein and zeaxanthin: two carotenoid antioxidants that improve eye health, help protect the eyes from ultraviolet rays, and reduce the incidence of age-related macular degeneration (the major cause of blindness in elderly Canadians).

→ Eggs have also been linked to a reduction in the risk of cataract development.

→ Americans consumed a total of about 66 billion eggs in 1998, more than 17 dozen a year per person, while Canadians consumed about 15 dozen a year. Although the egg is one of nature's near-perfect foods, it has one important drawback; its yolk contains about two-thirds of our total suggested maximum intake of cholesterol.[1]

Common Food Groups

Even though variations in diet traditions and food cultures have been shaped by differences in geography, agriculture, and climate, as well as by socio-economic factors, there are food groups common to the diets of most humans. These are the four groups we need to feed from: (1) grains, (2) vegetables and fruits, (3) milk products, and (4) meat and alternatives (such as poultry or fish). Consciously eating a balanced mix of these foods is still the cornerstone of a healthy diet.

Food Guide to Healthy Eating

The following guidelines and recommendations are adapted from *Canada's Food Guide to Healthy Eating* and the U.S. recommended daily allowance (RDA).[2]

→ Enjoy a variety of foods from each of the four main food groups: grain products; dairy products; vegetables and fruits; and meat and alternatives (such as poultry or fish).
→ Choose from whole grains or enriched grain products high in starch and fiber, with added vitamins and minerals.
→ Choose from low-fat milk products for calcium and proteins.
→ Choose from dark green and orange vegetables and orange fruit high in vitamin A and folacin.
→ Choose from leaner meats, poultry, and fish, or meat alternatives such as dried peas, beans, and lentils.
→ Achieve and maintain a healthy body weight by enjoying regular physical activity and healthy eating.
→ Limit intake of salt, alcohol, and caffeine, and prepare foods with little or no fat.

Recommended Servings from Each Food Group per Day from **Canada's Food Guide to Healthy Eating**

Grain Products	5-12 servings	
Vegetables and fruit	5-10 servings	
Milk products	Children 4-9 years: 2-3 servings Youth 10-16 years: 3-4 servings	Adults: 2-4 servings Pregnant and breast-feeding women: 3-4 servings
Meat and alternatives	2-3 servings	

Important notes on number of servings: A serving as defined in *Canada's Food Guide to Healthy Eating* may be much smaller than you are accustomed to eating. So check the guide on Health Canada's Web site (**www.hc-sc.gc.ca**) to see what you really need. Otherwise, you may be eating more servings than you realize. For example, a plate of pasta can count as three to four servings, one slice of bread equals one serving, while one bagel, pita, or bun equals two servings of grain products, and a juice box equals two servings of vegetables and fruit.

Heartfelt Veggies

In a large-scale study carried out over the past two decades, people who consumed at least three servings per day of fruits and vegetables had a 27-percent-lower incidence of stroke and a 42-percent-lower stroke mortality rate compared with those who did not eat this way. Their risk of death from cardiovascular diseases was also reduced by 27 percent. And men appeared to benefit more than women from frequent fruit and vegetable consumption.[3]

The research, part of the first U.S. National Health and Nutrition Examination Survey, involved prolonged follow-up of 9,608 adults aged 25 to 74, who were randomly chosen by gender, race, and sociological group.

Conscious Eating Is Cross-Cultural

Many cultures throughout history have recognized the need to consciously consume certain foods to maintain health. The ancient Egyptians, for example, promoted honey and milk as healthy foods. Similarly, the curative properties of soybeans were documented in the first Chinese book on herbal medicine, the *Agriculture Minister's Collection of Medicinal Herbs*, published in the third century B.C. In 1747, on board *HMS Salisbury*, naval surgeon James Lind gave lemon and oranges to seamen suffering from scurvy and cured them of the disease. For centuries, the Mayans and Mexicans used chocolate as a food-medicine to treat fatigue, before some of its medicinal properties were scientifically studied. And chicken soup has traditionally been hailed as a health-recovery food in many cultures.

Sweet Tidings: Chocolate for the Heart?

The use of chocolate as a medicine originated among the Mayans and Mexicans. More than a hundred uses have been documented in European texts, and treatments of mental and physical fatigue top the list. Even the flowers of cacao trees were used to treat fatigue. Chocolate can provide energy because of its sugar content and its large quantity of caffeine-like psychostimulants. And recently, studies from Harvard Medical School and the University of California have suggested that chocolate may be good for the heart because of the high content of flavonol in cacao beans.[4]

Unfortunately, not all commercially manufactured chocolate is high in flavonols, since flavonols have a slightly bitter taste that does not appeal to everyone. Generally, dark chocolates and European chocolates are likely to have a higher flavonol content than chocolates manufactured in North America.

Flavonols are also found in red wine and grape juice. So it's not surprising that the Harvard and University of California studies were presented at a symposium called "Dietary Flavonoids: Heart-Healthy Nutrients or an Excuse to Enjoy Wine and Chocolate?" sponsored by Mars, the chocolate manufacturer.

Wine and chocolates: what a way to pamper yourself! And they can even bring you health benefits. But don't forget that eating chocolate can also add pounds. As with any food or drink, moderation is the key.

Soybeans through the Centuries

Soy has been growing in China for more than three thousand years and was first exported to Europe in the 18th century. Used not only as food, but also as a medicine, the soybean was included in the first Chinese book of medicinal herbs, entitled *Agriculture Minister's Collection of Medicinal Herbs*, published in the third century B.C.[5] Then, during the late Han Dynasty (206 B.C. to A.D. 220), the *Records of Celebrated Physicians* indicated that soy was able to counter the retention of excessive tissue fluids. This was the first documented evidence that the soybean could serve as a remedy for edema.

Japanese life expectancy is the highest in the world, and the most notable diet component eaten throughout Japan is soy. Recently, research has shown that soy and its proteins (isoflavonoids, plant sterols, and saponins) may bring a wide range of health benefits, including lower cholesterol, hormone modulation, and antioxidant properties.

But of all these characteristics, soy's ability to lower cholesterol has been the most thoroughly researched. An analysis of more than 30 studies concluded that a daily intake of soy protein would lower LDL (bad) cholesterol by about 12 percent. Such data have prompted the U.S. Food and Drug Administration to consider a health claim for the capacity of soy protein products to lower cholesterol and prevent heart disease, based on 6.25 grams (0.2 ounces) of soy protein per serving and a 25-gram (0.9-ounce) daily intake. With attention like this, soy currently has a high health profile.[6]

Soy protein consumption also lowers total cholesterol and reduces LDL (bad) to HDL (good) cholesterol ratios. And it appears to have powerful antioxidant properties. Soy is one of the few foods that combine cholesterol-lowering and antioxidant properties.

But a problem connected with soy has been demonstrated in a recent study of 3,734 elderly Japanese-American men: those who had eaten the most tofu during mid-life had up to 2.4 times the risk of later developing Alzheimer's disease. Men who had consumed tofu at least twice weekly had more cognitive impairment, compared with those who had rarely or never eaten the soybean curd.

Higher mid-life tofu consumption was also associated with low brain weight. Brain atrophy was assessed in 574 men using brain scanning results and in 290 men using autopsy information. Shrinkage occurs naturally with age, but for the men who had consumed more tofu, an exaggeration of the usual aging patterns was observed.[7]

Good Old Chicken Soup

Chicken soup is known to have been prescribed as a cold and asthma remedy as early as the 12th century by physician and scholar Moses Maimonides. In Chinese food culture, it is also believed to bring many health benefits.

There are endless varieties of this traditional remedy, but the main ingredients in all are chicken and water.[8] Other popular ingredients include onions, sweet potatoes, parsnips, turnips, carrots, celery stems, garlic, pepper, and parsley. Apparently, this concoction may have some effect on thinning mucus and making breathing easier. Experiments in which chicken extract was fed to rats also demonstrated some heart-health benefits.

According to classical Chinese medical texts, it's important to remove the skin of the chicken before you prepare the soup, and ginger is often added with herbs or other ingredients.

Vitamins: Vital to Life

The launch of modern-day nutrition science may be traced back to the French chemist Antoine Laurent Lavoisier (1743–94), who maintained that life is basically a chemical process. But it's perhaps more accurate to say that life is an experience that may be enhanced and even extended through understanding life's chemical processes. And conscious eating and drinking can be promoted with this understanding.

Conscious eating developed into a systematic food and nutrition science about a hundred years ago. In 1906 British biochemist Frederick Hopkins demonstrated that foods contained necessary "accessory factors," in addition to proteins, carbohydrates, fats, minerals, and water, and in 1911, Polish chemist Casimir Funk coined the word *vitamine* (from the Latin words *vita*, meaning life, and *amine*, meaning nitrogen-containing chemical compound). The term soon came to be applied to many accessory factors, though it was later discovered that some vitamins contain no amines at all. Because of its widespread use, however, Funk's term continued to be applied without the final letter *e*. Today, the term *vitamin* refers to the catalysts that regulate chemical reactions in the body. There are 13 vitamins, and most of them are chemical substances that our body doesn't make. That's why we must obtain them through our diet.

In 1912, Hopkins and Funk advanced the vitamin hypothesis of deficiency, which proposed that the absence of sufficient amounts of a particular vitamin in a body system may lead to certain diseases.

Throughout the early 1900s, scientists succeeded in isolating and identifying the various vitamins recognized today.

But it was not until World War II (1939–45) that the United States began fortifying enriched white flour, cereals, pasta, and rice with thiamine, iron, niacin, and riboflavin. Soon after that, many other countries followed suit, and this food trend has helped eradicate some dietary deficiencies in the world population.

The Antiberiberi Factor. The discovery and development of vitamin B1 popularized the concept that a specific dietary deficiency leads to a particular disease. And vitamin B1 history is linked with a disease called beriberi, which is characterized by pain and swelling of the limbs. The first documented description of beriberi is found in the seventh-century Chinese classical text *General Treatise on the Etiology and Symptoms of Diseases* by Ch'ao-Yuan-fang and Wu Ching. Then, in about 1882, Takaki, a Japanese surgeon, dramatically decreased the incidence of beriberi in the Japanese navy by improving the sailors' diet. And in 1897, Dutch physiologist Christian Ejikman showed that symptoms of beriberi could be produced in chickens fed with polished rice and that these symptoms can be prevented or cured by using rice-bran feed instead.

In 1915, Elmer V. McCollum and Marguerite Davis proposed water-soluble vitamin B as the antiberiberi factor, and in 1936, Robert R. Williams identified the chemical formula and named it thiamine (now referred to as vitamin B1). The first commercial production of thiamine began the following year.

Today, sales of nutritional products—including supplements, natural health products, green teas, sports supplements, and especially vitamins—have ballooned into a multibillion-dollar industry. The U.S. market alone achieved sales of US$16.8 billion in the year 2000, with vitamins accounting for US$5.9 billion as the sales leader. An interesting side note is the historical concentration of market shares in this industry. For instance, Roche accounted for 40 percent and Germany's BASF accounts for 21 percent of global vitamin sales. Roche also manufactured 75 percent of the world's carotenoids, until February 10, 2003, when DSM announced its signed contract to acquire Roche's vitamins, carotenoids, and fine chemicals business.

How Vitamins Work

Proteins, carbohydrates, and fats combine in our bodies with other substances to yield energy and build tissues. These chemical reactions are catalyzed, or accelerated, by enzymes produced from specific vitamins, and they take place in specific parts of the body. The vitamins we need are divided into: *water-soluble vitamins* (the B vitamins and vitamin C) and *fat-soluble vitamins* (A, D, E, and K). They are best obtained from a balanced diet of foods.[9]

Water-soluble vitamins are absorbed by the intestine and carried by the circulatory system to specific tissues for use. B vitamins act as coenzymes—compounds that unite with a protein component called an apoenzyme to form an active enzyme. This enzyme then acts as a catalyst in the chemical reactions that transfer energy from the basic food elements to the body. It's not known, however, whether vitamin C acts as a coenzyme.

When we take in more water-soluble vitamins than we need, small amounts are stored in our body tissue, but most of the excess is excreted in urine. This means that we need a daily supply of water-soluble vitamins to prevent depletion.

Fat-soluble vitamins seem to have highly specialized functions. They are absorbed by the intestine, and the lymph system carries them to different parts of the body. They are involved in maintaining the structure of cell membranes and are also responsible for the synthesis of certain enzymes.

Our bodies can store larger amounts of fat-soluble vitamins than water-soluble vitamins. The liver is the main storage organ for vitamins A and D, while vitamin E is stored in body fat and to a lesser extent in reproductive organs. Relatively little vitamin K is stored. Excessive intake of fat-soluble vitamins (particularly vitamins A and D) can lead to toxic levels in the body and dangerous health consequences.

A vitamin or mineral in daily value (DV) is a standard that generally corresponds to the U.S. recommended daily allowance (RDA). DV indicates the minimum daily requirements of a vitamin or a mineral in order to prevent a deficiency disease.[10] It can serve as a general guideline in terms of how much of a vitamin or a mineral we need.

Many vitamins work together to regulate a number of processes within the body. And a lack of vitamins can upset the body's internal balance or block one or more metabolic reactions. On the other hand, excess catalysts in the body are not only useless but can sometimes seriously harm the body—including causing the growth of cancerous cells. Individual dietary needs must therefore be taken into account, and dietitians, nutritionists, and doctors must be consulted regarding supplements.

Pass the Popcorn, Dear

Whole-grain foods contain a natural combination of several nutrients important to overall health—such as a rich content of fiber, folic acid, vitamin E, magnesium, and potassium. But whole grains are currently low on the list of food items that North Americans eat.[10] Less than 5 percent of Canadians, for instance, consumed the recommended intake of whole-grain products in 2001.

Studies have shown that increasing the intake of whole grains to an average of 2.7 servings per day significantly diminishes the risk of high blood pressure and stroke. In addition, increased whole-grain intake has been associated with improvements in insulin sensitivity.[11]

There's a multitude of whole-grain foods to choose from: breakfast cereals, dark bread, wheat germ, brown rice, cracked wheat, graham flour, whole barley, popcorn, whole cornmeal, oats, rye, whole wheat, bran, and other grains such as kasha and couscous. Normally, breakfast cereals are considered to be whole-grain foods if 25 percent of their weight is made up of whole grains or bran.

Too Much of a Good Thing?

Food metabolism and the ways food and our bodies interact are chemical processes. As with any chemicals, natural or otherwise, and as with any chemical reactions, especially within the body, caution is advised.

There are 13 vitamins, and most of them are chemical substances that our body doesn't make. That's why we must obtain them through our diet.

Vitamins and minerals are known as essential nutrients because we cannot survive or thrive without them. Programs such as the addition of vitamin D to milk products; iodization of salt; and fortification of milk with vitamin C have improved public health significantly. But too much of a good thing can also be harmful. Calcium is a case in point: too little can cause fragile and malformed bones, but too much can lead to kidney problems.

Nutrient fortification needs to be fine-tuned, and most governments are now regulating the amounts of vitamins and minerals added to foods. In Canada, under proposed expanded food fortification policies, the public would be offered a wider range of "special purpose foods"—products formulated for groups such as pregnant women, seniors, and athletes, who have particular nutritional needs. Special purpose foods would also carry directions for use, including who should consume them, for what purpose, and how much is appropriate. New guidelines for levels of nutrient additions are also expected to be set.[12]

Food Fortification Milestones

Many medical conditions have become faint memories because of public health programs that promote food fortification. Here are a few examples:

→ Few children today suffer from the bone malformations of rickets because vitamin D has been added to evaporated and dried milks since 1940 and to fluid milk since the late 1960s.

→ The iodization of salt has virtually eliminated endemic goiter, an abnormality of the hormone-producing thyroid gland.

→ In remote communities, evaporated milk fortified with vitamin C eliminated infantile scurvy, which is associated with anemia, bleeding gums, and poor development of bones and teeth.

Not only is it important to be aware of intake for the purpose of food metabolism as energy, but it's also vital to keep an eye on intake that affects the workings of the digestive and absorption systems,[13] including stomach fluid acidity, intestinal bacteria flora, nutrition absorption rates, and intestine movements. Lack of dietary fiber, for instance, slows down intestinal movement and may lead to the production of cancer-causing agents, increasing the risk of colon cancer.[14]

Reliable information, knowledge, balance, common sense, and professional consultations with dietitians, nutritionists, and your doctors are all necessary parts of the successful gourmet wellness formula and are essential for a healthy Tao of nourishment.

The vitamins we need are divided into: water-soluble vitamins (the B vitamins and vitamin C) and fat-soluble vitamins (A, D, E, and K). They are best obtained from a balanced diet of foods.

Organic Foods

Pesticides and Farming. Farming has long been associated with the use of pesticides, and the first recorded use of pesticides actually dates back more than three thousand years. The ancient Romans used sulfur as a fumigant, and the Chinese later used arsenic to control garden pests, for instance. Arsenic in less toxic forms was also used until the 1940s in North America.

U.S. manufacturers currently produce more than 680 tonnes (750 short tons) of chemical pesticides a year, with a sale value of US$7 billion. About 72 percent of these chemicals are used in farming.[15]

Pesticides have been used to increase agricultural production, but pesticide residue can be a health risk. The British government's Pesticide

Residues Committee (PRC) recently published a study on these residues found on fruit samples collected between October and December 2001. The results showed that 64 percent of the 179 strawberry samples contained pesticide residue, with 4 samples containing residues that exceeded the maximum residue limit. Pesticide residues were also found in soft citrus fruits, peaches, and nectarines, at 94, 75, and 53 percent respectively. Even though the PRC assured consumers that none of the residues found were of concern for health and that "adverse health effects would be unlikely," it is a good practice to wash vegetables and fruits thoroughly.[16]

Organic Farming. Organic food growers use agricultural methods that harm neither farm workers nor the environment. The cornerstone of organic farming is crop rotation, but other methods are also used— including intercropping, planting of cover crops; rotational grazing; farm waste recycling; tilling; and adding minerals, compost, and biological amendments.

Organic meat, dairy products, and eggs are produced from animals that are given organic feed. Usually the animals also have outdoor access and can range freely. Organic livestock and poultry are given no antibiotics, hormones, or medication other than vaccinations unless they are ill. Since organic farming is more labor-intensive, and organic crop yields are often not as high as in regular farming, the price of organic produce is higher.

Worldwide sales of organic products are estimated at Cdn$20 billion (US$13 billion) a year, mostly in the United States, Europe, and Japan, and organic food production is the fastest-growing segment of agriculture in both Canada and the United States. The number of Canadian certified organic producers increased by 34 percent between 1999 and 2000. Most of Canada's organic produce is exported, largely to the United States, and Canada is one of the top five world producers of organic grain and oilseeds. Organic food sales in Canada are expected to grow by 20 percent annually to $3.1 billion by 2005; U.S. sales increased from US$78 million in 1980 to about US$6 billion in 2000, with a continuing growth of about 20 percent a year.

Organic foods are produced and processed under accreditation and certification systems in North America and Europe. But none of the certification systems for organic foods includes any standard referring to nutritional value, health claims, safety, or the quality grade of the foods certified.[17]

Food metabolism and the ways food and our bodies interact are chemical processes. As with any chemicals, natural or otherwise, and as with any chemical reactions, especially within the body, caution is advised.

It's interesting to note that the nutritional value of organic produce is not necessarily higher than produce that has been grown under non-organic conditions.

Opposition from Food Industry Associations. The Grocery Manufacturers of America (GMA) opposed the certification system after a U.S. government survey showed that more than 60 percent of consumers would likely interpret the U.S. Department of Agriculture (USDA) seal on organic foods as suggesting that these foods were "better in some way; safer; more healthy; and better for the environment" than other foods. The National Food Processors Association (NFPA) also pointed out that some organic foods could potentially be less safe than conventional foods because regulations prohibit the use of irradiation to kill bacteria and ban some seed treatments that provide effective prevention for mycotoxins.

> Lack of dietary fiber slows down intestinal movement and may lead to the production of cancer-causing agents, increasing the risk of colon cancer.

Genetically Modified Foods

What Is Genetic Modification (GM)?

Genetic materials such as DNA from a given species can be inserted into a host plant's genome. For example, daffodil genes can be placed into the genome of golden rice.

Most North Americans eat GM foods every day. In 1996, 3.2 million hectares (8 million acres) of GM foods were grown in North America, and by 1999 the crop had grown to more than 28 million hectares (70 million acres). Artificial genetic trait selection (AS) has been used for a long time. But there's a difference between GM and AS. With AS, farmers or researchers choose a desirable phenotypic trait (an appearance trait that is measurable) and allow it to propagate. With this method, it takes years to accomplish one desired dominating trait. With GM, however, genes are transferred across species to create a far greater variety of phenotypes in a shorter time.

A first generation of GM crops displays such manipulated traits as resistance to herbicides, insects, and diseases.

A second generation aims at enhanced nutrition (rice with added vitamin A precursors, for example) or reduced allergenicity or toxicity (such as a decaffeinated coffee crop). Some plants are also being developed to clean up wastes—by accumulating lead, for example.

Potential Health Risks of GM Foods

→ *Unintended and unexpected toxin production and/or changes in nutrient levels.* Genes can interact with each other in surprising ways. For example, unintended new toxins may emerge.

→ *Undesirable allergen production.* A study reported in *The New England Journal of Medicine* on modified soy plants and Brazil nuts showed that allergenic properties can be transferred from one plant species (Brazil nuts) to another (soybeans).[18]

Are GM Crops Good or Bad?

Evaluation must proceed on a case-by-case basis. Some GM crops will have significant health benefits, with few or no adverse consequences. Others will be problematic. The trick is to detect which is which. Scientifically rigorous risk assessment protocols need to be established, and better data disclosure is required. Just as importantly, public education and food label requirements need to be implemented.

The Amazing Food Trend Maze

Pesticides have been used to increase agricultural production, but pesticide residue can be a health risk. On the other hand, the nutritional value of organic produce is not necessarily higher than produce that has been grown under non-organic conditions.

As I work at developing the Tao of food and nutrition, I come across conflicting food trends that leave me puzzled. Today in the industrialized world, we have access to more food and nutritional information than ever before. Everywhere we turn, food tips and advice are presented to us. The media are always bombarding us with studies promoting, condoning, or condemning certain foods and eating behaviors, and the Internet provides 24-hour links to thousands of nutrition websites.

But professional and scientific opinions on the benefits and drawbacks of various foods and eating behaviors are numerous and at times even conflicting. It has become quite a challenge to understand what's good and to make decisions about what to have for dinner. I sometimes find myself lost in the information maze and exhausted by the overload.

In spite of all the available information and the fact that we all know nutrition is important and we want to eat well, we *don't* eat well most of the time. Even worse, as we're bombarded with increasingly thin, media-hyped body images, our North American society is marked by an almost epidemic proportion of overweight and obese people. There are times that I too have just thrown up my hands in frustration and headed straight to the fridge. When it becomes too hard to eat well and be thin, calories offer uncomplicated pleasure and escape.

Of course, fast foods and supersize portions don't help. The pace of modern life and the indulgence of an affluent society have shaped us and created major health concerns in North America.

So how do we forge our own way to gourmet wellness within this food trend maze? How can we enjoy both health and culinary benefits? Perhaps by getting back to the basics, and using a simple common-sense approach, we can take a look at why we eat, then what and how we eat.

What Happened to the Hamburger?

According to the U.S. National Cattlemen's Beef Association, the average American eats more than a hundred quarter-pound (113-gram) burger patties a year, and that number is climbing. This translates into more than 5.2 billion hamburgers and cheeseburgers sold in 1995, up 3.4 percent from 1994.

The burger is often considered to be an unhealthy food. But where does the hamburger come from, and is it really so bad?

Many conflicting claims exist as to who created the hamburger. Numerous hamburger historians have agreed on the origin of the meat patty, but not on who put the burger inside a bun.

The earliest ancestor of the burger was developed in medieval Russia. In the 13th century, when nomadic Tartars conquered much of that country and Eastern Europe, they introduced chopped raw beef. Inhabitants of the Baltic region began to season it with salt, pepper, and onion juice—creating the first steaks tartare.

About five hundred years later, in the 18th century, German sailors visiting Russian ports discovered this Baltic delicacy and introduced it to Hamburg and other German port towns. German chefs made some alterations to the meat, forming it into patties and sometimes adding an egg. Somewhere along the line, chopped onions were also thrown in for good measure, and the patties were lightly cooked.

It took about a hundred years for "Hamburg-style steak" to travel to North America, but once it arrived, eating stands along the piers of New York harbor began featuring it in order to attract German sailors and immigrants. Then, in 1834, the "Hamburger Steak" finally made a documented appearance on the menu at New York's famous Delmonico's Restaurant, selling for the stupendous sum of 10 cents!

Some say that when 15-year-old Charlie Nagreen of Seymour, Wisconsin, was selling ground beef at the Outagamie County Fair in 1885, he was the one who placed the beef between bread slices. Others claim that Fletcher Davis, of Athens, Texas, created the hamburger at the 1904 World's Fair in St. Louis, Missouri.

Whatever the history, by the late 19th century the burger had become a favorite food of industrial workers, the cornerstone of the first American drive-ins, and a standard item on the menus of North American restaurants.

Today, a typical fast-food burger meal consists of a quarter-pound (113-gram) cheeseburger with onion, lettuce, and tomato (about 270 to 1,000 calories), a glass of soft drink (0 to 140 calories), and fries (about 200 to 550 calories). The hamburger isn't a bad meal on its own; in fact with meat, vegetables, cheese, seasoning, and two slices of bread, it can be a rather balanced meal. But things can get *out* of balance, depending on how the burger is cooked, what calories are added between the two pieces of bread or bun (in the form of sauces and toppings), and what's in the accompanying drink and fries.

Why We Eat: Fuel for Life

To estimate your own "food fuel" needs and to understand the difference between a calorie and a Calorie, refer to the box "Fat Chance or Fat Arithmetic?" See also the table listing common activities and their corresponding energy consumption.

We depend on energy to sustain life and to function, and we derive this energy from food. To understand what food to eat and how much, we need to understand the wider picture of energy intake and consumption.

Energy use is at its lowest rate when we are at rest, and this is referred to as the resting metabolic rate. When the metabolic rate is measured at rest right after a person has been sleeping for eight hours in a fasted state, it's called the basal metabolic rate (BMR). Energy is consumed even in the basal state because our basic body functions require energy too.

Our total physical energy needs from food throughout the day include energy to maintain the basal state, as well as energy expended for activities. For an adult man, the daily energy requirement to maintain BMR is about 1,600 to 1,800 Calories, and for an adult female it's about 1,300 to 1,500 Calories.[19] The amount of additional energy you need depends on how active you are and varies from day to day.

Fat Chance or Fat Arithmetic?

How can we lose a pound (0.45 kilograms) of fat in a week? By doing our fat arithmetic![20]

A pound of body fat represents energy content of about 4,000 Calories (4,000 kcal). To lose a pound of fat in a week and balance your energy intake and output, simply follow the guidelines below. Note that a calorie is the amount of heat required to raise one gram of water one degree centigrade. Nutritionists use the term Calorie (capital C) or kilocalories (kcal) to represent 1,000 calories:

➜ Reduce your daily food intake by 571 Calories (4,000 divided by 7) from the intake required to maintain your basal metabolic rate and daily activities.

→ Or increase your caloric expenditure by increasing your daily physical activity so you use up 571 additional Calories.

→ Or do both: Reduce daily food intake and increase the level of physical activity.

→ Of course, the arithmetic also works the other way. If you consume 571 Calories daily in excess of your basic energy requirement, the excess will be stored mainly as fat. Do this every day for a week, and you will acquire one extra pound (0.45 kilograms) of fat.

To help manage your weight, keep a daily input-output journal. Do the following calculations:

Input:

→ Take note of your favorite foods, their Calorie counts, and food groupings.

→ List all the foods you consume daily, recording the weight/portion size of each food item eaten.

→ Calculate total daily Calorie input by working out the caloric value of each food item eaten first, then add them up. The caloric value of each individual food item can be calculated with information obtained from the nutrition label. Carbohydrates and proteins each have 4 Calories per gram, fats have 9 Calories per gram, and alcohol has 7 Calories per gram. Multiply Calories per gram by total weight consumed to convert food components into caloric intake values.

→ Compare your intake to *Canada's Food Guide to Healthy Eating* or to the U.S. recommended daily allowance (RDA) to make sure you are eating a balanced diet.

→ Choose which foods you would like to cut back on or keep in your diet without upsetting the balance in the food groups.

Output:

→ List the physical activities you enjoy.

→ Choose the physical activities you wish to spend more time on, in order to burn more Calories.

→ Record the amount of time you spend on each activity every day.

→ Estimate the caloric expenditure for each physical activity; then add the number of Calories you need to maintain basal metabolism.

Energy Input equals Energy Output:

→ When caloric intake equals caloric output, your weight will remain steady.

→ When intake exceeds output, you will put on weight, mainly as fat.

→ When output exceeds input, you will lose weight and fat.[21]

List of Activities in Calories per Minute of Participation

ACTIVITY	CALORIES/MIN
Basic	
Basal (male)	1.2
Basal (female)	0.98
Daily chores	
Washing face, brushing hair	2.47
Climbing ladder at 50° angle	7.7
Climbing stairs, 97/min	8.4
Walking, 6.5 km/h (4 mph)	8.2
Walking, snow shoes, soft snow, 6 km/h (3.6 mph)	13.8
Driving car	2.8
Desk work	
Calculating	1.8
Reading	1.98
Sports and physical activities	
Bicycling, 15.5 km/h (9.4 mph)	7.0
Swimming	10.9
Shoveling, 8 kg load, 1 m lift, 12/min	7.5
Sawing softwood	6.3
Stacking firewood	6.3
Football	9.07
Basketball	7.76
Rowing, 33 strokes/min	19.0
Felling trees	10.7
House work	
Kneading dough	2.04
Sewing sheets	1.18
Washing clothes by hand	2.69
Ironing clothes	1.69
Sweeping floor	1.85

Data from P. Altman, and D. Dittmar, **Biological Handbooks: Metabolism** (Bethesda: Federation of American Societies of Biological Sciences, 1968).

Calorie Consumption in Various Activities According to Body Weight

ACTIVITY	SPEED	45 KG (100 LB)	68 KG (150 LB)	90 KG (200 LB)
Bicycling	10 km/h (6 mph)	160	240	312
Bicycling	19 km/h (12 mph)	270	410	534
Jogging	11 km/h (7 mph)	610	920	1,230
Jumping rope		500	750	1,000
Running	9 km/h (5.5 mph)	440	660	962
Running	16 km/h (10 mph)	850	1,280	1,664
Swimming	12 m/min (25 yd/min)	185	275	358
Swimming	46 m/min (50 yd/min)	325	500	650
Tennis singles		265	400	535
Walking	3 km/h (2 mph)	160	240	312
Walking	3 km/h (5 mph)	210	330	416
Walking	7 km/h (4.5 mph)	295	440	572

Food fuel needs usually decline as we age, and a study has found that men aged 23 to 34 consumed foods with an average energy content of 2,700 Calories per day, compared to 1,800 daily Calories for men aged 65 to 74.[22] The reduced consumption is mainly the result of a lower metabolic rate and a less active lifestyle. On the other hand, a healthy 70-year-old woman will require about 20 percent more energy to walk at the same speed as a younger woman.

Food for Fuel

Foods consist mostly of carbon, hydrogen, oxygen, and in the case of protein, nitrogen as well. Food energy is stored in the high-energy compound adenosine triphosphate (ATP), which is produced by body metabolism. When we are at rest, our bodies derive energy almost equally from carbohydrates and from fats, but during short-term physical activities, energy is generated almost exclusively from carbohydrates.

We need fat to give us the energy to carry out prolonged physical activities. The fat reserve for energy is much larger than for carbohydrates, but fat is less accessible for metabolism because it must be reduced from the complex form of triglyceride to simple forms, in order to generate ATP.

Proteins are the building blocks for the body, so they are not metabolized until most of our fat reserves have been used up. When metabolism uses protein as fuel, the body is starting to take itself apart in an attempt to survive.

Carbohydrates. Carbohydrates are fuel for the muscles and the brain, and the energy from carbohydrate metabolism is used by our bodies first. Carbohydrates are broken down by enzymes during digestion and converted to glucose (blood sugar). Assisted by the hormone insulin, blood glucose is then transported into cells throughout the body, where it is either metabolized and used, or stored. Glucose is also stored in the liver.

As our muscles and liver store glucose in only limited quantities, it can be depleted easily. And when our muscles run low on muscle-stored glycogen, they start to use blood glucose. As our blood glucose levels drop, fatigue hits—and this will happen sooner when we're engaged in intense and prolonged activity.

Ideally, about two-thirds of our daily caloric intake should come from carbohydrates. They are found in grain products, fruits, vegetables, and sugar.[23]

Fat. Fat is an important fuel and energy source, providing about twice as many calories as carbohydrates and protein. It is essential for insulation, assists in the transportation of some vitamins, and helps regulate hormones.[24]

We have come to fear this food fuel, most likely because of an almost universal preference for a lean body image and because of the health risks associated with a high-fat diet, including heart disease, stroke, diabetes, and cancer. But in reality, a certain amount of fat is required for basic health, and some types of fats are actually good for heart health. It's now evident that the type of fat we consume is more important than the overall amount from all types. Nevertheless, recommended fat intake levels are limited to no more than 30 percent of total daily calories, including no more than 10 percent saturated fat.

In spite of all the available information and the fact that we all know nutrition is important and we want to eat well, we don't eat well most of the time.

As our blood glucose levels drop, fatigue hits—and this will happen sooner when we're engaged in intense and prolonged activity.

Good Fats, Bad Fats

Increasingly, research evidence is showing that the type of fat we eat is more important than the amount we take in. All fats have received a lot of bad press in recent years, but we now know that there are good fats and bad fats.[25]

Saturated fats increase bad-cholesterol levels and decrease good cholesterol. This type usually becomes solid at room temperature and includes butter, lard, coconut oil and meat, and palm oil.

Polyunsaturated fats can reduce total cholesterol levels and are found in oils that remain liquid at room temperature. They include corn, sunflower, and other vegetable oils. In particular, the omega-3 fatty acids—polyunsaturated fats found in fish, nuts, and seeds—are healthy for the heart.[26]

Monounsaturated fats are the preferred dietary fats because they both lower bad-cholesterol levels and increase good-cholesterol levels. They are found in olive, peanut, and canola oil.

In addition, fats can be either hydrogenated or non-hydrogenated. The process of hydrogenation changes liquid fat into solid form at room temperature, turning canola oil into margarine, for instance. This process creates trans-fatty acids, which increase bad cholesterol.[27]

As fats in food can be invisible, it's important to read nutrition or ingredient labels to make sure bad fats are not creeping into your diet unnoticed. Saturated, polyunsaturated, and monounsaturated fats are listed on food labels in North America. Trans-fatty acids are not listed, but they are identified as "partly hydrogenated" vegetable oil on food labels.

You may also want to become savvy about foods labeled "light," "reduced calories," and "no cholesterol." *Light* may mean the food is lower in calories or fat, but it may also only indicate that it's low in salt or even in color. *Calorie reduced* only means that the food is lower in calories when compared to similar foods, but total calorie count can still be high. And *no cholesterol* doesn't necessarily mean no fat. For example, foods made from vegetable sources can be extremely high in fat, even though they contain no food cholesterol. (Only foods from animal sources contain food cholesterol.)

Protein intake should be about one-sixth of total caloric intake.

Protein. Protein is essential for energy. The body breaks down dietary protein into amino-acid building blocks to make enzymes and cells. All of these are essential for muscle, hair, and tissue building and repair. Proteins also keep the immune system functioning, help transport nutrients around the body, and are important in the synthesis of hormones.[28]

Protein for Vegetarians

Most dietary animal protein contains all 20 essential amino acids, but plants do not. So if you're following a vegetarian diet, you need to combine various plant foods to make sure you're not missing out. For example, tofu should be eaten with vegetables, or rice with yams, in order to obtain complete proteins. But you do not need to eat the complementary proteins at the same meal. As long as you consume them all within 24 hours, they can be converted into the complete range of proteins the body needs each day.[29]

COMPOSITION OF RECOMMENDED ENERGY SOURCES		
	Average Person	Person In Training
Carbohydrate	50%	55-65%
Fat	35% or less	less than 30%
Protein	10-15%	15%

DAILY PROTEIN REQUIREMENT IN GRAMS PER POUND (0.45 KG) OF BODY WEIGHT	
Aerobic training	0.5
Strength training	0.7
Hard endurance & strength training	up to 0.9

GOOD SOURCES OF CARBOHYDRATES	
Banana	1 medium / 27 g
Apple	1 medium / 21 g
Raisins	quarter cup / 29 g
Corn, canned	half cup / 18 g
Rice, cooked	1 cup / 46 g
Baked potato	1 large / 51 g
Grape-Nuts	quarter cup / 23 g
Spaghetti	1 cup / 40 g
Baked beans	1 cup / 50 g
Pizza, cheese	2 slices / 42 g

GOOD SOURCES OF PROTEIN	
Beef, lean	4 oz / 24 g
Chicken breast	3 oz / 24 g
Fish	3 oz / 17 g
Cheese	1 oz / 8 g
Cottage cheese, 2%	3/4 cup / 16 g
Milk, skim	1 cup / 8 g
Yogurt, low-fat, plain	8 oz / 12 g
Chickpeas (garbanzo)	20 g

Although excess protein can be converted into fat, it's actually unlikely that this will happen. But foods that contain protein, such as meat and whole-fat dairy products, are usually accompanied by a large amount of fat, and this fat leads to weight gain. The recommended daily intake of protein is 0.36 grams of protein per pound (0.45 kilograms) of body weight—about 50 to 100 grams altogether every day. Protein intake should also be about one-sixth of total caloric intake. Foods high in protein include meat, fish, eggs, nuts, seeds, and beans.

Our total physical energy needs from food throughout the day include energy to maintain the basal state, as well as energy expended for activities.

What to Eat? Yesterday, Today, and Tomorrow

Studies show that the average adult needs about 1,500 to 2,000 Calories a day but the average North American adult consumes an estimated 1,800 to 2,700 Calories a day. In 2001, an estimated 61 percent of adult Americans between the ages of 10 and 74 were either overweight (34 percent) or obese (27 percent), and 48 percent of Canadians were reported to be either overweight (19 percent) or obese (29 percent). In the United States, an estimated 50 million people were obese in 2001. Approximately 13 percent of American children aged 6 to 11 are also overweight, and 14 percent of adolescents aged 12 to 19 are overweight. During the past two decades, the prevalence of those who are overweight has doubled among American children and tripled among adolescents.[30]

All indications are pointing to the fact that we are aware of the importance of eating well but somehow don't eat as well as we know we should. Research by the National Institute of Nutrition indicates that most Canadians consider nutrition important in food selection, but less than half rate their eating habits as very good or excellent.[31]A 2002 survey conducted by *The Globe and Mail* and the CTV network found that 73 percent of Canadians considered they ate nutritiously most or all of the time. But the same survey also reported that 60 percent had eaten one serving of junk food (sweets, candy, chips, or pop) in the previous day.

Canadians spent an estimated $78 billion on food and drink in 2002, with an average family buying $6,220 worth of such products each year. About 25 percent of that is spent in restaurants. In 1999, the average Canadian consumed 32 kilograms (70 pounds) of fat and oil, 12 kilograms (26 pounds) of cheese, 8 kilograms (18 pounds) of butter or

Popping Away ...

On average, every man, woman, and child in North America drinks approximately one 350-milliliter (12-fluid-ounce) can of soft drink every day. Statistics in 2000 also show that the average American drank about 216 liters (57 gallons) of soft drinks a year, while the average Canadian drank about 116 liters (30 gallons).

A total of 57 million hectoliters (15 billion gallons) were sold in the United States. These consumption rates are more than double those of the early 1970s. Today, soft drinks make up about 25 percent of all drinks consumed in North America.[32]

margarine, 9 liters (2.3 gallons) of ice cream, 63 kilograms (139 pounds) of red meat, 35 kilograms (77 pounds) of poultry, 15 dozen eggs, 41 kilograms (90 pounds) of sugar and syrups (of which 40 kilograms [88 pounds] was refined sugar), 89 kilograms (196 pounds) of grain products, 184 kilograms (405 pounds) of fruit and vegetables (of which 74 kilograms [163 pounds] were potatoes, with only 8 kilograms [18 pounds] of tomatoes and 10 kilograms [22 pounds] of lettuce), and only 9 kilograms (20 pounds) of fish and seafood. And what did Canadians drink? They downed 116 liters (30 gallons) of soft drinks, 102 liters (27 gallons) of coffee, 88 liters (23 gallons) of milk, 70 liters (18 gallons) of tea, and 68 liters (18 gallons) of beer. Not exactly a nutritious combination![33]

> According to the Canadian Heart and Stroke Foundation, only 17 percent of Canadians eat the recommended amount of vegetables and fruits, and only one out of seven pre-teenagers eats enough servings of vegetables and fruits.

Forging Your Own Path to Gourmet Wellness

Here are some simple guidelines for a common-sense approach to eating well:

→ Be aware of your energy intake and consumption. Estimate your own daily food fuel requirements in Calories. Then try to limit your caloric intake so it does not exceed your energy consumption.

→ Try to stay close to the recommended intake ratio of carbohydrates at least 55 percent, fat less than 30 percent, and protein about 15 percent.

→ Be aware of the kind of fat you're eating. Is it good fat or bad fat?

→ Select a variety of foods from all four food groups, and try to follow recommended daily serving amounts. Most people are not eating enough carbohydrates from whole grains, vegetables, and fruits. Try to increase intake from these sources.

→ Other important nutrients are fiber, vitamins, and minerals. Try to meet the recommended daily requirements. They are best obtained from foods, but supplements may be needed. Consult your doctor or dietitian for your own supplement guidelines.

→ It's important to realize that we're all different and that individual food needs differ.

→ Balance is the key. Consuming anything in excess will lead to adverse health consequences.

→ Drink enough fluid to make sure you do not become dehydrated.

Tomatoes and Broccoli: Two Anti-Cancer Stars

Lycopene is not just any antioxidant. Found in the highest concentrations in the testes, adrenal glands, liver, and prostate, it has been identified as an exceptionally potent scavenger of free radicals. This has resulted in a growing number of studies on its use to prevent or influence the development of certain cancers in humans.[34]

Unlike other carotenoids, lycopene is found in only a limited number of foods, the primary sources being tomatoes and tomato products such as ketchup, spaghetti sauce, and pizza sauce. Pink grapefruit, fresh guava and guava juice, watermelon, and fresh papaya are also good sources of lycopene. Of the total carotenoids within a tomato, lycopenes make up 60 to 65 percent. Research also shows that lycopene in tomatoes can be absorbed into the bloodstream 2.5 times more efficiently if it is processed into juice, sauce, paste, or ketchup.[35]

Regular consumption of cooked tomato products can lower the risk of prostate cancer by as much as 36 percent. And the health benefits are not limited to prostate health. Another study of more than one thousand men who had suffered a heart attack, compared to a similar group who hadn't, showed that those with high levels of lycopene appeared to suffer only half the risk.[36]

And then there's broccoli. Studies show that this vegetable can cause pre-cancerous cells to self-destruct. It contains compounds that have anti-carcinogenic properties, and when these are broken down, they stimulate cancer cells to "commit suicide." This appears to be a characteristic of a group of vegetables called brassicas, including Brussels sprouts, cabbage, and cauliflower.[37] They contain the potent anti-carcinogenic compound sulphorafane, which can dramatically reduce the number of malignant tumors and their reproduction, growth rate, and size, as well as delaying the onset of cancer.

Tipping the Grape Juice Balance?

Dark grape juice is noted for its ability to fight heart disease, but too much of it may inhibit the uptake of iron, and this could increase the risk of iron-deficiency anemia.[38]

A recent study conducted at the U.S. Department of Agriculture and Cornell University examined the effect of various juices—red grape, white grape, prune, pear, orange, apple, and grapefruit—on the capacity of intestinal cells to absorb iron. The researchers suggested that the polyphenols (antioxidants) in red grape juice might have inhibited the uptake of iron by 67 percent, while prune juice produced a 31 percent reduction. Light-colored juices, on the other hand, increased iron uptake. Pear juice produced the highest uptake levels, followed by apple, orange, grapefruit, and white grape juices.[39]

The Chinese System of Food–Body Compatibility

Classical Chinese texts about imperial court systems record that as early as the fourth century B.C., the second-highest official in command of health and medical affairs was the royal dietitian, who supervised the processing and preparation of different foods, balancing the nature of those foods and the seasons with the nature of the emperor's body.

Chinese medicine maintains that it is possible to understand how the characteristics of foods affect our health. Managing food–body compatibility is promoted for both healing and preventive health. In fact, food treatment is considered superior to treatment with medicines, especially in people who have already been weakened.

Dietary therapies to prevent and treat deficiency diseases were first documented in about A.D. 200 in the book *Systematic Treasury of Medicine* by the renowned doctor Chang Chi. But it was Hu Ssu-Hui, the imperial dietitian from 1314 to 1330, who described the complementary relationship between food and our bodies in his book *The Principles of Correct Diet*.[40]

Principles of Complementary Natures. The Chinese sense of complementarity is based on the belief that:

→ Everything has its own specific nature, including different predispositions, and inherited strength or weakness. This is true of humans and of foods.
→ Diseases are mainly the manifestations of an individual's overall health condition, which may be imbalanced.
→ The purpose of treatment is recovery, but if a treatment harms the body's nature so much that the patient is killed, the purpose of treatment has been defeated. Since balance is the key, food therapy (usually a milder form of treatment) is preferred to drugs.
→ Elements can be either *antagonistic* (inhibiting, retarding, confronting, eliminating), *neutral* (harmoniously co-existing), or *promoting* (intensifying, stimulating, adding) to the others.

By strategically manipulating elements of the body's nature as well as food items and disease, that disease can be treated or health can be maintained. Our body nature can be considered our *basic nature*, while *transient nature* may result from eating too much food of a certain type.

Managing food–body compatibility is promoted for both healing and preventive health in Chinese medical philosophy.

So traditionally the expertise of an experienced Chinese doctor was required to clearly determine a person's basic nature and advise food–body compatibility.

According to Chinese thinking, certain foods should be eaten at specific times of the day, and seasonal adjustments to diet are also considered essential. For example, it's considered unhealthy to eat cold foods for breakfast or to eat a heavy dinner before bedtime. Foods that are *cold* and *light* in nature are recommended for summer, and *heavier, more nutritious* foods are suggested for the winter. In this context, *cold* and *hot* refer to the nature of the foods, not to their temperature or taste. For example, crab is considered *cold*, so its preparation requires ginger, which is *hot* in nature, for balance. It's also considered good to serve crab with warm sake, which is *hot* in nature.

Here's a much simplified system that classifies people by their body's basic nature.[41]

→ Active (yang)
→ Inactive (yin)
→ Nervous (fluctuating yin-yang)
→ Fatter
→ Thinner

> According to Chinese thinking, certain foods should be eaten at specific times of the day, and seasonal adjustments to diet are also considered essential.

According to this matrix, body type and activity levels come into play, producing the six combinations that follow. These groupings are not exact, and there are subgroups and mixed natures, but for all body types, the food we take in can counterbalance our body's weaknesses or the tendencies created by our nature.

→ *Active and fatter:* Efficient digestive and absorbing systems. Limit *hot* foods, eat *cold* foods, avoid stimulating (e.g., spicy) foods.
→ *Active and thinner:* Slow function of spleen and inactive circulation of life energy, so energy fluctuates. Very sweet and salty foods aggravate these tendencies, and cold foods, which also irritate the body nature, should be avoided. Active people usually prefer rich foods, so moderation is recommended.
→ *Inactive and fatter:* Weak metabolism, sensitive to chills and indigestion. Eat foods to accelerate blood circulation and promote urination, including most organ foods, vinegar, and small amounts of stimulating foods. Avoid fried foods.

→ *Inactive and thinner*: For this body nature, it's essential to avoid very cold foods. Vegetables should be well cooked with ginger or meat. Rich and stimulating foods are recommended.

→ *Nervous and active:* Insufficient blood and life energy. Avoid gaseous and stimulating foods. Shellfish, slightly cooked vegetables, and citrus fruits are recommended.

→ *Nervous and inactive:* Weak digestion and internal organs, fatigue. Follow the "nervous and active" diet, adding a small amount of salt. Avoid toasted and roasted foods.

Cold, Hot, Heavy, Light. Here are some examples of *cold, hot, warming, cooling, neutral, light* (nourishing), and *heavy* (most nourishing) foods.

→ *Cold foods:* bananas, soft drinks, soybean milk, most shell foods, green tea
→ *Cooling foods:* apples, tomatoes, tofu, duck, beer
→ *Hot foods:* beef, butter, curry, chocolate, lamb
→ *Warming foods:* eggs, potatoes, ham, cheese, chicken soup
→ *Neutral foods:* chicken, rice, bread, milk, carrots
→ *Light (nourishing) foods*: honey, garlic, milk, wine, beef
→ *Heavy (most nourishing) foods:* chicken soup with medicinal herbs, ginseng and ginseng tea, pork liver, pigeon, shark fin
→ *Stimulating foods:* mangoes, pineapples, shrimp, eggplant, crab

It's important to consult your Chinese doctor before consuming these foods when you're having health problems. According to Chinese medicine, anything that nourishes the body may also nourish a virus, for instance.

Water: Life's Most Essential Nutrient

Like life, water just seems to be there—in us and for us. But it's the most important of the more than 50 nutrients that we require daily, and it's essential for all forms of life. Though we can survive up to several weeks without food, we can live no more than three or four days without water.[42]

Water is also the medium in which almost all metabolic reactions take place. It carries nutrients throughout the body, maintains body temperature, allows foods to be digested and absorbed, and is essential to the synthesis of energy-rich compounds in cells. Water also plays an important role in the elimination of toxins and the waste products of metabolism. And depending on lean body mass, it makes up from half to four-fifths of our body weight. Water is constantly being lost even in sedentary individuals, but it is used more rapidly during exercise. When fluid loss amounts to 1 percent or more of body weight, we are said to be dehydrated. Dehydration is mild when the loss is 1 to 2 percent of body weight, but at 10 percent, it is life-threatening.

Thirst is a poor indicator of how much water is needed and when, because most of us do not feel thirsty until fluid loss is already at levels of 0.8 to 2 percent of total body weight. So when we feel thirsty, we are already mildly dehydrated. Thirst response is also reduced by exercise and immersion in water, and the elderly have a less sensitive thirst mechanism than younger people. So urine color and quantity are the best indicators of hydration: normal should be pale yellow or straw-colored and in good quantity. Color charts are available for athletes to monitor their hydration status.[43]

When our bodies are low on water, both physical and mental performance are impaired. The early signs of dehydration include flushed skin; loss of appetite; headache; fatigue; dizziness; lack of concentration; dry mouth and eyes; a burning sensation in the stomach (often mistaken as hunger); possible joint and back pain; and dark, strong-smelling urine. Severe dehydration can lead to difficulty in swallowing; muscle spasms; dim vision; clumsiness; shriveled skin; painful urination; and delirium.

Water Requirements

Most of us do not feel thirsty until we are already mildly dehydrated.

The U.S. National Research Council recommends that fluid intake be geared to a person's energy expenditure. For example, a 70-kilogram (154-pound) adult male with an energy expenditure of 2,750 calories per day, living in average environmental conditions, requires about 2.75 liters (6 pints) of fluid per day (i.e., 1 milliliter per calorie of energy). Females have a lower daily energy requirement and need an average of 2.2 liters (4.6 pints) of fluid per day.[44]

In adults, even without noticeable perspiration, the daily loss of water is approximately 4 percent of total body weight, while in infants the loss is about 15 percent. To maintain the right hydration level, this water loss must be replaced on a daily basis.[45]

Water is replaced in three ways:

→ solid food provides about 1 liter (2 pints) — mainly from fruits and vegetables

→ metabolism provides about 250 milliliters (half a pint)
→ the remaining amount comes from intake of fluids (water, milk, fruit juices)

A pregnant woman requires about 30 milliliters (1 fluid ounce) of additional water intake per day, while a woman breast-feeding her child would need an additional 750 milliliters (25 fl oz) to 1 liter (2 pints) to replace the approximately 750 milliliters (25 fl oz) of milk she produces daily.

The recommended fluid intake for infants is 1.5 milliliters per calorie per day, which is higher than the rate for adults because infants lose a higher percentage of water in relation to their body weight.[46]

What Influences Our Hydration Levels?

Caffeine and alcohol are diuretics—substances that increase the rate and volume of urine excretion. A study of 12 coffee drinkers showed that 6 cups of coffee a day (equal to a total of 642 milligrams of caffeine per day) resulted in an average decrease in body weight of 2.7 percent due to fluid loss. And there was an important side note to this study: only 2 of the subjects experienced thirst even at this level of dehydration.

In a hot environment, sweating helps our bodies maintain normal body temperature because the evaporation of the water in sweat has a cooling effect. People engaged in hard exercise in conditions of high temperature, low humidity, or high altitude have been reported to have lost as much as 4 to 6 liters (8.5 to 13 pints) of fluid per hour![47]

Dehydration: A Risky Business

Dehydration may be connected with kidney stones and cancer, and it has a considerable negative effect on athletic performance. People who produce less than 1 liter (2 pints) of urine per day are more likely to suffer from kidney stones. There is also some evidence that high total fluid intake is related to a reduced risk of lower urinary tract cancers and colon cancer in women.

For athletes, even mild dehydration amounting to a fluid loss of 2 percent of body weight has been found to have a measurable effect on performance. Individuals who were dehydrated (using a diuretic) by about 2 percent of body mass were monitored in a recent study as they

For athletes, even mild dehydration amounting to a fluid loss of 2 percent of body weight has been found to have a measurable effect on performance.

ran 5 kilometers (3 miles). They performed more slowly than when they were normally hydrated—slower by an average of 6.7 percent. This level of dehydration was also shown to reduce arithmetical ability, short-term memory, and visuomotor ability.[48]

Water: Can You Drink Too Much?

A person performing an activity involving heavy sweating should limit fluid intake to 1 to 1.5 liters (2 to 3 pints) per hour.

Drinking too much water can result in water intoxication.[49] Decreased sodium concentration in body fluids leads to irritability, lethargy, and confusion, and when the condition worsens, convulsions and coma, and even death.

Most cases of water intoxication occur when 5 or more liters (11 or more pints) of water are consumed in a couple of hours. Current sports medicine recommendations indicate that a person performing an activity involving heavy sweating should limit fluid intake to 1 to 1.5 liters (2 to 3 pints) per hour.

Water intoxication has also been reported in infants who were bottle-fed with diluted formula or water, as well as in newborn infants whose mothers drank excessive amounts of water.[50]

From Gobbling Up to Gourmet Wellness to the Tao of Nourishment

Can any bodily activity be a total experience? Is there such a thing as spiritual eating?

Can any bodily activity be a total experience? Can it even be a spiritual experience done in the way of the Tao? Eating, for example. Perhaps we can find clues to the answers by looking at some common eating styles.

Fast Food: Fuel for the Machine. Fast food provides plenty of calories to keep the engine running at a low price. It's truly fast—in and out, a meal finished in 20 minutes ... a quick fuel stop, then back to the race. No problem about deciding what to order either: the menu is the same in all the chain restaurants, as is the taste, the price, and the decor. No surprises about anything. On a steady diet of fast food, we can efficiently stave off the hunger pangs.

Dining Out: The Restaurant Experience. Consider dining out at a posh restaurant. The table is covered with a crisp white linen cloth; a candle and a white rose are set in the center. You rest comfortably in a leather chair, original works of art hang on the walls, and a pianist plays unobtrusively in the background. You order from a menu with a wide selection of dishes you've never heard of before. When your meal arrives, the food is arranged on the plate like a work of art. After selecting the longer of the two sterling-silver knives (is it the "right" one?), you puzzle over which of the three forks to use. Speaking in near-whispers, you and your dining companion agree that the taste is truly exotic, but you wish the portions were a bit larger. When you leave 2.5 hours later, you feel that you've satisfied a bodily need and had a unique experience as well. The bill convinces you that you enjoyed it!

The fast-food and the posh-restaurant scenarios have the same basic aim: to supply the body with food fuel. But they are totally different ways of meeting this requirement. Is one closer to gourmet wellness than the other? What about another style of eating?

Home Dining. At home, the menu is limited only by your taste and imagination. You make whatever you want to eat or what you think will delight. You select the best of what is available at the market and plan dishes to complement or accentuate their effect on the palate. The aromas and the sizzling and bubbling sounds coming from the kitchen are part of the whole experience. The atmosphere is relaxing: you wear your favorite sweater with the hole in the sleeve, take off your shoes, and perhaps have a soulful and intimate conversation and a good laugh with your dinner companion. You can take as long as you like. It all feels very comfortable and secure.

> Cooking and eating make up a total experience: the coming together of senses and sensations, thinking, realization and remembering.

Now what about spirituality and eating? In many cultures some words of thanks are made to a God or Nature or the Earth for the gift of food that sustains life—an acknowledgment of our dependency, our fragile existence. In the ordinary meaning of the words, this prayer gives eating a spiritual aspect. But for me, the word *spiritual* also refers to an attitude that looks beyond appearances to the deep-down beauty in things.

Cooking and eating make up a total experience: the coming together of senses and sensations, thinking, realization and remembering, feelings within, awareness without, passion, and being and becoming. Like everything else in life, cooking and eating go best when we add the right amounts and kinds of spices, understand preferences, use lots of imagination, consciously enjoy the process, and create the most value for our bodies and souls. This is the simple recipe for gourmet wellness and the Tao of nourishment. Bon appétit!

Flavors in Favor

Today's consumers have developed such high expectations of their culinary experiences that they are demanding more than good tastes and aromas, and the food flavor and fragrance (F&F) industry is eager to comply. This has been especially true in Western Europe, North America, and Japan, but China is now the fastest-growing F&F market.

The F&F manufacturers have become very fashion-conscious, especially in the beverage industry. According to the European marketing consultant firm Frost & Sullivan, the alcohol and soft drink market accounts for about 30 percent of the flavoring sold in Europe. There seems to be a growing trend toward clear, healthy-looking drinks—soft drinks, herbal waters, and teas—with a baffling range of smells, tastes, and exotic names to choose from. The European flavoring market netted about $721 million (US$465 million) in sales in 2001, and the global flavoring market is expected to grow to an estimated $9.9 billion (US$6.4 billion) in annual sales by 2004.

There is also a growing trend away from synthetic F&F compounds to natural F&F. But natural F&F production is unpredictable and cannot meet world demand. For example, the world supplies of natural vanilla—even without disasters—can satisfy no more than the demands of a country the size of Germany.[51]

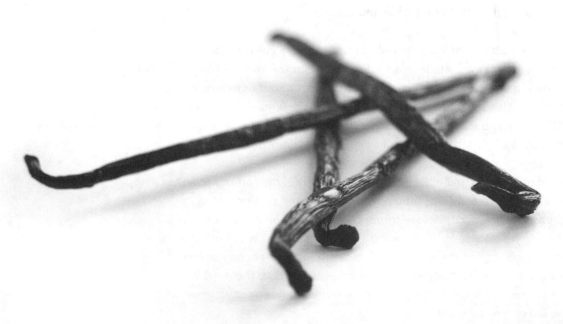

Natural vanilla

At Your Table:
Some Practical Pointers

Here are some practical everyday tips and recipes that you can use to help balance mood, counter the effects of aging, and boost your energy.

Food for Mood

A variety of journals have endorsed the idea that "you are what you eat" and recognize that it's important to "eat the right foods, in the right amounts, at the right times." Nutrition plays a key role in daily mood swings and affects the onset, severity, and duration of mood disorders such as depression.[42] Eating techniques that deal with poor appetite, low energy, and depression can be powerful coping tools for all of us, especially when mood problems exist.

B Vitamins. Although deficiencies in a variety of B vitamins can induce changes in behavior (see the table "Impact of Some Vitamin Deficiencies on Mood"), folic acid deficiency in particular has been associated with various psychiatric disorders, including depression, dementia, and schizophrenia. Low levels of folic acid have been noted in 31 to 35 percent of depressed patients and in 35 to 92.6 percent of elderly patients admitted to psychiatric wards. In fact, some investigators suggest that folate deficiency, with or without deficiencies in other nutritional factors, may predispose a person to, or aggravate, psychiatric disturbances, particularly depression.[52]

> Folic acid deficiency has been identified as a key element in various psychiatric disorders, including depression, dementia, and schizophrenia.

Folic acid promotes the synthesis of serotonin, and reduced serotonin levels have been associated with depression. Foods such as bananas, walnuts, and pineapples are good sources of folic acid.

Tryptophan. Nerve cells synthesize the feel-good brain chemical serotonin through a two-step process that begins with the essential amino acid tryptophan, which can be found in a number of common foods such as milk, turkey, chicken, fish, cooked dried beans and peas, brewer's yeast, peanut butter, nuts, and soybeans. Because tryptophan is such a large molecule, other more easily absorbed amino acids actively compete with it. To ease the absorption of tryptophan, you should eat these protein foods together with carbohydrates such as potatoes, pasta, and rice.[53]

Tyrosine. Tyrosine is an important amino acid that stimulates the production of norepinephrine, another essential neurotransmitter. This nutrient is especially important for people who are feeling excessive fatigue. Foods containing tyrosine include eggs, green beans, lean meat, peas, seafood, aged natural cheese, seaweed, skim milk, tofu, whole-wheat bread, and yogurt.

Simple, or refined, carbohydrates will induce surges in blood sugar. As the temporary boost in sugar levels declines, glucose levels drop, leading to dullness and fatigue.

Sugar, Alcohol, and Highly Sweetened Processed Foods. If brain serotonin levels are low, we're tempted to reach for a quick fix—such as table sugar, alcohol, or highly sweetened processed foods. But simple, or refined, carbohydrates will induce surges in blood sugar followed by more insulin as our bodies try to restore a sugar balance. As the temporary boost in sugar levels declines, glucose levels drop, leading to dullness and fatigue. Such imbalances may perpetuate the cycle of cravings and precipitate a state of depression. Normalization of serotonin levels is probably one of the most important ways to reduce binge-eating and drinking.[54]

Caffeine. Depression has also been associated with high caffeine intake. In a study of healthy college students, moderate and high-intake coffee drinkers scored higher on a depression scale than did low users. Other studies have shown that depressed patients tend to consume fairly large amounts of caffeine (more than 700 milligrams per day).[55]

Eating the Right Foods in the Right Amounts at the Right Times. Generally, foods containing protein will elevate tyrosine levels in the brain and boost dopamine and norepinephrine within minutes, increasing energy and alertness. Similarly, complex carbohydrates raise tryptophan and therefore serotonin levels in the brain, which will result in feelings of relaxation and pleasure.

To combat fatigue during the day, it's best to eat every three to four hours. Here's how it works. Without adequate amounts of the essential amino acid tyrosine, the body is unable to synthesize enough replacement dopamine. This dopamine depletion is thought to trigger fatigue, mood changes, and intense cravings for sugar and addictive substances. But regular small portions of protein-rich foods taken at frequent intervals can restore dopamine balance. Fatigue and depression will also set in if serotonin is not replaced for a long period of time. Increasing complex carbohydrates in conjunction with protein at the right time will restore brain chemistry balance.[56]

Trish Decker of the Centre for Addiction and Mental Health in Toronto has proposed a sample meal pattern that maximizes neurochemical responses in the brain.[57] The menu is based on the concept that we should start with an energizing power breakfast (high-protein) and have a protein-rich morning snack for energy, then eat more protein-rich foods at lunch for energy and a protein-rich afternoon snack for mental stamina. At dinnertime, a carbohydrate-rich meal will help you relax and promote sleep. And the day can be finished off with an after-dinner carbohydrate snack to further promote sleep and relaxation.

Impact of Some Vitamin Deficiencies on Mood[58]

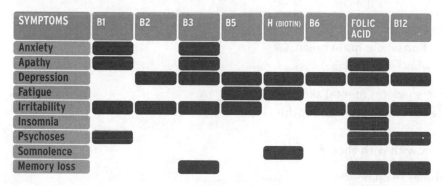

SYMPTOMS	B1	B2	B3	B5	H (BIOTIN)	B6	FOLIC ACID	B12
Anxiety	■		■					
Apathy			■				■	
Depression		■	■	■	■	■	■	■
Fatigue				■	■			
Irritability	■	■	■	■		■	■	■
Insomnia							■	
Psychoses	■						■	■
Somnolence					■			
Memory loss			■				■	■

Antioxidants for Anti-Aging?

About 1 to 3 percent of the oxygen we breathe in goes to generate free radicals. These electrically charged molecules steal electrons from other substances, causing damage in the process to critical cellular elements such as membrane lipids, nucleic acids, proteins and enzymes, and DNA.[59] They help kill bacteria and fungi, and make viruses inactive. But excessive free radicals lead to chronic inflammation, pain, cancer, blood vessel damage, nervous system impairment, increased likelihood of sickness, and death.

Normally, our bodies have adequate antioxidant mechanisms to safeguard against excess free radical damage. But when these mechanisms are weakened, the changes can lead to disease. Excessive free radical generation is also associated with an impaired immune system. And antioxidants such as beta-carotene and vitamins A, C, and E have been shown to increase natural killer-cell activity, improve immune response, reduce infection-related illness, and enhance recovery from infection.

Eat Your Way to a Better Mood and Stay Healthy Too: A Sample Menu[60]

1. Power breakfast for energy:
→ whole-grain cereal with low-fat milk
→ scrambled egg with whole-grain toast
→ fresh fruit and/or juice

2. Protein-rich morning snack for energy
   (small portions, three to four hours after breakfast):
→ 8–10 pieces of nuts
→ cheese plus 2–3 crackers
→ low-fat milk

3. Protein-rich lunch for energy:
→ tuna or lean roast beef on whole-grain bread, OR
→ skinless chicken on a whole-wheat bagel

4. Protein-rich afternoon snack for mental alertness
   (small portions, three to four hours after lunch):
→ non-fat yogurt, OR
→ half a whole-grain sandwich with cheese

5. Carbohydrate-rich dinner to relax:
→ pasta with tomato sauce, OR
→ a stir-fry with rice

6. Carbohydrate-rich night snack to promote sleep:
→ a low-fat muffin, OR
→ fresh fruit, OR
→ hot cereal with honey, OR
→ a bagel with honey

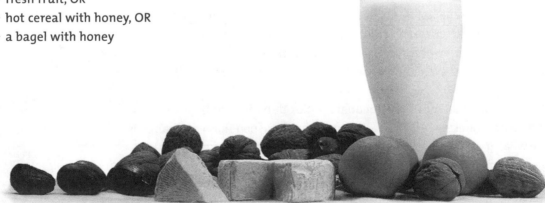

Some evidence also suggests that antioxidants can potentially delay the aging process and protect against the development of age-related diseases. Most antioxidants are vitamins that are naturally found in many fruits and vegetables. That's why it's recommended that we eat five to nine servings of fruits and vegetables each day.[61]

Herbs as Antioxidants

Researchers with the U.S. Department of Agriculture have found that herbs are an abundant source of antioxidants and could provide potential anti-cancer benefits when supplementing a balanced diet.[62] The herbs with the highest antioxidant activity belong to the oregano family. On a per-gram, fresh-weight basis, oregano ranks higher in antioxidant activity than fruits and vegetables, which are known to be high in antioxidants: oregano has 42 times more antioxidant activity than apples, 30 times more than potatoes, 12 times more than oranges, and 4 times more than blueberries.

Energy Nutrition

If you are physically active, you may need to consume a high-carbohydrate training diet that fuels better performance. This diet aims to give you 55 to 65 percent of your energy in the form of carbohydrates—eight or more servings a day from each of the grain products, vegetables, and fruit groups. (For the meaning of *serving*, refer to *Canada's Food Guide to Healthy Eating* or the U.S. recommended daily allowance.)

This training diet should also be low in fat, and it should include enough protein to build and maintain muscle tissue. But don't eat excessive amounts of protein. Though it's sometimes thought that more protein will stimulate greater muscle growth and development, extra protein is actually converted to fat or excreted in the urine. This will increase fluid requirements and risk for dehydration. Active individuals need about 15 percent of their energy intake from protein: two to four servings a day from the meat/alternatives group and two to six servings of dairy products.[63]

To obtain all the essential vitamins and minerals, it's important to include a wide variety of foods. Calcium and iron are especially important for the physically active. But water is the most essential nutrient for peak sports performance. It's vitally important to drink adequate amounts of fluids before, during, and after exercise.

> Most antioxidants are vitamins ... that are naturally found in many fruits and vegetables. That's why it's recommended that we eat five to nine servings of fruits and vegetables each day.

> See Chapter 4, "How Are You? Feeling Bad, Feeling Good," for more on mood.

If you are physically active, you may need to consume a high-carbohydrate training diet that fuels better performance.

Energy Drinks. Other than water, the principal ingredients in energy drinks are carbohydrates, for a quick energy boost, and caffeine, to stimulate the nervous system.[64] They may also contain a variety of other ingredients. Before using an energy drink, check the ingredients and check with your doctor, especially if you have a known health condition or are at risk of cross-medication side effects. Energy drinks are also not normally as effective if you exercise for a short period of time because the body has enough sugar stored in the muscles to last about two hours.

Here are a number of things to consider when you're choosing a sport drink:[65]

→ Be aware that exercise and certain stimulants (e.g., Ephedra, Kava) can be a deadly combination.

→ Mixing alcohol with an energy drink further complicates the potential health consequences.

→ Check health and performance claims and verify that all the ingredients are safe and legal. Consult your nutritionist or your doctor.

→ Look at the type of sugar used. Glucose, glucose polymers (also called maltodextrins), or sucrose are better, as fructose in large doses can slow absorption of the fluid and cause cramping and diarrhea.

→ Energy drinks usually contain a sugar concentration of 2.5 to 10 percent. A 6-percent solution may be the best. A concentration greater than 10 percent will slow down absorption of the fluid and can cause nausea and stomach cramping.

→ Always test energy drinks during your training. Race day or game day is not the time to experiment with a new sports drink.

Energy Bars. Energy bars can be classified into four basic groups:[66]

→ high carbohydrates (70 to 85 percent), to provide a steady release of energy
→ high protein (more than 26 percent), to prevent hunger and to help process sugar
→ balanced (40 percent carbohydrates, 30 percent protein, and 30 percent fats)
→ supplemented, with added vitamins or with vegetable proteins.

When choosing an energy bar:

→ Consider low-fat content (less than 5 grams of fat per bar).
→ Consider high fiber (3 to 5 grams of fiber per bar).
→ Check the caloric value on package.
→ Consume some real food with the energy bar.

Energy bars are good replacements for foods high in sugar such as doughnuts, but they are not complete meals. They should not be consumed as a total substitute for real foods.

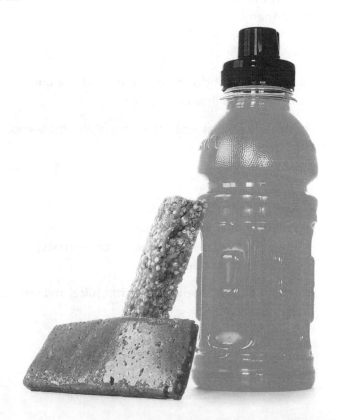

Water Recipes

We need to drink plenty of water every day, but may find this a chore. These gourmet water recipes are designed to help us enjoy drinking more water. Water is the main ingredient, to which we add rose petals, jasmine flowers, orange blossoms, ginger, cinnamon, a splash of juice or tea ... anything that gives the water some zip and contributes to wellness—in the spirit of the Tao of nourishment!

Gourmet Water Recipes

In praise of gourmet wellness and water, water recipes are created using pure, sophisticated water as the main ingredient.

1. Cinnamon Water
(serves 4)

→ 3 cups water
→ 3 cinnamon sticks
→ some peppermint leaves
→ ice cubes

Add cinnamon sticks to water and bring to a boil.
Simmer for 20 minutes.

Pour over ice cubes. Garnish with peppermint leaves.

2. Rose Water
(serves 4)

→ 3 glasses of sparkling water
→ 1 glass of pink grapefruit juice
→ 4 teaspoons of rosewater (edible concentrate)
→ a dozen tea-rose buds

Mix sparkling water, pink grapefruit juice, and rosewater concentrate, sprinkle with tea-rose buds, and serve.

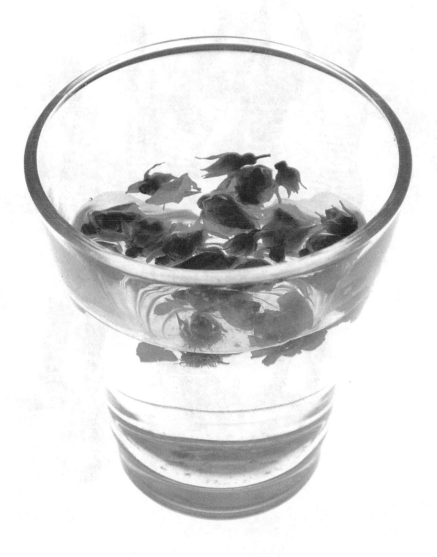

Rose water

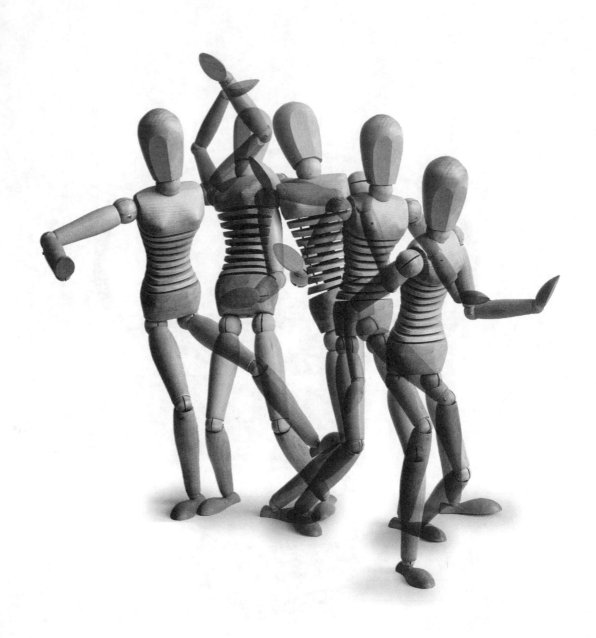

9 Our Bodies in Motion: *Forward to Wellness*

Humans would not have survived if they hadn't been able to withstand long stretches of heavy work. Physical activity is therefore evolutionarily linked to health, pleasure, and longevity.

It's amazing how many uses there are for the exercise equipment in the average household: something to sit on while talking on the phone, something to hang your plants (and pants) on, something to let the kids play on (this one is risky). Furniture designers are even starting to borrow the "look" and "feel" of exercise equipment to add a sense of familiarity and comfort to some of their more garish creations.

We obsessively buy fitness gadgets over the phone, on the Internet, or from TV infomercials. It could be called *telebycganphilia* (*tele* [afar; Gr] + *bycgan* [buy; OE] + *philia* [love of; Gr]). Why do we keep ordering all these fitness pieces, only to keep sitting on the couch or at the computer?

Evolution has hardwired us for physical activity.

Evolution has hardwired us for physical activity. For hundreds of years, humans would not have survived if they hadn't been able to withstand long stretches of heavy work: hunting, gathering, defending, or attacking. Physical activity is therefore evolutionarily linked to health, pleasure, and longevity. Bodies in movement are poetry in motion—graceful, full of vitality and energy. But how can we keep our bodies in motion? How can we move forward to wellness?

Most people are convinced that physical fitness is important for health and well-being. According to the *Physical Activity Monitor 2001*, issued by the Canadian Fitness and Lifestyle Research Institute, and data from the 1998/99 Canadian National Health Survey, Canadians believe regular physical activity improves one's ability to cope and reduce stress (88 percent); improves productivity (87 percent); helps speed up recovery from minor illness (85 percent); and improves job performance in areas such as concentration (83 percent). The main reason Canadians are active is to gain a sense of physical and mental well-being.[1]

Two in five Canadians indicated that tight work deadlines are preventing them from being more active.

Canadians want to be fitter. In fact, 78 percent of Canadians want to increase their physical activity participation level; they just somehow haven't followed up on their wish. And the stats reveal these sedentary ways: 57 percent of Canadian adults aged 18 and over are considered insufficiently active for optimal health benefits, and 25 percent of all adults are not active at all. The trend toward inactivity increases with age and is more common among women than men, and among those who are less educated and have a lower income.[2]

Physical Activity and Our Sense of Well-Being

Physical activity is now being recognized for its ability to improve our sense of well-being. The runner's high, a euphoric state associated with endurance activities, is based on the release of morphine-like chemicals into the brain. These neurochemicals, called endorphins, are thought to be the body's natural painkillers.[3] But as more research becomes available, it is becoming clear that the mental health benefits of exercise extend beyond the runner's high. According to Jack Raglin of Indiana University, an authority on exercise and depression, "We find mood improvements and psychological benefits occurring in exercise doses that are too mild to result in much endorphin production. This is good because not everyone has the motivation or skill to train for a triathlon. In fact we now know that as little as 30 minutes of brisk walking a day has very profound effects on health and sense of well-being and these effects can be felt, even immediately in some cases."[4]

The hypothesis is that physical activity affects our sense of well-being in many ways, probably raising the levels of all neurotransmitters and thus increasing our energy, motivation, drive, focus, pleasure, and self-control.

Support for this can be seen in a recent study conducted at Duke University Medical Center, Durham, North Carolina. The researchers assessed adult patients who were suffering from major depressive disorders. They found not only that exercise was as effective as medication, but also that the people who exercised were significantly less likely to relapse into depression than the group who only took medication.[5]

The Young and the ... Inactive?

Nearly half of young people in Canada aged 12 to 21 are not vigorously active on a regular basis, as physical activity declines dramatically with age during adolescence. Teenaged girls are also much less physically active than their male counterparts. In high school, enrolment in daily physical education classes dropped from 42 percent in 1991 to 25 percent in 1995. Only 19 percent of all high school students are physically active for 20 minutes or more in physical education classes every day during the school week.[6]

How Do We Get the Ball Rolling and Keep It Rolling?

What stops us from being more "physical" when we say that's what we want? The most important factors are these:

→ Two in five Canadians indicated that tight work deadlines are preventing them from being more active.
→ Two in five quoted lack of time.
→ One in four cited lack of pleasant places to walk, bicycle, or be active near work.
→ One in four reasoned that roads near work are too busy for safe walking or cycling.

Sound familiar?

"Exercise!" you might say. "When I think of doing something for myself, I don't think of hopping on the treadmill; I think of eating ice cream!"

Exercise may also take a back seat to the infinite number of other things we want to do for ourselves: read, listen to music, take a bath, meditate, express our creativity ... but exercise? "Exercise!" you might say. "When I think of doing something for myself, I don't think of hopping on the treadmill; I think of eating ice cream!"

But what if the only kinds of ice cream you'd ever tried were "dirt" and "fish-tank-water" flavored? Would you run to the ice cream container every time you wanted to treat yourself? The fact is that most of us have only tried exercise in those flavors known as "blood, sweat and tears" or "boring, repetitive movements." But many activities actually exist that meet most of our fitness needs, and we might actually grow to *like* some of them or even come to *love* a few. And they can easily become part and parcel of the many things we do every hour of our regular days.

Popular Activities: The Canadian Top 20

Activity	%	Activity	%
Walking for exercise	69%	Bowling	8%
Gardening, yard work	48%	Exercise classes, aerobics	7%
Home exercise	29%	Baseball, softball	7%
Swimming	24%	In-line skating	6%
Bicycling	24%	Skating	5%
Social dancing	22%	Basketball	4%
Golf	13%	Hockey	4%
Jogging, running	12%	Tennis	4%
Weight training	11%	Volleyball	3%
Fishing	11%	Alpine skiing	3%

Data from Canadian National Population Health Survey, 1998/99.

The Mindset: To Enjoy

Much of the time we see exercise as a goal-oriented activity. Even if we discover a routine we enjoy, it's easy to slip into thinking about the outcome instead of getting pleasure out of the activity as it's unfolding. An obvious example is walking, which is the most popular activity for Canadians (69 percent).

Some people walk to get from point A to point B. And it's a good choice to walk, as opposed to driving your car. But some people walk with a slightly different *quality*. It's not that they're strolling around with their heads in the clouds, but while they're going to their destinations, they take the opportunity to appreciate their own walking. They have a little "spring" in their steps—because every step brings them to a slightly different vantage point and new and interesting things to see.

Have you ever seen any of these people? If you look for them, you'll most likely find that they walk by you every day. These people *are just like you*. They have an unused exercise bike at home, they have a job that stresses them out, they have all kinds of obstacles in their lives. But what they've done differently from us grumpy walkers is this: they've made a wellness choice. Whether they know it or not, whether they've just had a good day or made a lifetime commitment, by enjoying and appreciating their walk, they are choosing to enjoy and appreciate *be*-ing well. Does it sound too easy?

The Rationale: Wellness Benefits

What are the health side effects of physical activities? The *Physical Activity Benchmarks Report* completed in Canada in 1997 showed that the health of two-thirds of Canadians is seriously at risk because of inactive lifestyles.[7] The report also indicated that a quarter of all deaths from heart disease in 1993 in Canada were a direct result of physical inactivity and could have been avoided. Another report on physical activity and health by the U.S. surgeon general indicated that by increasing regular physical activity, people could decrease their risk of heart disease *to the same extent that they would if they quit smoking*. This landmark 1996 report synthesized decades of research on physical fitness and health and concluded that regular physical activity reduces the risk of some of the leading causes of illness and death in North America.

According to Normand Gionet, chair of the Canadian Fitness and Lifestyle Research Institute, "gradual functional decline does not have

> By increasing regular physical activity, people could decrease their risk of heart disease **to the same extent that they would if they quit smoking.**

"Even 10 minutes of physical activity three times a day improves mental outlook by easing tension, depression, and/or anger."
—American Psychological Association

to be part of the aging process ... as much as half of the decline between the ages of 30 and 70 can be attributed not to aging itself, but rather to a sedentary lifestyle."[8] And a study released in 2002 by the American Psychological Association indicated that even 10 minutes of physical activity three times a day improves mental outlook by easing tension, depression, and/or anger.[9]

Regular physical activity has been shown to improve your health in the following ways:

→ reduces the risk of premature mortality
→ reduces the risk of heart disease
→ reduces the risk of developing diabetes
→ reduces the risk of developing high blood pressure
→ helps reduce blood pressure in people who already have high blood pressure
→ reduces the risk of developing colon cancer
→ reduces feelings of depression and anxiety
→ helps control weight
→ helps build and maintain healthy bones, muscles, and joints
→ helps older adults become stronger and better able to move about without falling
→ promotes psychological well-being and mental health
→ helps burn calories and preserve lean muscle mass
→ helps improve glucose metabolism and can prevent late-onset diabetes
→ helps improve self-esteem
→ can increase energy and improve relaxation

Exercise has also been shown to improve sleep patterns and sleep quality. Thirty to 45 minutes of moderate-intensity exercise should be performed three to six times a week before early evening. It should preferably be aerobic, at 50 to 70 percent of maximum heart rate, and appropriate for one's age. Exercise too late in the day can be overstimulating or alter glucose patterns.[10]

The Canadian Physical Activity Guide [11]

The increasing amount of research over the past 20 years on the beneficial effects of exercise spurred the Active Living Unit of Health Canada to develop Canada's first physical activity guide. It follows in the footsteps of *Canada's Food Guide to Healthy Eating*, and can be found on the Internet at **www.hc-sc.gc.ca/hppb/paguide**.

Moving Away from Disease

Physical activity is important in disease prevention, but it is also a powerful ally when it comes to curing and managing diseases. Its effects are striking in cardiac rehabilitation, and Sandra O'Brien Cousins and her research team at the University of Alberta report that physical activity also plays an important role in dealing with cancer, diabetes, arthritis, osteoporosis, hormonal problems, and lung disease.[12]

Cancer. Sedentary people tend to have a higher risk of colon cancer and breast cancer than active people. And for cancer patients, physical activity leads to a reduction in symptoms such as nausea, vomiting, tiredness, and fatigue. It also results in pain reduction through muscle strengthening and helps cancer patients deal with depression and anxiety symptoms. Researchers have also demonstrated that moderate aerobic exercise improved immune system function in a cancer group by improving the function and activity of natural killer cells.[13]

Diabetes. The type of diabetes that starts in adulthood can be controlled totally or in part with a regular exercise and nutrition program.[14]

Arthritis. Do you suffer from arthritis and think that physical activity may only make things worse? Recent research on osteoarthritis suggests that *not exercising* aggravates joint pain and stiffness by allowing muscles to grow weaker and joints to become more painful.[15]

Osteoporosis. Current evidence suggests that exercise retards the rate of bone loss. Without exercise, bones tend to weaken with age and can reach a critical level in older adults, leaving individuals susceptible to fracture.[16]

Hormonal Problems. There are more and more indications to suggest that regular exercise helps slow down the loss of hormone functions. Growth hormone, a builder of lean tissue, decreases with age but is released during exercise in young and old alike. Higher levels of cortisol, insulin, and norepinephrine (a waistline-destroying hormone) also increase with age, but can be kept in check to a great extent through physical activity.[17]

Lung Disease. Exercise cannot restore damaged lung tissue but it can greatly improve lung endurance. For people suffering from chronic

Sports and Osteoarthritis

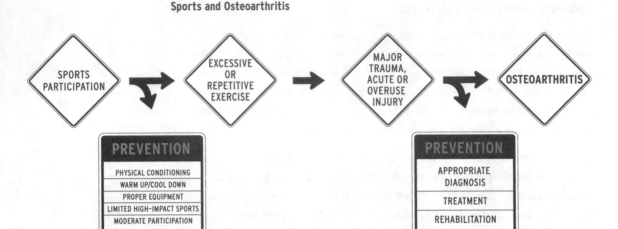

obstructive pulmonary disease (which is strongly linked to smoking), the best exercise is to walk for short periods with adequate rest intervals and to do supervised breathing exercises, as well as resistance training, to strengthen other weakened muscles.[18]

The Motivation to Continue

Luc Pelletier and his colleagues at the University of Ottawa have done research suggesting that we are most motivated when we do things for fun, enjoyment, or stimulation; a feeling of accomplishment; the pleasure of learning; or a well-identified benefit such as sleeping better and feeling calmer.[19] So to keep up an activity, you must enjoy it! For a feeling of accomplishment, pursue an activity you know you can do. When you succeed, you will feel competent and your motivation will increase. If you enjoy learning, try a new activity or build new skills. Make whatever benefits you seek—companionship, a feeling of well-being, heart health—part of your physical activities.

It's also important to do things that are convenient. Many activities are accessible right from your front door—walking, running, jogging, in-line skating, cycling...Take every opportunity to be active: walk for short errands, jog or run during your lunch hour.

For a feeling of accomplishment, pursue an activity you know you can do.

Research has identified two different types of motivation. *Intrinsic motivation* occurs when performing a physical activity is its own reward. *Extrinsic motivation* is motivation too, but it is short-lived. Factors outside of you provide reasons for being physically active (rewards, money, and prizes, for example). These may get you started, but lasting motivations need to come from within.[20]

How do you create motivation from within? First, see if you can identify things that make you feel as though you are not in control or that you tend to rebel against. For example, if you start lots of physical activity based on external rewards, you might eventually find them stifling because they are controlling you. You may also find yourself controlled by others. A teammate may become upset at your performance and make you feel nervous or, worse still, incompetent. The pressure could also come from you. You may focus too much on performing well, and when you fall short of your expectations, you could end up browbeating yourself and feeling miserable.

To counteract this, move from feeling pressured to observing what's going on. Here are some dos and don'ts to help you achieve this:[21]

→ **Do** focus on enjoying the experience—the movement, the surroundings, the company, or the landscape.
→ **Do** monitor your physical responses in a relaxed manner. Study the strategies for a game; practice the skills.
→ **Don't** push yourself too hard. You may rob yourself of the feeling of enjoyment you need to be regularly active.
→ **Don't** let others push you too hard. If you don't feel comfortable with one leader, find another who can provide the positive feedback and encouragement you need.
→ **Don't** "should" yourself! Instead of saying "I should exercise," say *"It would be better for me if* I went for a walk today because I could take in some fresh air." Or *"It would be fun if* I went for a walk because I could enjoy the scenery."
→ **Do** engage in physical activity to reward yourself. It will improve your mood, reduce your anxiety, and help you relax.

Don't push yourself too hard. You may rob yourself of the feeling of enjoyment you need to be regularly active.

Thinking about Moving?

Who ever said contemplation was for wise men in the mountains only? Many of us contemplate, and for a long time, whether to exercise or not. Are you a contemplator? Try finishing these two sentences:

→ I ought to exercise because ...
→ I don't exercise because ...

If you are a true contemplator, your list of cons will outweigh your list of pros. Part of you dishes out orders and says "Exercise!" but another part rebels and says "No way!" Guess which part usually wins at that game?

The good news is that permanent changes in lifestyle usually begin with contemplation and mental preparation. Then action kicks in, followed by maintaining an "action habit" (the "maintenance" stage).

Which stage lasts the longest time? Contemplation. Ambivalence can keep us stuck in that stage for years. To move on, we must ensure that the advantages outweigh the disadvantages. Here are ways to make this happen:

→ Write down the pros and cons of being active. If you list only 5 or 10, keep looking. There are more than 50!
→ Think of ways to enjoy activities with someone else—a fun walk or an activity night. Whatever strikes your pleasure chord.
→ Imagine a flow of fresh air and energy circulating inside your body. Think of loosening those stiff joints and filling your lungs with life-giving air.
→ Think of 3 ways you could reward yourself for increasing your activity level.

When the pros become more powerful than the cons, you'll move from contemplation to preparation. But beware! Contemplators don't need immediate action; they need more insight. If you are a contemplator, take the time in the next month to find out more about the benefits of an active, healthy lifestyle. Make the most of your contemplation experience!

> Imagine a flow of fresh air and energy circulating inside your body. Think of loosening those stiff joints and filling your lungs with life-giving air.

Light Exercise Boosts Immunity

There is now evidence that exercise intensity may be a key factor in determining whether exercise boosts the immune system. New research from Denmark suggests that light to moderate exercise enhances immune responses, therefore reducing susceptibility to infections such as the common cold or flu. Intense exercise, on the other hand (such as marathon running or a period of very heavy training), seems to suppress immunity, thus increasing the risk of upper respiratory tract infections. This is especially true of competitive exercise, which creates stress.[22]

Safe Motions

Once you know you are *mentally* ready to adopt an active lifestyle, you may need some reassurance that you are *physically* ready for it as well. Becoming more active is *very safe* for most people. However, according to the Canadian Fitness and Lifestyle Research Institute, more than half of the Canadian population believe that participation in physical activity leads to injuries. In addition, 42 percent believe that participation leads to ongoing pain and stiffness in joints, and 27 percent have said that physical activity makes people too muscular.[23]

The PAR-Q questionnaire developed by the Canadian Society for Exercise Physiology can help you assess whether you are ready for physical activity. Besides answering these questions, you should check with your doctor before you start an exercise program.

Test Your Physical Activity Readiness (PAR-Q)[24]

→ Has your doctor ever said that you have a heart condition and that you should only do physical activity recommended by a doctor?

→ Do you feel pain in your chest when you do physical activity?

→ In the past month, have you had chest pain when you were not doing physical activity?

→ Do you lose your balance because of dizziness or do you ever lose consciousness?

→ Do you have a bone or joint problem that could be made worse by a change in your physical activity?

→ Is your doctor currently prescribing drugs for your blood pressure or a heart condition?

→ Do you know of any other reason why you should not do physical activity?

If you answered YES to one or more questions, consult your doctor before you start becoming a lot more physically active.

If you answered NO to all questions, you can be reasonably sure that you can start becoming more physically active right now. But start slowly and progress gradually. And if you have any doubts, consult your doctor.

Source: **Physical Activity Readiness Questionnaire** (PAR-Q) © 2002. Reprinted with permission from the Canadian Society for Exercise Physiology. http://www.csep.ca/forms.asp

Here are a few more things to keep in mind before you launch into more activities:[25]

→ Wear the proper shoes and clothing to increase your comfort and reduce the chance of strains or injuries.
→ Use proper equipment, wear protective gear, and follow safe procedures, especially if you take up higher-risk activities. For example, if you opt for cycling, wear a bicycle helmet and obey the rules of the road.
→ Do warm-ups and cool-downs to prevent muscular damage. If you participate in team sports, make sure you've built up enough strength to handle sudden, pivotal movements. Learn and use the proper techniques for each sport you participate in.
→ Begin to exercise gradually; don't start vigorous activities cold. Increase activity time, frequency, and intensity slowly.

A Little Bit of Movement Goes a Long Way

For health benefits, moderate activity will do the trick: 30 minutes of walking, swimming, or gardening most days of the week, for example.

Randy Adams, manager of partnerships with the Fitness/Active Living Unit of Health Canada, says that many people have been in the "'no pain–no gain' mindset: if it wasn't hurting, it wasn't good." Now guidelines clearly indicate that for health benefits, moderate activity will do the trick: 30 minutes of walking, swimming, or gardening most days of the week, for example.[26] Activities like this can be done in longer bouts or broken up into short stints throughout the day. Lower blood pressure is just one of the benefits of even a little exercise. Cardiovascular fitness begins to improve with just 20 to 30 minutes of any activity three times a week, as long as it involves increased oxygen consumption. That averages out to less than 10 minutes of your time each day!

Moving around the House

Here are a few suggestions of enjoyable activities you can do around the house. Feel free to explore and make up your own. If you're already an active person, look for ways to get more enjoyment out of your exercise.

→ Create a new morning routine. Wake up to some relaxed stretching or walk around your backyard in your pajamas. Feel the grass under your feet and see the smile on your neighbor's face. If you're not already starting your day with exercise, begin by adding just 10 minutes of movement.

→ Trade in your power lawnmower for an old-fashioned manual one. This will provide an added fitness benefit to your gardening chores.

→ Start taking a "daily check-in" walk with your spouse or children when you all get home from work or school. This is a great way to catch up on what's happening in each other's lives while getting some exercise.

→ Try to make sure that you do not sit in one place for long periods. Just stand up and stretch or move around at least once every half hour.

→ If you have kids, go and play with their toys. Chances are, you bought them. Children use up a lot of energy playing. Just a little bit of that for adults can be tremendously rewarding.

Working Out at Work

About 15 million Canadians spend more than half their waking hours at work. Given the fact that physical activity improves health, increases productivity, and reduces stress, it makes good sense for employees and employers to find ways to increase activity during the workday.[27] From an organizational perspective, many useful ideas and an abundance of background research can be obtained from this Health Canada Web site: www.activelivingatwork.com.

About 15 million Canadians spend more than half their waking hours at work, so it makes good sense to find ways to increase physical activity during the workday.

Playing Your Moves

The child we once were still lives inside all of us, and if you let him or her out to play more often, the health benefits will follow.

Try some of these:

Fun Activities. Walking around: sightseeing, taking photos, walking to the corner store, checking out garage sales, heading over to the neighbors', canvassing for a charity, walking through a museum, going to theme parks and standing in line ... Picking seashells on the beach, flying a kite, playing catch, playing Frisbee, having sex ... The list is endless.

Fun Sports. Rollerblading, roller skating, rock climbing, hiking, archery, fencing ...

Team Sports. Football, soccer, basketball, hockey ...

For simple yet effective work exercises, see the "Activities" section at the end of this chapter.

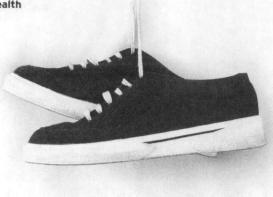

Variations on a Moving Theme

Fitness is generally divided into three activity groups: endurance activities, flexibility activities, and strength activities.

1. *Endurance Activities.* These activities help your heart, lungs, and circulatory system stay healthy and give you more energy. Examples include walking, golfing (without a ride-on cart), yard and garden work, propelling a wheelchair ("wheeling"), cycling, skating, continuous swimming, tennis, dancing.

2. *Flexibility Activities.* These activities help you move easily, keeping your muscles relaxed and your joints mobile. Regular flexibility activities can help you live better and longer, also improving your quality of life and independence as you get older. This category includes gentle reaching, bending, and stretching of all your muscle groups. Some examples: gardening, mopping the floor, yard work, vacuuming, stretching exercises, tai chi, golf, bowling, yoga, curling, dance.

3. *Strength Activities.* These activities improve your posture, help your muscles and bones stay strong, and help prevent diseases such as osteoporosis. They make you work your muscles against some kind of resistance, as when you push or pull hard to open a heavy door. Possible strength activities include heavy yard work (such as cutting and piling wood), raking and carrying leaves, lifting and carrying groceries (not to mention infants and toddlers!), climbing stairs, exercises such as abdominal curls and push-ups, weight/strength-training routines, wearing a backpack to carry books.

To ensure good overall strength, try to do a combination of activities that exercise the muscles in your arms, midsection, and legs. Strive for a good balance—upper body and lower body, right and left sides, and opposing muscle groups (e.g., both the front and back of the upper arm).

Total Fitness Programs

A single fitness activity may not always provide you with all health and fitness benefits.[28] Activities such as jogging, cycling, and skating promote cardiorespiratory fitness but don't really improve muscle strength, posture, or body alignment. Weightlifting is great for building muscle mass, but does little to improve your flexibility and range of motion. Some forms of mind–body exercise, such as yoga or Pilates-based exercise, offer increased flexibility, isometric strength, and mental focus but do little to improve your aerobic capacity or to burn body fat.

A more balanced program that includes a wider variety of activities is known as "cross-training." Different types of exercise can be performed in the same workout or alternatively on successive days. For instance, a cyclist could also do stretching exercises every day of the week, strength training twice a week, and intense running sprints one day of the week.

Cross-training can:

→ reduce the risk of injuries by preventing repetitive stress on specific joints
→ help prevent boredom by adding variety to workouts, thus keeping you motivated
→ develop the entire body, rather than specific areas.

A cross-training exercise program should include:

→ *Cardiorespiratory (aerobic) exercise*—walking, jogging, running, cycling, swimming, aerobics, aqua aerobics, cross-country skiing, rowing, skating.
→ *Anaerobic conditioning*—the same activities as above, but done at much higher intensities for shorter amounts of time. These short bursts of intense muscle activity are known as "sprinting."
→ *Muscle strength*—strength training (weightlifting), calisthenics (push-ups, sit-ups, pull-ups), isometric exercise (contracting the muscles against a fixed object that provides resistance, such as pushing against a wall).
→ *Muscle endurance*—the same activities as above, but using lighter weights or less resistance, together with more repetitions.
→ *Flexibility*—passive and active stretching, such as yoga, tai chi, or other flexibility training techniques.

Note that cross-training is often not recommended for serious athletes. In order to achieve the highest possible level in a sport, their training requires specific focus.

Meditative Movement Options

Yoga, qi gong, and tai chi share the common goal of awakening the life force and spirituality of the participant.

Eastern fitness perspectives have gained a lot of attention due to the great popularity of the meditative movement of yoga, qi gong, and tai chi. The fundamental principles and physiological effects of these activities are vastly different from those of other approaches to exercise. Meditative movement exercises, for instance, emphasize extremely slow movements and breathing techniques. Where traditional sports and exercise focus on competition, strength, and youthfulness, for instance, the meditative disciplines aim for self-sufficiency and longevity. Traditional exercise may also tend to be more social and team-oriented; meditative movement nurtures the self or emphasizes one-on-one training.

To learn some yoga positions, qi gong techniques, and tai chi movements, see the "Activities" section at the end of this chapter.

Although very different in some respects, yoga, qi gong, and tai chi share the common goal of awakening the life force and spirituality of the participant through physical activity that involves development of the mind, body, and soul in unison.

Meditative Movements and Options

FEATURES	SPORTS AND EXERCISE	MEDITATIVE DISCIPLINES
Motion	Fast	Slow
Stillness	Not desirable	A prevalent goal
Musculoskeletal system	Tense	Relaxed
Cardiovascular system	Speeds up	Slow and dilated
Breathing	Abrupt	Gradual
Metabolism	Increased	Reduced
Awareness	External	Internal
Skills taught and learned	Public	Esoteric
Motivation	Competition, youthfulness	Self-sufficiency, longevity
Group dynamics	Team, social	Private, one-on-one

Yoga, qi gong, and tai chi are done in many different styles and forms. At the introductory levels there are some commonalities, but as we progress to intermediate and advanced levels, the differences in technique become more apparent. Many individual schools emphasize these differences in order to promote their particular style or discipline, but spiritual enlightenment and physical fitness are the ultimate goals for all.

Relaxation Exercise and Emotional Flow[29]

"Relaxation exercise" may sound like an oxymoron, but it's actually a method of releasing tension and gaining awareness of the body, our emotions, and even our spirituality, through systematic stretching and movement of our muscles. Lee Strasberg, the famous New York acting teacher who died in 1982, originally developed this type of exercise based on the theories of Russian director Konstantin Stanislavsky. The goal was to help actors eradicate tension in their bodies, to make sure their creative impulses were not impeded. Strasberg's techniques have been used by the likes of Marlon Brando, Al Pacino, Marilyn Monroe, Dustin Hoffman, Ellen Burstyn, Robert De Niro, and Shelley Winters, among thousands of others.

Tension accumulates by the day, week, and month throughout our lifetimes. Thanks to the 21st century's accelerated pace of daily living and social conditioning, we habitually hold back anger, sadness, and even joy, adding to our stress levels, increasing emotional constipation, and creating more and more muscular tightness and tension.

For simple relaxation exercises, see the "Activities" section at the end of this chapter.

Relaxation exercise is about finding tension in our bodies and releasing it through movement, breath, and vocalization. Although this process is quite different from meditative movement, the principles behind it are similar in many respects. In this context, the flow of life energy is expressed as the flow of emotion through the body. As with blocked or stagnant energy flow, blocked emotions can damage both our bodies and our psyches.

How Hard, How Often? In spite of the immediate and long-term benefits of regular exercise, too much exercise can lead to fatigue and risk of injury. And compulsive exercise can take over your life in an unhealthy way.[30]

There's a simple way to find out how much aerobic exercise you need. It's called the FIT formula, and it was developed by the American College of Sports Medicine (ACSM).[31]

F = Frequency: 3 to 5 times per week

I = Intensity: 60 to 90 percent of maximum heart rate (This range is also known as your target heart rate range)

T = Time: 20 to 60 minutes of continuous activity (excluding warm-up and cool-down periods) or a minimum of two 10-minute bouts in a day

Intensity plays an important role in the FIT formula, and it's the most difficult factor to judge. But you can determine the intensity of an activity by monitoring your heart rate and staying in your target heart rate range.

You can also use the Rating of Perceived Exertion, or RPE, scale developed by exercise researchers.[32] It asks you to rate on a scale of 1 to 10 your answer to the simple question "How do you feel?" Zero means you are not exerting yourself at all; 10 means you have reached your maximum possible exertion.

Use this scale to gauge how hard you're pushing yourself in your workout. Every five minutes or so ask yourself, "How do I feel?" Aim for an RPE of between 4 and 5.

The talk test is another simple way to gauge your intensity. While performing any aerobic activity, you should be abe to carry on a casual conversation without becoming breathless.

Now that you've learned how to monitor your intensity, which level is best?

A few years back, a popular theory held that aerobic exercise performed at the low end of the target heart rate zone for a longer time would burn more fat than a higher-intensity, shorter workout. For example, 75 minutes of exercise at 60 percent of your maximum heart rate would burn more fat than 40 minutes at 80 percent. Why would this be? At lower intensities, our bodies use fat as their primary fuel; at higher intensities, they use glycogen, the major carbohydrate stored in our cells. So if fat burning is your goal, it seems to make sense to exercise longer at lower levels. But that's only half the story: since fewer calories are burned at lower intensities, not as much total fat is burned.

Exercise for Yourself

Exercise can be woven easily into your life if you do it for yourself and not to meet the expectations of others. Many of the intense exercise routines we sign on for aren't actually necessary for maintaining health, and when we take on too much, our exercise programs are usually short-lived and no longer enjoyable. Instead of loading more guilt on your overburdened self ... have fun! Get involved in activities. Move and stretch. Feel your life and your living in your body. You are a work of art in progress, in motion. Nourish the person within, as well as the person without. Find a balance. Enjoy wellness today and for the rest of your days.

The key is to find individualized activities that are fun and relaxing. Then your mind, heart, soul, *and* body will enjoy them with you.

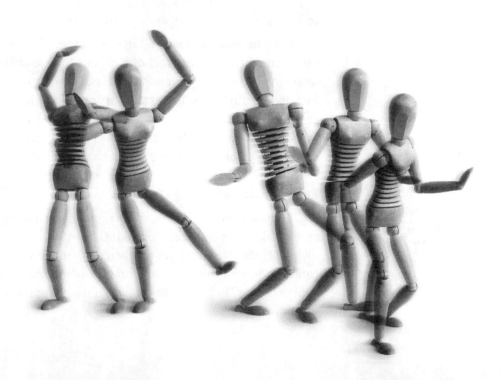

Activities

Moving Right at Home

Many simple yet effective exercises can be done at home or even at the office without special equipment. If you're not accustomed to doing movements like these, start slowly—and choose the ones that you enjoy!

Bottom Blast

Most of us probably take for granted the fact that we can stand up from and sit down in a chair. But this apparently simple activity requires coordinated efforts on the part of a whole group of muscles, including the hamstrings and the muscles of the back, thighs, and buttocks. As we age, we lose muscle mass. That, combined with a more sedentary lifestyle, can ultimately make everyday activities such as getting up out of a chair more difficult.

Regardless of your age or fitness level, take a few minutes every day, if possible, to perform the following exercises. They can keep you aware of your muscles and will invigorate you if you spend long hours sitting down.

Stand and Sit: Modified Squat. Sit in the middle of your chair with your torso straight. Place your feet directly beneath your knees, a little wider apart than the width of your shoulders. Put your hands on your thighs, just above your knees. Then stand up, pressing into your thighs as you come up. Sit back down, leading yourself down by pointing your tailbone back toward the chair. Repeat 10 to 15 times, and finish by standing up. Take a small break and then do another set.

Ergonomics and Worksercises

Ergonomics is the study of your work environment and how you adapt to it. It takes into consideration your comfort level at your workstation. Invariably, we twist or strain to reach the keyboard or sit in odd contortions, creating neck, back, or wrist pain. Posture awareness, chair consciousness, and some simple workstation modifications can help prevent problems.

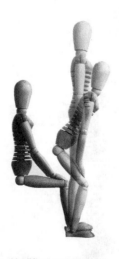

Modified squat

→ Lower the height of your chair so your back touches the back of the chair and you are comfortable.

→ Your feet should rest firmly on the floor, slightly in front of you.

→ Center your keyboard in front of your monitor. Your eyes should be at the same level as the toolbar.

→ Keep the keyboard and mouse close to the edge of the desk.

→ The keyboard and mouse should be positioned so your arms fall naturally at your sides, with your wrists straight out in front while typing/using the mouse.

→ Support your wrist and forearms with a gel pad or wrist support.

→ Avoid repetitive gripping of the mouse.

→ Keep frequently used items close. Avoid reaching for anything!

→ Do frequent wrist, finger, and hand exercises.

Sitting in a chair places 400 pounds per square inch of pressure on your lower back. If your back is unable to support your body, the strain will affect other areas of your body as well, including your hands, arms, and wrists. Here are a number of tips to help you reduce strain as you work:

→ Your desk posture: Be sure to sit with your back leaning against the back of your chair. If your chair is too deep, you may need to roll up a towel or buy a lumbar roll to maintain the natural curve of your spine. Be sure the back of your head is lifted, your breastbone is lifted, and your lower back is supported. Your back should be angled backward a few degrees to widen the angle between the torso and the thighs: this increases blood flow and reduces the compression of your spine. Your shins should be at a right angle to your thighs.

→ Your arms should be relaxed and loose at your sides, with your forearms and hands parallel to the floor. The correct wrist and hand position should create a 90-degree angle with the arm; your wrists should be in neutral position, not flexed or extended.

→ Be sure to change your position frequently, and avoid using excessive force while typing. Over time, a heavy typing style could aggravate hand, wrist, or finger pain symptoms by placing joints and tissues under continual stress. Consider the use of ergonomic devices such as back supports, mouse wristpads, and keyboard gel wristpads.

Worksercises for Your Back. It's important to exercise only in the pain-free range. You should consult your doctor about any exercise if you are in pain. As a general rule, stretch in the opposite direction to the position

Invariably, we twist or strain to reach the keyboard or sit in odd contortions creating neck, back, or wrist pain.

you habitually take while working. If you sit a lot at work (flexion), stretch in extension; if you stand a lot at work, stretch in flexion (bending).

1. *Side-Bending Sitting* (for people with standing jobs)
   Sit on a chair with your arms at your sides. Lean your upper body to the right, keeping your buttocks on the chair. You'll feel the stretch on your left side. Repeat, leaning your upper body to the left. Alternate sides. Hold 10 seconds. Repeat 5 times.
2. *Trunk-Rotation Sitting* (for people with standing jobs)
   Sit down on a chair and cross your arms at shoulder height. Turn your head, shoulders, and upper trunk to the right side. Hold 5 seconds. Repeat to the left. Do this pair of exercises 3 times.
3. *Standing Back Extension* (for people with sitting jobs)
   Stand face to a wall, with your feet a few inches from the wall. Exhale and lean into the wall until your abdomen touches the wall. Hold 30 seconds. Rest 5 seconds. Repeat 5 times.
4. *Standing Side Bending* (for people with sitting jobs)
   Standing with your back against a wall, exhale and tighten your abdominals. With your right arm overhead against the wall, put your left hand on your waist. Hold 5 seconds. Repeat on the opposite side. Alternate this pair of exercises 3 times.
5. *Hip Flexor Stretch* (for people with standing or sitting jobs)
   This exercise stretches the muscles on the front of

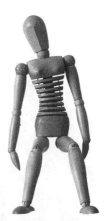
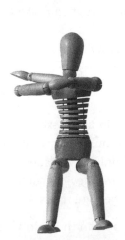
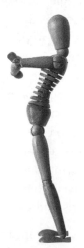
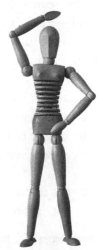

1. Side-Bending Sitting

2. Trunk-Rotation Sitting

3. Standing Back Extension

4. Standing Side Bending

your thighs that are used in lifting. Stand facing a wall and support yourself by placing your right hand on the wall. Bring your left knee back, grasping the ankle with your left hand. Pull until you feel a stretch on the top of your thigh. Hold for 20 to 30 seconds. Repeat on the other side (with your left hand on the wall).

6. *Hamstring Stretch* (for people with standing or sitting jobs)
This exercise increases flexibility in the muscles at the back of your thighs. A low chair, support, or step is needed for this stretch. Place one heel on the chair or step. Then bend your supporting knee slightly, keeping your back straight. Lean forward from your hips, with your hands folded behind your back. Hold 20 to 30 seconds. Repeat on the other side.

7. *Wall Slide* (for people with standing or sitting jobs)
This one strengthens the muscles on the front and sides of your thighs and buttocks. Stand with your back against a wall, shoulder-width apart. Relax your shoulders and exhale. Place your hands on your thighs and slowly slide down the wall. When you are at about a 45-degree angle, hold for 15 to 20 seconds. Then slowly slide back up the wall, keeping your back against the wall. Inhale and relax. Repeat twice.

8. *Backward Bending* (for people with standing or sitting jobs)
This exercise increases the flexibility of your spine. Stand with your feet shoulder-width apart. Place your hands on the small of your back and keep your head upright, not bending back. Then bend from the waist backward. Hold for 15 seconds. Repeat 2 to 3 times.

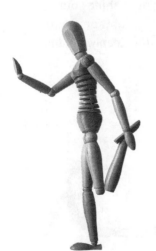
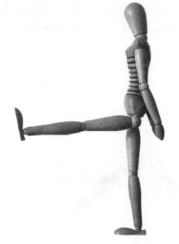
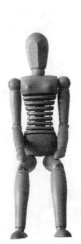
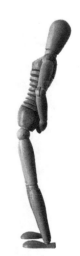

5. Hip flexor stretch

6. Hamstring stretch

7. Wall side

8. Backward bending

Yoga

Yoga means to yoke, to focus, and to unite; it addresses the development of both the body and the mind. Doing the postures becomes both a mental and physical exercise. It is not something to achieve or conquer, just a surrendering to the postures as you release stress. An important realization is how to interpret pain or discomfort; rather than tightening the body in response to pain, use breathing to help ease it. Understanding when pain is the "wrong" kind of pain is also important so as not to overstretch and cause damage.

Here are some yoga poses. It's best to perform them in bare feet on a surface such as a yoga sticky mat, to keep you from slipping.

1. *Child's Pose*
   Bend your knees and sit down on your feet with your big toes touching. Bend your torso forward over your knees, placing your forehead on the floor and trying to keep your sitting bones on your heels. Drop your arms along the outside of your legs, and if possible, grab the bottom of your heels. Breathe in and out smoothly. If you are uncomfortable on your knees, place a pillow under your bottom. Hold this pose for 5 to 30 breaths.

2. *Downward-Facing Dog*
   With your feet parallel and as far apart as the width of your hips, bend over and walk your hands forward so your body is in an inverted *V* position. Think of pushing your tailbone up and of pushing your chest through your arms. If your hamstrings feel too tight for you to straighten your legs, keep them slightly bent. Breathe deeply. Hold for 10 to 25 breaths.

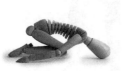
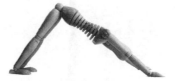
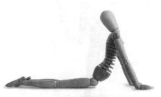

1. Childs's pose   2. Downward-facing dog   3. Upward-facing dog

3. *Upward-Facing Dog*

Lie face down on a mat and place your hands palms down just under your armpits. Engaging your abdominals to support your back, press into your hands, inhale, and lift your head and chest up. If you feel no discomfort in your lower back, continue to press up, straightening your arms. If possible, lift your hips and upper thighs off the floor, resting the weight of your legs on the arches of your feet. Hold for 3 to 5 breaths.

4. *Lunge*

Bend both legs and then step one leg back into a lunge. The knee of your front leg should be at a right angle, directly over the ankle joint. Your hands should be on either side of your front foot, either with the palms down or with the weight on your fingertips. Your extended leg reaches back while your chest and front knee pull forward. Repeat on the other side. Hold for 5 to 10 breaths per side.

5. *Triangle Pose*

Start in standing position, with your feet placed wide and parallel. Reach your arms out to your sides, with your palms facing forward. Turn one foot to the side and then lower the arm of the same side down and place your hand on the arch of your foot. Reach your other arm up. Think of pulling your chest away from the belly area, and the tailbone in the other direction. Repeat on the other side. Hold for 10 to 15 breaths per side.

6. *Tree Pose*

Stand with your feet together and your arms by your sides. Lift one foot and place it on your inner thigh, with your knee pointing out. If it is not possible to balance your foot there, place it on the calf muscle. Avoid putting your foot on the knee area. Lift your arms up over your head. Repeat other side, 10 to 15 breaths per side.

Yoga means to yoke, to focus, and to unite.

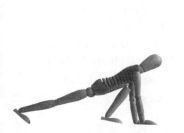

4. Lunge

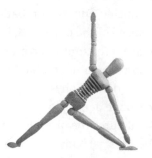

5. Triangle pose

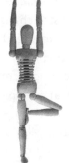

6. Tree pose

7. Relaxation

7. *Relaxation*

Lie on your back with your arms by your sides and your legs as far apart as the width of your hips. Close your eyes and notice whether you feel any tension or discomfort anywhere in your body. If so, try to let it go. Open your mouth as wide as you can and stretch your tongue toward the ceiling to release any tension in your mouth or jaw. Then simply relax, breathing normally and allowing your body to sink into the floor. Stay there for at least 5 minutes. When you are ready to come out of this, roll your body to the right or left, into a fetal position, and then slowly come to a standing position.

Tai Chi

Tai chi refers to ultimate extremes or infinite polarities.

Tai chi is a special kind of Chinese martial art that is unique in style, principle, method, and philosophy. It originated with Taoist Master Chang San-Feng, who came from the Wu Dong Mountains. Tai chi incorporates weapons training, including the sword, blade, and pole, but it is the slow-motion "fist" (*chuan* in Chinese) or bare-handed technique that gave tai chi its singular reputation. Today when we say "tai chi," we are referring to *tai chi chuan*—the slow-motion hand technique. When we refer to weapon techniques, we specify which kind, such as tai chi sword.

Tai means "the ultimate, the be-all," and *chi* means "extreme," or " the end-all," so *tai chi* refers to ultimate extremes or infinite polarities. The concept of polarity as the driving unit of energy is very scientific. Electricity requires positive and negative polarities, and magnetism requires north and south poles. Our whole universe is based on polarities; tai chi aims at mastering the polarities, to direct life energy or qi to flow vividly and smoothly.[33]

This unique physical exercise consists of slow, continuous movements, and stretching and balancing. During combat, tai chi aims at moving with, or ahead of, the speed of the opponent, but the real purpose of slow motion is to build up qi energy through continuous, fluid, circular, yin and yang forms. The big-circle form emphasizes stretching and breathing.

Many people have experienced physical benefits from tai chi, including improved muscle tone, bone density, organ function, healing, and even younger looks. Tai chi nurtures the qi, which improves mental balance, and in turn affects the physical body.

Tai chi movements take into detailed account the body's natural posture, its center of gravity, and its own comfortable limits of mobility.

It incorporates ergonomic, chiropractic, and physiotherapy principles, among others. A description of the tai chi stance, the most basic posture, illustrates this point.

We've all been told to stand up straight but we have not all been taught how. Tai chi uses analogies such as: "Stand like the scale in perfect balance" to impart the qualities of the desired stance—one that is vertical yet balances on the natural curvature of the spine. Tai chi uses words such as "Empty the neck" and "Hang from the peak of the head" to describe the state of alleviating the weight of the head on the neck. Students learn to assume correct standing posture for 5 to 15 minutes as part of their tai chi training.

The benefits of a correct standing posture are multifaceted:

→ minimization of the gravitational stresses that begin to affect our bodies from the moment we get out of bed
→ decreasing the demand on our muscles and tendons to counteract the force of gravity
→ relaxation of the muscles, which leads to improved circulation of all body fluids and qi energy
→ reducing the risk of constriction and inflammation of muscle fibers and tendons (fibromyalgia, fibrositis, tendonitis)
→ a healthier musculoskeletal system and improved flexibility
→ improved alignment of the spine, which helps to prevent pinched nerves, leading to healthier organs and organ functioning
→ facilitating proper expansion and compression of the rib cage and diaphragm, making for easier breathing; decreased stress on the cardiopulmonary system results not only in better exchange of oxygen and carbon dioxide, but also in a more relaxed mental state

Relaxation Exercise

Muscle Relaxation. When doing muscle relaxation exercises, it is important to remember that you are not just tensing muscles and then returning them to their original state. Resting between tensing is the key.

Muscles are made of fibers that need blood and oxygen. Blood is pumped around the body by the heart, and the rate at which it's pumped depends in part on how fast you're breathing. The amount of oxygen in your blood also depends on your breathing—whether it is slow or fast, deep or shallow. When you tense your muscles, they require more

Many people have experienced physical benefits from tai chi, including improved muscle tone, bone density, organ function, and healing, and even younger looks.

oxygen, which is carried to the muscles in the blood. The muscles send out signals that they require more oxygen, so the heart beats more quickly, in order to increase the blood flow rate. When you relax that muscle group, the demand for oxygen goes back to normal. Your heartbeat slows down, and so does your breathing.

Things go one stage further, however. After you have tensed and then relaxed a muscle group, the muscles relax even more. This opens the door for further relaxation of those particular muscles.

The following is a self-help technique, in two parts, that alleviates accumulated stress in the body and muscles. It involves progressively and gently contracting and relaxing (and resting in between) the major muscle groups that store tension.

Part 1. Lie on your back in a quiet, warm, and preferably dark room. Make sure that your body is comfortably supported. If necessary, use pillows or cushions for additional support. Position your arms so they're comfortable by your sides and ensure that your legs are not crossed and are also in a comfortable position.

Take a few long, slow, deep breaths, closing your eyes as you do so, and let your mind go blank. Breathe slowly and deeply at all times when performing this exercise.

Take your time. When you're ready, gently, very gently, tense every muscle in your body. Hold this for about 2 seconds and then release.

Relax for a moment and this time, gently, again very gently, stretch every part of your body. Then release and rest again for a few moments.

Part 2. Starting with your head and working your way down, think of all the body parts that can store tension, and as you think of each part, simply let go of the tension and allow the body part to relax.

Start with the top of your head, the scalp, and as you think of your scalp, simply relax your scalp and let go of the tension.

Repeat this for the following areas in turn: forehead, jaw muscles, shoulders, arms, hands, fingers, large and small muscles of the back, the chest muscles, hips, thighs, calves, ankles, feet, and toes.

If you find it difficult to relax any one area, try tensing and stretching that area as outlined above or try gently shifting your position to make yourself more comfortable and so on. It can sometimes be very difficult to relax our faces. If this is a problem, try smiling, yawning, pulling faces, and sticking your tongue out.

Once you have covered all the tension-storing body parts, stay in position for between 10 and 14 minutes, perhaps listening to your favorite piece of relaxing music. Avoid jumping straight back up again, as this will counteract the benefits of the relaxation.

Breathing Exercise. The mainstay of many breathing techniques is abdominal breathing. And the best way to learn this technique is to sit up straight on a chair with your hands resting on your lap and your feet placed firmly on the floor.

When you're ready, close your eyes and begin to concentrate on your breathing. Pay attention to the depth of your breath and its rhythm and pace. Next, pay attention to which muscles you use when you breathe. It might help to place one hand on your diaphragm (just under your ribs, at the top of your stomach). Place the other hand on the upper part of your chest. Keep breathing normally and become aware of which hand is moving in or out as you breathe.

You may discover that you are doing abdominal breathing already—that is, the majority of movement is under your bottom hand. If not, adjust your breathing slowly until only your bottom hand is moving. When this happens, it means that you are using your diaphragm to control your breathing. This may take some getting used to.

It's best to breathe through your nose while keeping your mouth closed. Avoid clenching your teeth, as this generates stress in your jaw area. When you first begin, you may be surprised at the time distortions that can occur. For instance, you might spend two minutes on an exercise but believe you have spent a quarter of an hour doing it, or vice versa.

Qi Gong Breathing. A simple method of turning this breathing exercise into a qi gong exercise is to press your hands together and position them in front of your heart about 8 centimeters (3 inches) from your body. Look down at the tips of your middle fingers while pressing the bottoms of your palms together. Breathe slowly and deeply, counting 1, 1, 1 in your mind as you exhale. Part your hands slightly, and feel the warmth/heat between your palms. This is your energy flow.

Raise your head to a comfortable position and continue with the breathing exercise and the counting. Now you'll be conscious of your breathing and your energy flow while limiting, or even emptying, your thoughts by just repeatedly counting 1.

"Be flexible in appearance, but maintain harmony within," says Chinese philosopher Chuang Tsu.

After you have tensed and then relaxed a muscle group, the muscles relax even more. This opens the door for further relaxation of those particular muscles.

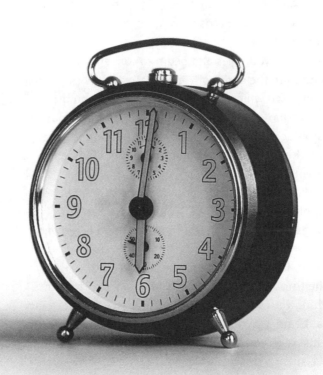

10 From Daily Hassles to Spiritual Fitness

It's the very first moment of the day.
The clock is screeching.
The bedroom and outside are still dark.

Seems like the snow has stopped.
I stumble to shut off the alarm ...
Am I glad to be starting a clear day
or unhappy because I missed the pleasure of waking up naturally?

My lips are cracking ... the humidifier must be out of water ...
I feel foggy ... shouldn't have stayed up so late.
Need a shower, a cup of hot tea, maybe a piece of toast to clear my head.
Ah, I've got to take the car in for a tune-up ...
What color shirt should I wear?

It's the very first moment of the day.
The past and the future, the external and internal worlds,
all dawning in the present ...

So many little things every day.

It's the cumulative
effect of small daily
hassles that takes a toll
on us.

The cumulative effect of small daily hassles takes a toll on us.

While most people accept the fact that major traumatic life events affect physical health, many find it surprising that our mental, emotional, and spiritual well-being depends less on major events than on our response to daily happenings and stress. It's the cumulative effect of small daily hassles that takes a toll on us.[1]

Initial research on the effects of stress on health began with Hans Selye at the Montreal Neurological Institute in the 1960s and 1970s.[2] His work indicated that catastrophic events and major life changes could induce psychological, mental, and emotional stress, weaken the immune system, and cause direct damage to major organs. Both positive and negative major changes in life situations cause stress. These events include marriage; relocation; an addition to the family; the death of a loved one; job promotion or change; separation from family members; and natural disasters. For example, on the day in 1994 when there was a major earthquake in Los Angeles, there was also a five-fold increase in sudden-death heart attacks.[3] After the Hanshin-Awaji earthquake in Japan, there were also increases in blood pressure and deaths from heart attacks over the next several months.[4]

The developing fields of behavioral medicine and psycho-neuro-immunology are now mapping the links between everyday events, emotional stress, mental health, and the immune system. And the implications for our well-being are enormous.

Studies have shown that people who endure the hectic pace of urban living and overcrowded neighborhoods have much higher rates of hypertension and other stress-related health problems.[5] Following the collapse of socialism in the former Soviet Union, for instance, life became less predictable, and goods and services became more difficult to obtain. The added daily hassles have led to an increase in stress-

They Add Up ...

Daily hassles that cause us grief and wear and tear include all sorts of small, irritating, annoying, or frustrating everyday situations. Examples include rush-hour traffic, misplacing items we use every day, waiting in line-ups, having mechanical breakdowns, searching for a parking spot, meeting deadlines, forgetting groceries, missing a bus, being put on hold for a long time on the phone, having a bad-hair day, or not being able to find the right thing to wear.

related illness and have taken an estimated five years off the life expectancy of Russian men.

Research linking heart problems to stress is impressive. One study, recently published in the *International Journal of Epidemiology,* involved eight years of testing.[6] It was carried out in the Whitehall district of London and involved a huge test group (73 percent of all civil servants working in 20 government departments). A variety of stress factors, such as marriage or other family problems, work-related issues, and monetary concerns, were considered. In this group, the men who were highly stressed were 83-percent more likely to have coronary heart disease. The situation was better for women, but they still had a frightening 51 percent increase in heart problem risk compared to the less-stressed group.

> In one study, men who were highly stressed were 83 percent more likely to have coronary heart disease.

To cope with stress, many people resort to the psychoactive drugs in alcohol and tobacco (the most popular self-prescribed psychoactive drugs for stress). But these drugs have harmful physical effects. Even medically prescribed drugs can lead to dependency and often have negative side effects.

There are other ways of handling the pressures. For one thing, we can learn to recognize stress symptoms and control response. Coping techniques include avoiding stressors and stressful situations; changing thinking, expectations, and attitudes; practicing relaxation techniques; taking time for yourself, perhaps even a vacation; getting a pet; and improving your general health and well-being. (More details on coping techniques appear later in this chapter.)

Some emotion-arousing aspects of our everyday living can be dealt with directly. For instance, research shows that reducing average daily commuting time to less than 30 minutes resulted in a 21 percent decrease in the number of lost workdays per year.

> Reducing average daily commuting time to less than 30 minutes resulted In a 21 percent decrease in the number of lost workdays per year.

Better management of simple daily activities can reduce a lot of stress: having hooks near the door for your keys or purse will cut down on the hassles associated with misplaced items; shopping early (or very late) cuts down the annoyance of long lines. Sound-deadening ear protectors will reduce noise and unnecessary interruptions. Scheduling your daily tasks realistically will decrease the panicky feeling that you have too much to cope with.

What Is Stress Anyway?

Noted Canadian stress researcher Hans Selye defines stress as the non-specific, automatic, generalized, and immediate response of the body to any demand made upon it.[7] The demand can be a real or imaginary threat, a challenge, or any change that requires the body to adapt. The stress reaction is the fight or flight response of the body associated with the production of adrenaline, cortisol, and other stress hormones. The purpose of this reaction is to generate large amounts of energy instantly in the face of potential danger, to prepare us for required actions. However, the dangers and stresses faced by primitive humans were of the high-threat and short-duration type—such as spotting a bear nearby. Stresses today tend to be of the lower-threat, longer-duration type—such as an unhappy marriage. However, our bodies have not evolved to the point where they can tell the difference, and we still respond as if there were only two options: fight or flight.

Both of these reactions require the full commitment of the cardiovascular system: our heartbeats speed up to increase blood flow and to transport oxygen to our muscles and organs, and our blood-clotting mechanisms work at full force to prepare for possible injury.[8] The increase in metabolic rate and blood pressure are produced by the activities of stress hormones. A sustained stress response is exhausting, and chronic stress can cause heart problems, especially if other risk factors exist—such as lack of exercise, hypertension, smoking, diabetes, obesity, or a genetic predisposition to heart problems.

Stress has physical, mental, emotional, and behavioral symptoms. It can generate either good stress responses, which foster growth, action, and solutions, or bad responses, which interfere with body functions and lead to physical, mental, and emotional distress. It may be generated by social situations; personal and work relationships; crowds; strangers; or unreliable, moody, or competitive people. It may be environmentally based, including noise, clutter, temperature, light, height, or natural disasters. It may also be organizational: rules, restrictions, red tape, formalities, deadlines, and office politics. Internal stressors include feelings of sadness, anxiety, anger, or resentment. Stress manifests itself in more than 125 symptoms and in different combinations. However, for most of us, it shows up with about 5 to 10 characteristic symptoms that we can learn to recognize in ourselves. Managing stress is about taking that first step of getting to know when we are feeling unhappy or unwell and then starting to do something about it. The impact of stress on your health depends more on the way you perceive it than on the type or amount you experience.[9]

Physical, Emotional, Mental, and Behavioral Symptoms of Stress

1. *Physical symptoms*
→ heart beats hard and fast
→ muscles tense, shoulders are raised, fists are clenched, breathing is faster

→ sweating starts, mouth goes dry, a knot is felt in the stomach

→ sudden onset of lightheadedness; feel shaky

When stress goes on for a long time (chronic stress), other symptoms show up:

→ headaches, lightheadedness, or dizziness

→ clenching of the jaw or grinding the teeth

→ tightness or soreness in the muscles of the neck or across the tops of the shoulders

→ low back pain, chest pains, or a feeling of pressure in the chest

→ palpitations, rapid breathing, or feeling as if you have to take a deep breath (described as "air hunger")

→ abdominal symptoms such as nausea or vomiting, heartburn or indigestion, abdominal cramps, constipation and/or diarrhea, and more frequent urination

→ cold hands and feet or sweating palms, soles, or other parts of the body

→ fatigue (one of the most common symptoms)

→ loss of appetite or increased appetite

→ sleep disturbance, trouble falling asleep due to anxiety, trouble staying asleep or early morning wakening (these are also symptoms of depression)

→ loss of interest in sex

2. *Changes in mental function*

→ difficulty concentrating on mental tasks

→ more forgetful

→ indecisive or slower to make decisions

→ feeling that the mind is racing or going blank

→ excessive negative thinking

→ losing a sense of humor

→ worrying or being preoccupied

3. *Emotional symptoms*

→ nervous, anxious, tense, jittery, racing inside, "on edge" or restless, irritable, impatient, short-tempered, frustrated, slowing down, flat, apathetic, depressed, sad

4. *Behavioral symptoms*

→ fidgeting, getting up and pacing back and forth, nail biting, compulsive eating, smoking, drinking, talking loudly or shouting, blaming, swearing, crying, or nervous habits such as fiddling with jewelry or twisting locks of hair

→ problems in relationships or being argumentative; decreased productivity; drug abuse or dependence; feeling insecure; low self-esteem

Positive emotions associated with daily events can also offset the negative effects of others. Technically referred to as uplifts, these are just everyday events, such as getting adequate rest, completing a task, eating out, resolving or avoiding conflicts, getting love and affection, petting a friendly cat or dog, or relaxing with a book, movie, or game. Each uplifting episode contributes to reducing harmful stress.[10]

Simple strategies can be used; for instance, you might want to set aside 15 or 20 minutes each day to improve something about your living conditions: rearrange your office, tidy up your closet so you can locate things, or make a list before you go shopping. Remember that every little thing either adds to, or subtracts from, your sense of well-being.

Emotional Disturbance

Emotional disturbances, whether generated internally or linked to interactions between the individual and the environment, can be just as detrimental to health as physical stresses.[11] And the evidence linking emotional disturbances to heart disease is accumulating. According to a study published in the *Journal of Cardiovascular Risk*, specific emotions such as anger, irritation, impatience, and hostility increasingly appear to have an impact on both the slow development of coronary artery disease and the incidence of sudden heart attacks.[12]

The initial studies on stress and heart disease were done mostly on men, but more recent studies show that women reporting high levels of mental stress are also more than twice as likely to die from stroke and heart disease over the following eight years, compared to their more laid-back peers. This is true even when they are not subjected to other risk factors.

> Anger increases muscle tension and stress hormones by a factor of eight, and this increases blood pressure. Anger also seems to make the blood stickier and more likely to clot.

The strongest association between emotions and illness is between anger and heart attacks. Researchers J.E. Williams and colleagues found that fatal heart attacks are two to three times more likely in those with the highest anger scores.[13] Specifically, heart-attack risk doubles during the two hours after an angry episode, suggesting something specific about anger that may trigger the heart attack cascade. Another study, published in the *European Journal of Applied Physiology,* suggested that the effects of anger may be manifested through many different mechanisms simultaneously.[14] Anger increases muscle tension and stress hormones by a factor of eight, and this increases blood pressure. Anger also seems to make the blood stickier and more likely to clot.[15]

Do anger-related risks lie in our response to stress or in having an angry personality? A recent study suggests that a strong, angry temperament (not anger in reaction to criticism, frustration, or unfair treatment) places middle-aged persons at increased risk for cardiac events and may confer a heart-disease risk similar to that of hypertension.[16]

Other studies have shown that the emotional environment that existed during childhood predisposes an individual to experience depression and anxiety as an adult. Similarly, lack of emotional connections during childhood increases the development of eating disorders and low self-esteem.[17]

Emotional Fatigue = Burnout

"Burnout" is another term for emotional fatigue. It refers to fatigue or exhaustion that causes a decline in the ability to experience joy or to feel and care for others. There is a flatness and lack of emotional response. Emotional fatigue develops over time—taking weeks, sometimes years, to surface. It is caused by a constant output of emotional energy over time without adequate input for balance.[18]

Sometimes people who witness a lot of trauma as part of their jobs—such as law-enforcement agents, paramedics, peacekeeping forces, and firefighters—suffer from long-term emotional fatigue. One version of this—compassion fatigue—occurs after a great deal of energy and compassion is expended on others over a period of time, without enough assurance that there is reason for hope in the world. It can also affect those who are actively engaged in taking care of a family member, especially during a crisis period when there is a greater need to give out feelings of compassion and sensitivity. If the crisis doesn't pass quickly and the individual continues functioning at this level, he or she is just as susceptible to compassion fatigue over time as those in high-risk professions.

The most critical need for the emotionally fatigued is to acknowledge the experience. To recover from burnout, we have to redirect ourselves away from the draining focus and back to ourselves. Simply getting plenty of rest and becoming more aware of dietary and recreational habits to improve physical health will help. Some people may opt to leave the emotional surroundings, and other people may take a while before they are comfortable enough to feel emotions again. Vacations may help. And it's important to know that it takes time to regain emotional balance.[19]

Mental Fatigue

Mental fatigue is the
perception and/or
reality that one is
increasingly unable to
maintain a predetermined
level of behavioral
efficiency when
continuously facing
demands to do so.

Mental fatigue is any state of fatigue that has no apparent physical reason such as overexertion or lack of sleep. It is the perception and/or reality that one is increasingly unable to maintain a predetermined level of behavioral efficiency when continuously facing demands to do so.[20]

Mental fatigue is the most dangerous type of fatigue, as it can result in serious errors of judgment. It is typically associated with tasks demanding intense concentration; rapid or complex processing of information; and other high-level cognitive tasks. The causes of mental fatigue may include prolonged mental activities—particularly those requiring sustained alertness—and boredom resulting from repetitive or monotonous activity, excessive working hours, and sleep deprivation.

Symptoms and Consequences of Mental Fatigue[21]

→ reduced attention span
→ increased difficulty in communicating
→ slowness in comprehending or responding
→ inability to concentrate
→ mental confusion and disorientation
→ obvious forgetfulness
→ significant changes in mood
→ increased irritability and apathy
→ carelessness and poor work output
→ decreased vigilance—especially during monotonous tasks or in tedious
  environments
→ difficulties in processing information
→ hallucinations or frequent daydreaming
→ irrational thoughts and delusions
→ faulty short-term memory
→ degraded ability to make judgments
→ inability to grasp even simple instructions
→ slowed perception
→ loss of sense of humor
→ physical symptoms: headaches, blurred vision, micro-sleep

Bored and Tired of Life?

On the other hand, a life that is too easy, without any stress, can also be detrimental to health. We've all had those days when nothing interesting is going on and we feel bored, vaguely dissatisfied with life, and too tired to move or do anything useful. There is even a common word for this condition. It's *ennui* and it's often used to describe the weariness we feel when we are just plain bored with life.[22]

A life that is too easy, without any stress, can also be detrimental to health.

Why should boredom make you tired? This is actually a sort of psychological protective device that has developed as we've evolved. If we are experiencing nothing dangerous, interesting, or relevant to our well-being, our brains shut our bodies and minds down to conserve energy and to allow time for rejuvenation. But psychologically, this often leads to feelings of dissatisfaction and depression.

Since lack of stimulation is part of the problem, you can solve this by doing simple things that provide pleasant stimulation to the senses. Light up the place, listen to music, watch television, take a shower (not a bath, since you want the stimulation of the water hitting your skin), or eat something that is spicy, very sweet, or contains exotic flavors.

If you have done all of this and still feel weary, you probably need social stimulation. Call a friend or relative or maybe just play with your pet dog or cat. You can also start making a list of things to do and start taking action. If you have actually been doing things all day and are tired, this is not *ennui*, but a signal that it's time to rest.

The Heart–Mind–Body Link: How It Works

Hans Selye was the first stress researcher to demonstrate the direct impact of stress on physical health.[23] He showed that exposure to various stressors causes a substantial decrease in the number of lymphocytes (small white blood cells) in the blood and leads to the shrinkage of the thymus (immune gland). More recent studies have confirmed that stress is associated with reduced natural killer-cell activity, lower antibody and cytokine production, and reduced lymphocyte proliferation.[24]

The brain and the rest of the body can effectively communicate with and influence each other.

Modern molecular tools have also made it possible for researchers to identify biochemical linkages between the nervous system and the endocrine system. And one of psycho-neuro-immunology's surprise findings was that the mind–emotion–body connection is a two-way street. Our thoughts and feelings affect our bodies via the nervous system—that is, the brain is hardwired to all parts of the body by an extensive network of nerve endings linking sensory organs, tissues, the immune system, internal organs, the walls of blood vessels, the endocrine glands, and so on. In addition, the brain produces thousands of chemicals and releases them into the bloodstream. Our thoughts and feelings affect our bodies through the circulation of these chemicals, which include both neurotransmitters and neuropeptides.

Many immune cells throughout our bodies have receptors that communicate with neuropeptides. In addition, the brain can produce cytokines (key immune messengers) to carry messages to immune cells. Thus, the brain and the rest of the body can effectively communicate with and influence each other.

Linking Environmental Sensory Cues

Emotionally coded peptides travel throughout the body, creating a line of communication between our environment, our senses, our brain, and the rest of the body.

Candace B. Pert, a neuroscientist at Georgetown University in Washington, DC, and author of the bestseller *Molecules of Emotion*, has suggested that we pick up changes in our environment through sight, smell, taste, touch, hearing, and pattern recognition. This input travels to nerve bundles throughout the body, which release specific peptides into the bloodstream.[25] There are probably 50 known peptides, each with a particular shape, representing a specific emotional message. These emotionally coded peptides travel throughout the body, binding to receptors on specific cells in the immune system, the endocrine system, and all our organs, thus creating a line of communication between our environment, our senses, our brain, and the rest of the body.

At the same time, emotionally coded peptides might also originate from the surface of cancer cells, inflammatory cells, or infected cells, carrying messages to the brain in a feedback loop and affecting our moods, drive, energy level, concentration, coping mechanisms, behavior, and general health.

This system thus transforms environmental energy into blood-borne chemicals that link the mind and the rest of the body in what Pert calls a "psychosomatic network."[26] The implication of this network is that—even though we may not be aware of their workings—environmental cues, physical sensations, emotions, immune responses, mental states, and behaviors are all linked in feedback loops that constantly affect each other.

One recent study on eating disorders demonstrated the application of this network. A group of girls with bulimia were asked to make a tape with a selection of songs that they found to be soothing. They were instructed to carry a portable tape recorder and to play the songs whenever they felt tempted to purge. This affected them so much that without any other intervention, the girls reduced their purge eating behavior by 75 percent, an effect greater than would be expected from any type of medication or counseling.[27]

What about Spirituality?

The features that distinguish us from other animals are always both blessings and curses. We're self-aware, so we can project into the past and the future, learn from experiences, and build on predictions. But we are also burdened with past regrets and future worries, and this adds to the stress of everyday living. We're able to create with what we have on hand and take advantage of our surroundings, but we are now paying the price of diminished resources and dubious health for our inventions of convenience. We have the mental capacity to perceive wholeness and to integrate, or to differentiate and separate. But we are also continuously struggling between right and wrong, good and evil. We are able to share joy and laugh with others, but sometimes we also have to agonize over their pain. Being human requires us to be more than biological beings; we have the added dimensions of the intellect, emotions, culture, creativity, and spirituality.

> Being human beings requires us to be more than biological beings; we have the added dimensions of intellect, emotions, culture, creativity, and spirituality.

In the past 20 years, medical and psychological journals have been reporting on an increasing number of studies about the health effects of spirituality.[28] The traditional mechanistic biomedical model is finally being complemented with medical investigations into mind–heart–body–spirit interactions and interconnectedness.

What Is Spirituality?

Spirituality may be described as a central philosophy of life that guides personal views and behaviors and expresses a sense of relatedness to something greater than and beyond the self. It is at the core of a person's existence, integrating and transcending the physical, emotional, intellectual, and social dimensions.[29] Definitions of spirituality often include two elements: (1) It is a universal and natural human desire;

> Spirituality and religious devotion are associated with increased resilience to stressful life events.

(2) It involves an awareness beyond ordinary physical limitations that enables a person to gain new perspectives and experiences.[30] Religion is an expression of a particular spiritual perspective that refers to an external, formal system of beliefs, values, rules of conduct, and rituals.[31] It often requires public participation in a faith community, but spirituality is a broader umbrella concept under which religion falls.

Research has shown that spirituality and religious devotion are associated with increased resilience to stressful life events.[32] They are important variables in coping with illness, and researchers have noted that they bring overall positive influences to health and well-being.[33]

How Spirituality Affects Your Health

Unhealthy spirituality and religion associated with abuse and neglect, blind obedience, intergroup conflict and violence, and authoritarian control can have serious negative implications for physical and psychological health.

Research investigating the influence of spirituality on health suggests that while spirituality and religion usually play positive roles, this is not always the case. Positive effects were found among participants of all ages and both genders in a number of geographical regions (including North America, Asia, and Africa) who followed a variety of spiritual practices or religions, including Catholic and Protestant Christianity; Judaism; Buddhism; and Islam.

The positive effects on health were based on the assumption that the spiritual or religious experience itself was positive and healthy. But unhealthy spirituality and religion associated with abuse and neglect, blind obedience, intergroup conflict and violence, and authoritarian control can also have serious negative implications for physical and psychological health.[34]

The Effects of Spirituality and Religion on Physical Health[35]

HEALTH MEASURE	EFFECT	HEALTH MEASURE	EFFECT
Heart disease	lowers rate	Stroke	lowers rate
Systolic blood pressure	lowers	Kidney failure	lowers rate
Diastolic blood pressure	lowers	Cancer mortality	lowers rate
Cirrhosis	lowers rate	Cardiac surgery mortality	lowers rate
Emphysema	lowers rate	Overall mortality	lowers rate
Myocardial infarction	lowers rate	Surgery-related stress	lowers
Chronic pain	decreases	Positive health habits	increases
Cholesterol levels	lowers	Longevity	increase

The Positive Impacts of Spirituality and Prayer

Some researchers have suggested that spirituality affects health positively through various physiological mechanisms. The immune system fights invading organisms, affects brain-control functions such as sleep, body temperature, and metabolic rates, and its signals also reach the thinking and feeling centers of the brain.

Our thoughts and feelings influence the types of hormones and neurotransmitters we produce, and this, in turn, affects our ability to protect ourselves against both outside threats (viruses and bacteria) and internal abnormalities (malignancies). Spirituality promotes positive emotions such as forgiveness, hope, contentment, love, and calmness, and these reduce stress responses, increase immune competence, and restore physiological stability. This may explain why mental calm, emotional cheerfulness, and spiritual peace and hope affect health positively.[36]

Expectant faith may also be seen in the workings of the placebo effect—that is, healing or improvement resulting from the trust that a medication or other remedy can cure or improve a health condition. Placebos work because they mobilize the patient's inner resources for healing. When the element of hope is destroyed, the body's resistance to disease decreases, and the probability of cure is diminished.[37] If even inert substances can have profound effects on the body, simply because of the trust and faith elements, obviously there is a connection between how we think, what we feel, what we believe, and how our bodies function. The reverse is also true: our physical conditions affect how we think and feel.

Some studies have shown that everyday spiritual practices—especially prayer—have positive effects on health. For example, people who pray regularly and have positive spiritual experiences during prayer are more likely to be satisfied with life. This finding is independent of age, income, gender, educational level, and race. The same study also suggested that the determining factor was the depth of intimacy with the divine, not the frequency or types of prayer performed.[38] The act of praying may involve neuro-immunological, cardiovascular, and brain electrical changes leading to slower metabolic rates and muscle relaxation.[39] Studies also show that prayer as a healing factor is not nullified or limited by time or distance—and that prayer seems to work when

> When the element of hope is destroyed, the body's resistance to disease decreases, and the probability of cure is diminished.

intended for the healing of other people as well, though the mechanism of how this works is not yet clear.[40]

In a 1988 study of the effectiveness of prayer for others, American researcher Randolph Byrd studied 400 coronary-care-unit patients who were randomly assigned to either receive or not receive prayers.[41] Neither the patients nor their physicians knew that some of these patients were prayed for. Prayers were sent by persons who had no connection with any patient, doctor, researcher, or hospital personnel. Those who prayed were given only a patient's first name and diagnosis, and some simple information on the patient's current condition. Byrd found that the patients who were prayed for had fewer serious side effects and stayed fewer days in the hospital than those who were not prayed for. A similar subsequent study in 1999 by American researcher William Harris and his colleagues also found that patients prayed for had fewer serious side effects. But their hospital stays were not found to be substantially shorter.[42]

Health and healing seem to consist of "a dynamic, integrated state of balance and communication with regards to body, mind, and spirit; the physiological systems of the body; other individuals; the external environment; and God," according to researchers K. Bakken and M. Hofeller in their book *The Journey towards Wholeness*.[43]

Meditation

The purpose of meditative techniques is to relax and to rejuvenate ourselves. And central to most meditation is the concept of the life force. This concept appears in different personal, cultural, and spiritual variations, but the term *the whole spiritual being*, together with all of its connotations, probably best describes it. In other words, the life force is the sum total of who we are, including our relationship with the universe and other people. For example, we can say that a person's life force is low or weakened in illness. Prayer is the most common way to direct good wishes and rejuvenating energy to oneself or to others in order to strengthen a life-energy condition. Both Eastern and Western meditative techniques help calm and energize the life force.

The practice of meditative techniques can earmark the beginning of spiritual awareness, and some may start a spiritual journey from this point. Others regard meditation as a relaxation technique for a healthier lifestyle. Either way, as we build up our life force, health becomes a natural consequence.

Indian yoga and Chinese qi gong are similar in many respects.[44] Both include warm-up stretching exercises followed by motionless meditation. Both maintain that the exchange of life energy between a human body and the universal energy is similar in many ways to air exchange between the body and the atmosphere. We can master breathing rate and airflow volume by consciously practicing the desired breaths. Likewise, we can master life-energy flow by being consciously aware of this flow within the body and then moving it.

Beginning with breath training, meditation can move us into a state where thoughts dissipate. Homeostasis is restored as our bodies are allowed time to inspect, balance, and restore themselves. Our life force is nurtured as our minds abandon undue everyday stress. Gradually, the life force can grow so strong that we can actually feel its presence and its movement throughout our bodies.

According to the philosophy of Chinese medicine, *qi* is the vital life energy that activates every function and drives every process in the human body, voluntary as well as involuntary. It is a form of bioelectric energy stored in the body's essence. When qi is balanced, the entire organism flourishes and, conversely, when qi is disrupted, vital functions fail. Through digestion, the body extracts vital nutrients and transforms them into energy.

Qi gong is the cultivation of the qi through meditation, breath work, and/or stretching. When you practice qi gong, tai chi, or yoga diligently, you may eventually become more self-aware and therefore also aware of the flow of your life energy. This is called qi sensation. These meditative-movement disciplines teach us to become aware of our body and breathing, in stillness and in motion. Awareness of first our body, second our energy, third our surroundings, and finally other people is seen as a prerequisite for enlightenment. This is the spiritual side of advanced qi gong or yoga.

In the 1970s, Herbert Benson first described how breathing techniques work physiologically: deep diaphragmatic (belly) breathing signals the brain to turn off cortisol, slow down brain waves, and re-establish nurturing functions such as digestion, healing, sleep, and libido.[45]

Here are the steps of a simple breathing meditation:

Stop the Chatter. Combining deep breathing with the repetition of a word, phrase, or activity occupies the noisy part of the brain, allowing deeper levels of stillness. Anyone can meditate anywhere and

> The exchange of life energy between a human body and the universal energy is similar in many ways to air exchange between the body and the atmosphere.

Sometimes greater awareness can increase anxiety—especially if there are repressed emotions. Acceptance helps us reframe the past in a new light, re-examine old beliefs, and release repressed emotions.

anytime—while walking, folding laundry, or waiting in line-ups. It is not a must to sit with crossed legs or wear a robe!

Be Restfully Aware. Even in the midst of everyday chaos, we have the power of intention and self-direction. This means we can consciously and willfully remain calm and restful but still aware.

Let Yourself Be More Observant. With a decrease in stress hormones, a more rational view of the world becomes possible, allowing us to be a more detached observer of a situation, rather than only a participant or victim of it.

Experience Heightened Self-Awareness. Experience new clarity and gain new perspectives from which to address problems.

Accept Yourself. Sometimes greater awareness can increase anxiety—especially if there are repressed emotions. Acceptance helps us reframe the past in a new light, re-examine old beliefs, and release repressed emotions. This allows us to refocus our attention and energy positively on the self.

Cultivate Positive Thinking. The simplest way to promote emotional, mental, and spiritual wellness is to manage stress and consciously address our emotional, intellectual, social, creative, and spiritual needs, as well as our physical needs. Recognize and identify your feelings; enjoy nature, art, or music; develop meaningful relationships; think positively; take time to nurture your inner self; take care of your physical health; manage your time; and maintain balance in all aspects of your life as much as possible.

Reflections on Spiritual Fitness

Happiness is possible for a broken heart, peace is attainable for a tormented soul, and faith lost can be found again.

This is the most difficult part of the book to write. So many wise counselors and spiritual sages have already taught us about spiritual fitness, and I have no systematic spiritual lessons to share. But I know something about hope. I know happiness is possible for a broken heart, peace is attainable for a tormented soul, and faith lost can be found again. Perhaps some of the realizations that have helped me could be useful to you.

So many encounters have shaped my life and created momentum for my happiness and total wellness: life situations; dialogues; physical, emotional, and spiritual interactions with other people, with nature, with things, with the world, with myself. Here are some reflections on a few of those encounters.

One Autumn Day. It was a beautiful autumn day in October 1993. I was attending the opening ceremony of a photo exhibition at the Asian Centre of the University of British Columbia in Vancouver. The photographer was a Japanese philosopher-writer named Daisaku Ikeda. His remarks lasted 30 seconds, and apart from acknowledging a number of people, all he said was: "I'm not a professional photographer. I take pictures because I see something beautiful. And when I put everything in that moment, I capture the moment, and eternity with it."

I felt as though someone had just struck me, and it suddenly dawned on me that I had never really participated in life. I had only been an observer. Even in the midst of a crowd at a gala party, I had always felt apart and alone, as if I did not belong. I watched and analyzed. I prided myself on being always in control, above and beyond, and I took for granted that loneliness was a reasonable price to pay for superior aloofness and the safety of calm intellect.

It wasn't just what he said. It was also how he said it. He lived it and it was so simple. If he could live like that, I wondered if I could live that way too.

A Roomful of Starry Nights. Just before my son moved out of our house, he changed the color of his room to black: walls, carpet, and blinds. He cleared everything out of the room except for the mattress, the stereo system, and a single black light. Then he put glow-sticker stars everywhere. He had created a hideout for me filled with music under the stars.

As I lay there in the dark, gazing at the starry night and immersed in soul-stirring music, I started the journey of healing from a serious illness. This was the same starry sky under which my father had told me stories, the same starry sky under which I had walked with my son on the beach when he was small, and the same starry night as the one out there. Whenever, wherever, they were all part of me. Had always been, and would always be. They are me. I need never be lonely or afraid.

There is no life except in the living, says bioethics specialist Guy Bourgeault of the University of Montreal. And as American author Greg Anderson advises, there is no journey to healing: healing is the journey.[46] By the same token, there is no now or here except when we are

> "Eternity contains the polarity of infinities. From which 'this' and 'that' were begotten."
> —The I Ching

"Heaven and earth exist together with me, and the ten thousand things and I are one," —Chuang Tsu.

in them to perceive them as such. And we are nowhere, except *now here*, positioned in this moment amidst all there is, was, and will be.
Tao had no name before words. It is only because of words that there are distinctions …

Everything can be a "that"; everything can be a "this."

No being can see as another being, so one being sees "this," which is also "that," and sees "that," which is also "this." But "this" and "that" come from each other …

Before any distinctions between "this" and "that," there is only the all-encompassing point of eternal infinities and spontaneities—at once the biggest and the smallest (太).
—Chinese philosopher Chuang Tsu[47]

* (太) is the Chinese character meaning the biggest and the smallest, eternally
inseparable within each other.

A Conquest. As soon as I went into the restaurant, it caught my attention. The haunting sounds of the Andean flutes with accompanying Spanish guitar filled the place with magical tunes. The air was cooler inside, and I sat next to the corridor that opened onto a garden of flurry-colored flowers in full bloom everywhere. A patch of rich blue sky with no trace of cloud served as a backdrop. Happy loving couples strolled past from time to time. The whole setting was at once exotic and simple, hot and humid, yet so calm and peaceful.

Being alone and being lonely were not the same. I could only better my life when I was enough of a companion to myself.

I asked about the music. It was by a band playing at the resort at the time. So I ordered one of their CDs at the restaurant. It was called *La Conquista* (The Conquest). How appropriate. It was October, five years after the divorce and the pancreas incident I mentioned at the beginning of this book. I'd come alone to this resort, which was famous as a place for couples, to see how I'd fare if I were to be uncoupled for the rest of my life. My performance was mixed, but it was a conquest in many ways. Most of the time I was able to quietly enjoy everything around me—the lemon tree outside my room, the bright moon against a blanket of stars, and the peach margaritas. Only once in a while an uneasy sadness would sneak in, surprising me as if I'd just spotted a vaguely familiar stranger.

I opened the CD and stared at the picture inside. In the shadow of a dark mass of magnificent mountains, dimly lit by a bright full moon, was desert ground covered with skulls and bones. The words said: *"La Conquista is a dedication to all those people who have come out from any struggle to better their lives."*

Then I understood. My heart could have been hurt, or it could even have died a thousand times over the course of many lives, but there was only one lesson to learn. Being alone and being lonely were not the same. I could only better my life when I was enough of a companion to myself.

Mastering Our Minds. How can we master our minds except through our own beings? We are so trained to think that it's difficult *not* to think. And we also assume that if we think hard enough, we'll be able to figure out solutions. But only the *being* can master the mind. Why? The logical mind has at least two fundamental weaknesses:

→ It is only a subset, not the universal set equal to the entire being that is us.
→ The logical mind and its thinking process depend on language and symbols as tools, and these are sequential, linear, and one-dimensional. By nature, they are therefore inadequate for dealing with life situations, which are multi-level and multi-dimensional.

For example, thinking alone will not work when we try to resolve life issues or emotional and relationship problems using logic. There is no path to the heart except through feeling. Mental capability is a tool; failure to use it properly and overusing it both lead to stress and fatigue.

So we need to take time off from the world to listen to our own hearts. When we follow our hearts, we are following more than logical thinking, instinct, conscience, feelings, knowledge, decisions, or behaviors. We are following the total awareness and drives of life itself. This approach is also the basis of wise perspectives and effective timing. Solutions to life's problems often depend on how focused and sensitive our total awareness is.

What Next? To effectively deal with what is going to happen next, a 50 percent is an important perspective.

When I went to my Chinese herbalist during the pancreatic incident mentioned in the introductory chapter, he advised, "Give yourself a 50 percent chance for the next moment to live, instead of whatever the statistics dictate. Then you'll have as good a chance as anybody else to live at any time. We never know what's going to happen next. Just do the best you can, and enjoy living until you die. Or you're already

> "Become the master of your mind rather than let your mind master you."
> —Shakyamuni Buddha as quoted in the **Six Paramitas Sutra**[22]

> Solutions to life's problems often depend on how focused and sensitive our total awareness is.

dead before you cease living," he said.

Are we facing death? Or are we facing life? The challenge is not in facing death. The challenge is, and has always been, in facing life, in the realization of the value of life including its many difficulties, potentials, and joys. We live the percentage that we allowed ourselves.

Maximum Positives. If Einstein is right in his Theory of Relativity, then space–time is a dynamic, changing, and expanding continuum. While we make changes to cope and to grow, we are also changing our relationships with other people and with our surroundings. It's necessary to respect this basic interdependent relationship of all things and to maintain a dynamic equilibrium of give and take.

How?

There are many things in the works that I'm not aware of and that I cannot control in life. What I can control best is myself. By praying that I create maximum positive value out of any encounter and any relationship, I can effect maximum positive energies around and within me. This way, even if there are negatives, they can be used to create more positives. Even if there are obstacles, they will eventually be turned into blessings. When the universe is contained in the universe, there is no room to lose.

For example, if I encounter an unfriendly salesperson when shopping, I can react in one of three ways:

→ get upset (adding a negative to a negative, creating more negatives);
→ be indifferent (adding zero to a negative, still resulting in a negative); or
→ send a silent goodwill prayer to the salesperson (canceling a negative with a positive). That person never needs to know about this, but I'll feel much happier because I'm in control of the situation in a positive way.

Total Wellness

How do I enjoy the maximum value of things or of any encounter, for that matter?

Perhaps I can start with a simple, quiet prayer of "thank you" and appreciate all my encounters. For instance, the cup I happen to use has a special "relationship" with me. Since I encounter this and not any other cup, I can appreciate this chance relationship. Then it doesn't matter

"Dream as though you'll live forever. Live as though you'll die tomorrow."
–James Dean

Create your own spring.

what the outcome of the encounter is—whether I use it again or it ends up slipping from my hold and hitting the floor. By the same token, appreciating each day, whatever it is going to bring, is more likely to make it a special and a great day.

To me, spiritual fitness is total wellness. It is choosing to be well, creating maximum life value from moment to moment, for ourselves and for all. Without help, we will not be able to live to our full potential. But the potential for maximum value has always been within us, and it can be realized through merging with the goodness in us and around us.

Everything has its own nature and its own use. Nothing is without nature or use. To realize one's own nature is to be useful. Realizing one's own nature is happiness ...

Live so that you are at ease, full of joy, and in harmony with the universe. Day and night, create your own season by sharing the spring with all ...

Be all that the heavens grant you.

—Chuang Tsu

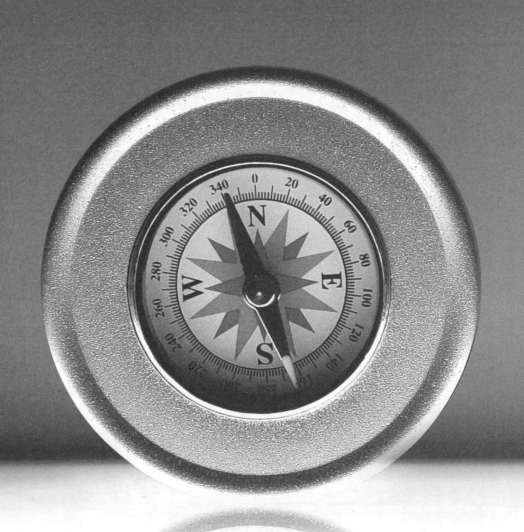

Traditionally, most of our information about health matters has come from medical professionals. Increasingly, though, we are looking for information from multiple sources. There is no lack of readily accessible information. Health information and opinions abound in print and broadcast media, and on the Internet. For example, just type the word "menopause" in the search box of Google.com, and in 0.07 seconds you will be swamped with 928,000 referrals to websites that offer something on this subject. But how useful is the information? We need to determine the following:

→ how reliable and accurate it is;
→ what it means;
→ how it should be used, if at all.

How to Evaluate the Accuracy and Reliability of Information

Even the experts in a particular area may find this question difficult to answer at times, but here are some important criteria that can help you make judgments about the health and wellness information you discover.

1. Find out who has generated the information.

a. Author

What are the author's professional and/or academic credentials; what is the author's experience or knowledge base on the subject; is the author a member of relevant and authentic professional organizations? Many good publications include a profile of the author, which will provide this information.

→ Is the information source referenced?
→ Has the information been reviewed? By whom? Are the information sources and reviewers credible?

b. Sponsor

The reputation of the organization producing or sponsoring the information can be a useful (but not always reliable) criterion for judging accuracy and reliability. Some print publications and websites, for instance, are owned by or affiliated with purveyors of health products, and the "articles" appearing in such media are actually advertisements for the owners' products, disguised as objective reports.

Appendix

How to Evaluate Health and Wellness Information

For websites, as well as print media, a list of the sponsoring organization's advisory board members and their professional affiliations can be a useful guide to judge the quality of content in a general way.

Consider the Source

Authors of health articles in books and magazines and on websites usually fall into one of three categories:

Recognized experts in a field. They usually report their findings and opinions in professional journals, using terminology and alluding to published work familiar only to others in the field. Their articles are most likely to be accurate and up to date, but may not always be readily understandable to the layperson or even to some health professionals who do not work in the same area of study.

Professional writers and editors. For the most part, information on medical and health subjects appearing in various media comes from people who are not first-hand experts in the area. But responsible publishers, media, and websites employ writers and editors who have had some training in the fundamentals of biological and medical science. This prepares them to understand and evaluate primary materials. They also have the writing skills to present this information accurately and clearly to the general reader.

Mixture. In too many instances, a mélange of excerpts from various articles is presented without any effort made to integrate or present the information in a clear and understandable fashion. Sometimes this happens because writers themselves fail to gain an in-depth understanding of the material.

2. Take into account the references cited.
Any report, whether in print or in the electronic media, should cite the books and other materials the author used in preparing the article. At least some of these sources should be in recognizably authoritative publications (e.g., *The New England Journal of Medicine, The Lancet,* the *Canadian Medical Association Journal,* the *Journal of the American Medical Association,* the *British Medical Journal, Science Magazine,* the *Mayo Clinic Health Letter,* newsletters of various schools of medicine, and websites of all these organizations and publications). If no source is cited or if the only sources cited are newspaper or popular magazine articles or websites, one should be wary of the content until its information can be confirmed in other professional publications.

3. The information should be current.

Health research is taking place today at a faster rate than ever before. So to be useful, the information must be current and reflect the most up-to-date research. New discoveries usually result in radically new drugs and procedures. But sometimes the latest studies also show that an older drug or procedure is more effective than one that had replaced it.

4. Verify information of special interest to you.

If you are thinking of using information as the basis for some plan of action, for example dieting, forgoing surgery, taking 10 grams of vitamin C per day, or giving up a certain medication, it is essential to consult other, reliable sources to check the facts and gather other opinions. It is also essential to consult your health professionals before taking action directly related to your health. As you verify information, make sure you check its completeness, to see whether there's another side to the story. For example, an article may have correctly reported that Product G was effective in 77 percent of the subjects tested, but it may have failed to mention that it had adverse side effects or that Product K was effective for the same condition in 89 percent of the subjects. Don't be satisfied with just two or three accounts of a particular piece of information.

5. Find out how the data were collected.

It's important to know the methods used to obtain information. Were data collected in an unbiased fashion? Are the data based on observations of a significant number of subjects or only a few? Were the studies done on humans or animals only?

Biomedical information can be obtained through a number of different procedures, not all of which have immediate relevance or significance for human health. Here are some of the procedures used:

In vitro studies. In vitro means "in glass" and refers to the fact that this method involves the use of cells or tissues removed from a human or animal and grown in glass or plastic Petri dishes. This technique is often referred to as "tissue cultures." These studies can provide valuable information and stimulus for other studies, but cells in a tissue culture may not behave exactly as they do in the intact body where they are subjected to other influences, such as neighboring tissues and circulating hormones.

In vivo studies. *In vivo* means "in the living organism." Studies of drugs for potential use by humans or of the effects of substances such as tea, fats, and vitamin E are done on experimental animals—usually mice, rats, pigs, dogs, or monkeys. Such animal studies can provide important information as to the potential effectiveness and side effects of the drugs or other substances when used by humans. But the results obtained with animals are not always directly applicable to humans. It may be difficult to find animals with similar disease conditions, and animals may not metabolize experimental drugs in the same ways as humans. Nevertheless, in May 2002, the U.S. Food and Drug Administration announced that certain drugs useful for serious or life-threatening conditions may be approved on the basis of information gathered from animal studies alone when well-controlled studies in humans are not ethically feasible.

Human studies. The best test of a treatment or other intervention for use in human medicine is to study its effects in humans. There are two basic procedures for doing this.

a. Intervention studies

→ *Randomized clinical trials.* In general, randomized trials can be used to answer a question such as this: Is one drug (or procedure) more effective for treating a certain condition than no treatment or another drug (or procedure)? In testing the efficacy of a drug (or a procedure), the subjects, all of whom have a certain health condition, are randomly divided into two groups. One group receives the drug being tested while the other group, the control group, may receive nothing at all or a placebo (a pill or capsule or liquid that looks like the ones given to the treatment group but has none of the drug in it). At the end of the treatment period, the investigators determine the outcome for each individual. A large number of subjects should be enlisted in the study, and it should be carried out over a sufficient period. Ideally, the two groups should be matched in age, sex ratio, race, socio-economic status, etcetera, so that any differences at the end of the trial can be associated with the difference in treatment and not attributed to other factors.

→ *Randomized clinical trials may be single-blinded.* In this case, the volunteers do not know whether they are receiving the genuine drug (or therapy) or the placebo. This is done to eliminate the possibility of bias on the part of the subjects as they report their reactions to treatment. But since the investigators know which people are getting the drug and which are not, there is still a possibility of bias.

→ *Double-blinded randomized trials*. In such trials, neither the subjects nor the investigators know whether a subject has received the treatment or the placebo because a third party has assigned the treatment or placebo to each subject in a coded form. Only after the investigators have recorded the final data is the information decoded. This procedure can eliminate investigators' biases.

b. *Observational studies*

→ Often the effect of a drug on human health cannot be investigated ethically or practically using intervention methods. For example, to study whether cigarette smoking is related to cancer, it's not necessary to find volunteers willing to take up cigarette smoking for the next 10 or 20 years because large numbers of people have already had the habit for those lengths of time. People exposed to cigarette smoke can be observed for the occurrence of cancer and compared with a similar group of people who have never smoked. These are called epidemiological studies—studies of factors controlling the presence, distribution, and control of a disease in a population.

These are the main types of observational studies:

→ *Cohort studies* are a valuable type of observational study. One of the most famous was done in England beginning in 1951: it demonstrated the causal relation between cigarette smoking and ill health, including lung cancer. About 40,000 doctors not diagnosed with lung cancer were divided into four cohorts (groups): heavy, moderate, and light smokers, plus non-smokers, and their health was studied for 10 years. It was found that death from all causes and from lung cancer specifically was in significant excess among the smokers compared to the non-smokers.

Cohort studies usually result in a measure called the *relative risk*, which relates the likelihood of a disease in one group to the likelihood in another.

→ *Case-control studies*. These are usually concerned with trying to discover factors involved in causing a relatively rare medical condition.

In these studies, a group of people with authentic cases of a particular condition is compared to a control group of people who do not have that condition but are matched with regard to gender, race, age, and socio-economic background. The subjects are interviewed about their lifestyle; exposure to chemicals; medical history; and whatever else the investigators may consider pertinent. In addition, their medical records are examined. By comparing the data for both groups, investigators may find some common element associated with the disease condition that is not present in the control group. The analysis depends in part on the ability of the subjects to recall past events, which may not always be accurate.

→ *Case reports*. In a case report, a physician will relate the details of his or her observations of a single patient or a few patients who show some unusual aspects of symptoms or treatment. Though such reports may lack the statistical validation of case-control studies, they can alert investigators to possible problems (or solutions) that can be investigated more thoroughly in controlled studies.

→ *Meta-analysis*. This is a statistical analysis that reviews a number of published, primary studies, such as clinical trials, related to the same condition; for example, 16 independent studies about the effects of drinking black tea on cardiovascular health may be analyzed. In terms of medical statistical value, randomized clinical trials top the list, followed by cohort studies, case-controlled studies, and then case reports.

Evidence for Complementary Treatments

For the past 10 years or so, mainly in North America, the medical profession has moved toward emphasizing evidence-based medicine (EBM). EBM advocates the use of procedures whose effectiveness is supported by data from randomized controlled clinical trials (RCT) and it tends to downplay the intuition and experience of the physician. Certain drugs and procedures routinely accepted by the profession as useful and effective have been found to be ineffective when evaluated using rigorous scientific, experimental criteria—especially RCT.

As more and more people in the Western world have chosen to use complementary treatments and products, conventional practitioners have become more vocal in raising questions about the safety and efficacy of these remedies. According to many conventional practitioners, most of the evidence for the usefulness of these remedies is anecdotal or, at best, comes from case reports, which are seen as lower in the evidence hierarchy than randomized clinical trials.

Conventional practitioners contend that if these treatments were really useful, clinical evidence would show it. On the other hand, complementary practitioners argue that evidence-based medicine regards the results of clinical trials from a statistical perspective and disregards the success of the minority of cases. Many complementary treatments are tailored to individual patient conditions and needs, and therefore may not be able to withstand the clinical trial demands of a successful application to a large patient population. Furthermore, complementary approaches to treatment are usually holistic, using more than one modality simultaneously. Isolating each treatment factor for the purpose of study would lead to ineffective treatment.

In Canada and many other countries, drugs prescribed by physicians must be approved by a government agency that requires evidence of efficacy and safety based on clinical trials and other tests. Similar standards do not usually exist for the herbs, dietary supplements, vitamins, and other preparations used in complementary medicine, as long as the label on the package makes no health claims. Herbal preparations, for example, are treated as food products and must meet standards that are quite different from those governing conventional prescription drugs. While the manufacturer must sell a herbal product as a "food," complementary health practitioners may legally recommend the same product as a medicinal preparation.

Because of increased consumer use of natural health products (NHP) during the last 10 years, Health Canada took steps in 1999 that led to the formation of a Natural Health Products Directorate. This agency is dedicated to the regulation of NHPs, in order to provide Canadians with "safety, quality and freedom of choice" in their use of NHPs. To achieve this objective, in early 2003 the directorate was in the process of producing a regulatory framework that would allow NHP producers to make health claims without having these claims subjected to all the provisions of the regulations that govern prescription drugs.

Definition of a Natural Health Product

This definition of a natural health product is from Canada's Natural Health Products Directorate:[1]

Substances that are manufactured, sold or represented for use in:

- (i) the diagnosis, treatment, mitigation or prevention of a disease, disorder, or abnormal physical state or its symptoms in humans;
- (ii) restoring or correcting organic functions in humans; or
- (iii) maintaining or promoting health or otherwise modifying organic functions in humans.

Conventional Medicine: How Much Is Based on Scientific Evidence?

How much of conventional medicine (i.e., most medicine practiced by M.D.s) is actually based on scientifically derived evidence of efficacy, and particularly the ultimate in evidence—randomized clinical trials (RCT)? Critics of conventional medicine and some non-critic M.D.s often cite an estimate of 10 to 20 percent—a figure frequently repeated without reference to its source. However, a recent survey of studies on this question concluded that an average of 76 percent of medical interventions are based on some form of evidence (RCT, cohort studies, case control), with 37 percent based on RCT. Not all areas of practice come close to the RCT average, though. Burn therapy, pediatric surgery, and retinal break treatment have lower percentages, for example.[2]

Communicating the Results of Research

Scientists have always communicated the results of their studies to colleagues in two major ways—through presentations at conferences and publication in journals. Each of these methods has its own purposes. Data presented at meetings is often of a preliminary nature, the unpublished results of work in progress. But publication in a journal serves, or *should* serve, a different function. In this case, the researcher is reporting new, previously unpublished data that have withstood rigorous and repeated testing. This work is discussed and interpreted in relation to what others in the field have published, and peer-reviewed by experts in the field. One disadvantage of the peer-review process is that it is difficult for completely new areas of works with no previous peer reviews to be accepted for publication.

Medical Information and the Media

The mass media are a major source of information on medical matters for the general public and, to some extent, for the health professional.

Much of the information they report is based on news releases, which usually come from pharmaceutical companies; universities and institutes; sponsors of medical journals; or meetings and conferences, including those sponsored by foundations concerned with specific diseases (e.g., the Canadian Cancer Society or the Canadian Cystic Fibrosis Foundation).

A British study looked at the kinds of medical research that two British newspapers (*The Times* and *The Sun*) considered to be newsworthy during 1999 and 2000. Their stories were based on news releases for 517 out of 1,193 journal articles published during these two years by two internationally prominent British medical journals, the *British Medical Journal* and *The Lancet*. The news releases were equally divided between "good news" and "bad news" and between observational studies and randomized control studies.

The newspapers reported on only 81 of the 517 news releases. There were no stories at all on any of the 676 published journal articles that had no news release. This suggested that, at least for these two newspapers, reporters did not actively search the journals for stories. Bad news stories were more likely to be reported, and the randomized control studies were less likely to be covered than observational studies.[3]

In the case of conferences, the media usually neglect to point out the fact that information reported at conferences is often preliminary, may not be conclusive, and has not been published or reviewed.

It is apparent that, at least in newspapers, stories of new developments in medical research are based almost exclusively on what is covered in news releases, and that these releases cover only a fraction of the actual work being done. Another study concluded that news releases do not always call attention to the deficiencies of a study. In addition, they sometimes exaggerate the significance of studies and do not always indicate when the funds for a study come from parties with a vested interest in the results.[4]

Potential Trouble at the Source of Medical Information

Biomedical research is the ultimate source of conventional medical information. In most developed countries, it is carried out in universities and medical schools, by pharmaceutical companies, by research foundations supported by private funds or money donated by the public, and at government-supported research institutes.

While most scientists at these institutions are dedicated to their work, they do it for more than the noble purpose of understanding nature and using their findings to benefit humanity. They are also interested in career advancement, prestige, financial reward, and status—perfectly normal desires that make scientists no different from people in other jobs. Unfortunately, as in other professions, some researchers intentionally take a shortcut to achieve these legitimate ends by publishing outright fraudulent data, by selecting only those data that "prove" a favored outcome, or by withholding data that demolish the basis for a long-standing practice.

The scientific enterprise depends on the honesty and integrity of its practitioners, and although relatively few violate this fundamental code of ethics, those who do can cause significant damage. Fortunately, over time, science is self-correcting and false information is eventually ferreted out when other scientists try to use or repeat these flawed results. But in the meantime, progress is retarded, resources are wasted, and in the case of clinical medicine, the health of people may be compromised.

An additional and growing concern about the integrity of biomedical research relates to the increased links between academic researchers and pharmaceutical and biotechnology companies. This trend is particularly prominent in the clinical research that is essential for studying the efficacy and safety of new drugs and procedures. Such studies are designed, organized, and carried out by clinicians at medical schools and at the hospitals affiliated with those schools, but pharmaceutical companies fund almost all of these clinical studies. In the United States, it's estimated that the cost of developing one new drug is US$300 million to $600 million on average and that each year about $3.3 billion is spent by the U.S. pharmaceutical industry to support clinical trials. This represents about 70 percent of all the money spent in the United States for this purpose, the rest coming primarily from the government.

Clinicians generally agree that the industry-academic arrangement has on the whole benefited the public, but that there are also negative aspects. Some agreements require that an investigator receiving support from industry cannot publish data without the permission of the industry partner. This restricts the free flow of information that characterizes science. Potential conflicts of interest may also arise from academic-industry agreements. Some scientists, for instance, have been involved in clinical trials sponsored by companies in which they had a financial interest.

Contract-research organizations (CROS) represent an even more worrisome alliance, one that developed about 10 years ago between the pharmaceutical-biotechnology industry and for-profit companies. These CROS are displacing academic institutions as industry's collaborator in clinical trials.

In the academic world, an arrangement between the investigator and industry has to conform to the university's standards with regard to both financial matters and research protocol. CROS, however, manage clinical trials for drug companies from beginning to end: devising the trial protocol, enrolling investigators and patients, analyzing the data, preparing applications for government approvals, and writing the manuscript for publication—a chore traditionally regarded as a sacred obligation of the researcher. In some instances, CROS have invested in the drug company whose drug is being tested in the trial. And CROS seem to be on the rise. It has been estimated that in the United States in 1998, 40 percent of the money spent by drug companies for clinical trials went to academic centers, compared to 80 percent in 1991.[5]

Searching the Web for Reliable Health Information[6]

Let's focus on one concern—dietary supplements—for an example of how to search the Web for reliable health information. In January 2002, the Center for Food Safety and Applied Nutrition of the U.S. Food and Drug Administration published an article entitled "Tips for the Savvy Supplement User: Making Informed Decisions and Evaluating Information," from which the following pointers have been adapted. Note that the tips can be applied to searching the Internet for other health information, and that the article is available in its entirety at **www.cfsan.fda.gov.**

1. Tips on searching the Web for information on dietary supplements

Try to use directory sites of respected organizations, rather than doing blind searches with a search engine. Ask yourself the following questions:

a) Who operates the site?

Is the site run by the government, a university, or a reputable medical or health-related association (e.g., the Diabetes Association, the Heart Foundation, Health Canada)? Has the information been written or reviewed by qualified health professionals and/or experts in the field—in academia, government, or the medical community?

b) What is the purpose of the site?

Is the purpose of the site to educate the public objectively or to sell a product? Be aware of practitioners or organizations whose main interest is to market products, either directly or through sites with which they are linked. Commercial sites should clearly distinguish scientific information from advertisements. Most non-profit and government sites contain no advertising, and access to the sites and materials offered are usually free.

c) What is the source of the information, and does it have any references?

Has the study been reviewed by recognized scientific experts or has it been published in reputable peer-reviewed scientific journals such as *The New England Journal of Medicine*? Does the site say "some studies show …" or does it state where the study is listed so you can check the authenticity of the references? For example, can the study be found in the U.S. National Library of Medicine's database of literature citations?[7]

d) Is the information current?

Check the date when the material was posted or updated. Often new research or other findings are not reflected in old materials (e.g., side effects or interactions with other products or new evidence that might have changed earlier thinking).

e) How reliable are e-mail solicitations and the Internet?

While the Internet is a rich source of health information, it is also an easy vehicle for spreading myths, hoaxes, and rumors about alleged news, studies, products, or findings. To avoid falling prey to such hoaxes, be skeptical and watch out for overly emphatic language with UPPERCASE LETTERS and lots of exclamation points!!!! Beware of such phrases as "This is not a hoax" or "Send this to everyone you know."

2. More tips and to-dos

a) Ask yourself: Does this information sound too good to be true?

Do the claims for the product seem exaggerated or unrealistic? Are simplistic conclusions being drawn from a complex study, in order to sell a product? Be skeptical about anecdotal information from people who have no formal training in nutrition or botanicals, or from personal testimonials (e.g., from store employees, friends, or online chat rooms) about the incredible benefits of using a particular product.

b) Think twice about chasing the latest headline.

Sound health advice is generally based on a body of research, not a single study. Be wary of results claiming a "quick fix."

What Does It All Mean?

Having gathered information and evaluated its accuracy, you will next face the question "What does it all mean?" The materials you read probably present more than just facts. An article may tell you, for example, that serum cholesterol above a certain level was found to present a *risk for heart disease*. But to fully understand and appreciate this fact requires knowing what cholesterol is, in what foods it is found, how it brings about its effect on the function of the heart, and even what is meant by the word "risk."

It is possible to achieve a basic, accurate, and useful understanding of factors such as these without becoming a medical student. Consulting a textbook on human physiology will give you the fundamental information you need. You'll be surprised at how much you can learn by yourself when the matter directly concerns you. Understanding how things happen (e.g., the mechanism of a disease) eliminates a lot of the mystery surrounding the disease and can, at the same time, dispel fear. Textbooks are peer-reviewed and go through so many editions that the information they contain should be quite reliable. Some background understanding will also help you learn about treatment strategy and may motivate you to participate actively in your own health management.

Using Information about Health

How do you use the information you've collected? In the first place, it can help you formulate questions to ask your physician about the nature of a condition, its treatment and prognosis, and questions that touch on matters the practitioner may not usually discuss with you.

The information you collect may stimulate you to try therapies or preparations that you have confirmed are beneficial to your health. But before you go ahead and act on what you've read, even if you are convinced that you have pertinent, accurate information and understand it all, you must obtain the opinion of a medical expert.

While the doctor–patient relationship has traditionally been based on the notion that "doctor knows best," this interaction is now undergoing radical change for two major reasons. First, patients have easier access than ever to medical information and opinion through various media. Second, if data are available to and understood by the patient, the patient can play a greater role in making treatment decisions and is no longer simply left to approve or disapprove of the course selected by the physician.

To act wisely on the basis of the information you've collected, you must seek the advice of trained medical professionals. A course of treatment involves more than just technical information, and many of us do not have the training and experience to know all the factors affecting therapy application.

Health professionals should be consulted to diagnose, to provide data, to act as a check on the patient's understanding of the data, and to serve as a guide and reference for decisions on treatment, even though the final health decision ultimately rests with the patient.

Can Patients Discuss Their Research with Doctors?

A survey of 212 cancer patients and about 400 oncologists carried out in Toronto provides some interesting data about the attitudes of both groups toward health information in the media and on the Internet.

More than 85 percent of the patients wanted more information about their medical condition, and 54 percent of these felt that their current physicians and health-care personnel were not providing it. About 71 percent of the patients searched for information on their own, mostly on the Internet, and on the basis of the information collected, about 30 percent of these requested specific treatments, while 6 percent refused the treatment prescribed by their physician. The survey showed that almost 90 percent of the patients found their physicians were willing to discuss information from the media or the Internet, and the majority of doctors even spent what the patients regarded as a moderate to a great amount of time discussing the information with them.

The majority of patients (62 percent) and physicians (86 percent) said that seeking information from sources other than the physician had no negative consequences for the patient–doctor relationship. This should encourage patients to approach their physicians with questions about information they have garnered from other sources.

About 60 percent of the physicians surveyed thought that the information in the media and on the Internet was accurate only *sometimes*, while 24 percent thought it was *rarely* or *never* accurate. When asked about the patients' understanding of the information they'd collected, 46 percent of the physicians said it was *sometimes* correct, while 48 percent thought the patients *rarely* or *never* had an adequate understanding of what they had read.[8]

Acknowledgments

My first words of thanks go to my husband, Michael, who created a path with me where there wasn't one, and turned *WellnessOptions* into a reality; to my son, Yee Jee, who taught me what love is by being who he is and who carried me through some of life's darkest moments; and to my brother, Billy, whose faith in life and its endless potential returned hope to me.

I'm grateful to those who believe in *WellnessOptions*. So many people lend helping hands: Michael's family and friends, especially my mother-in-law, who provided the bulk of the financial support to publish the magazine; and members of the honorary advisory board who set the standards for excellence and provided editorial guidelines.

My special and fondest thanks go to our working comrades, especially my creative partner, Moses Wong; co-editors Dr. Manny Radomski, Dr. Michael Filosa, and Dr. John Kellen (who, unfortunately, passed away in February this year), and all the other *WellnessOptions* team members listed on the facing page. Without their faith in the project and their passion, efforts, enthusiasm, creative contributions, and professionalism, *WellnessOptions* would not have developed its unique brand identity and editorial personality so successfully. Their help was also instrumental in the making of this book.

Former publisher of Penguin Canada, Cynthia Good, understood the vision and initiated the book project. Editorial Director at Penguin Canada, Diane Turbide, gave me confidence and provided me with a crystal-clear focus. Kathryn Dean patiently improved both structure and substance; Cheryl Cohen went through the details thoroughly; and Lorraine Kelly taught me the business side of things. Thanks to Catherine MacGregor, Kathrine Pummell, Julie Traves, Colleen Clarke ... and, especially, Managing Editor Tracy Bordian, who guided and organized every step of the making of this book efficiently and intelligently.

I'm indebted to my mother, Gala, and many friends who have stood by me in good times and bad: Swee Teh, Yuriko Skillan, my sister-in-law Sufumi, Robert Fashler, Mikey and Akiko Masuda, Harry and Mia Phillips, Colleen McGuinness, Ian Richardson, Jon Festinger, Gary Forget, Mike Audet, Donna Skeffington, and K.S. Tso.

There are many other people whom I have encountered and have learned from. Some of them I have come to know, some are strangers who just happened to be there to show me the way, some caused me pain or took advantage of my good will but made me stronger ... the list is too long; nevertheless, I'm thankful to them all.

Finally, my special thanks to three wise men: my father, who taught me how to question and to dream; Zhou EnLai, who inspired me to believe and to persevere; and Daisuku Ikeda, who wrote simply and sincerely, "You're worthy of respect ... have courage, I will see you smile across the rainbow where your tears have been."

Thank you.

The *WellnessOptions* Team

Y. Michael Chan *PhD, CChem, FRSC(UK), FACB*
Michael Chan is a clinical biochemist in Toronto. He began his career in the pharmaceutical industry, followed by an overseas university appointment. His current interest is in laboratory techniques for monitoring health and diseases.

Manny W. Radomski *PhD*
Manny Radomski is the former director general of the Defence & Civil Institute of Environmental Medicine, National Defence Department of Canada. He is also professor emeritus in the Faculties of Medicine and Physical Health and Education at the University of Toronto. He has published extensively in the areas of enviromental stress, sleep, and growth hormone and exercise.

Michael F. Filosa *PhD*
Michael Filosa has been a faculty member at the University of Toronto for more than 30 years. He has published many articles on his research in cell biology.

John Kellen *MD, PhD*
John Kellen was professor emeritus of Laboratory Medicine and Pathobiology at the University of Toronto, and an honourary staff member at Sunnybrook and Women's College Health Sciences Centre. He was editor-in-chief of Modern Medicine of Canada and was active in diagnostics and research on cancer.

Ariel K. Dalfen *MD*
Ariel K. Dalfen, a graduate of Princeton University, holds an MD from McMaster University. She is now a psychiatry resident at the University of Toronto. She also writes and lectures about the impact of the Internet on psychiatry and mental health.

Alykhan S. Abdulla *MD, CCFP, DipSportMed*
A.S. Abdullah started in genetic and biochemical engineering then moved on to family and sports medicine through the Universities of Calgary and Toronto. Presently he is a specialty consultant in sports and community medicine.

Michael Zitney *MD*
Michael Zitney received his training at the University of Toronto. He is currently the director of the Headache and Pain Relief Centre in Toronto. Michael Zitney practises a multi-disciplinary approach to pain management, combining conventional and complementary treatments.

Stanley Coren *PhD, FRSC*
Stanley Coren is a Professor of Psychology at the University of British Columbia. He received his doctorate at Stanford University and has published widely in professional journals. His psychological research includes studies on sleep, human vision and hearing, effects of birth stress, creativity, handedness, behaviour genetics, and human–canine relationships.

Anthony M. Ocana *RDN, MD, CCFP*
Anthony Ocana is a family doctor, registered dietitian and physician psychotherapist. He is a frequent reviewer for the *Canadian Medical Association Journal* and an instructor at the University of British Columbia. He has a special interest in mental health, eating disorders and addiction. He now works for the Health Smith Wellness Group.

Doris Cheung *MSc(Pharm)*
Doris Cheung holds a masters degree in pharmaceutical science from the University of Toronto and has extensive practical experience in hospitals, the pharmaceutical industry, and retail drug stores. She was the editor of the Ontario Pharmacists' Association Drug Information Centre Exchange newsletter.

Yee Jee Tso
Yee Jee Tso is a professional actor and freelance writer based in Toronto. His film, stage and TV series credits include: *Antitrust, Dr. Who, Da Vinci's Inquest, Madison, Wild Abandon, The Highlander and Outer Limits.*

Tamara Harth *MA*
Tamara Harth is the Information Manager at the Toronto Sunnybrook Regional Cancer Centre, where she provides health database and research support, Web content management, as well as training to clinical and medical staff.

Paul Saunders *PhD, ND, DHANP, CCH*
Paul Saunders is the Chair Materia Medical of the Canadian College of Naturopathic Medicine, and editor of the *Canadian Journal of Herbalism*. He holds a doctorate degree in plant ecology, and he is a naturopathic doctor.

Lawrence (Larry) Chan *ND, DC, Dipl. Ac.*
Larry Chan is a naturopathic doctor and a chiropractor. He has a Diploma in Acupuncture from Shanghai Research Institute. His specialization is in anti-aging medicine. Larry Chan is a certified member of the American Academy of Anti-Aging Medicine.

Jonathan E. Prousky *BPHE, ND*
Jonathan Prousky is an assistant professor of Clinical Nutrition with The Canadian College of Naturopathic Medicine.

Rebecca Bell
Rebecca Bell, a graduate of York University's Dance Department, has been a fitness instructor for more than 18 years. She has also published and appeared on television as a fitness expert.

Erika Ebbel
Erika Ebbel majors in Chemistry and minors in Music at the Massachusetts Institute of Technology. Her interest in antiviral natural products isolated from a Chinese herb led to her involvement with many institutions including Stanford University and the U.S. Department of Agriculture.

Dianne E. Hinch-Moroz *MSc*
Dianne Hinch-Moroz has served as a fitness consultant for McMaster Hospital, the Deparment of Kinesiology at McMaster University, the Department of National Defence Canada, and Redeemer University College.

F.H. Abdulla *CDA*
Faiza Abdulla started in dental and medical nursing and is now the director and owner of Kingsway Health Centres. She has written for medical and consumer publications.

Moses Wong
Moses Wong graduated in graphic design at the renowned Rhode Island School of Design in the United States. He has designed for several award-winning magazines in New York and Toronto.

Book design and photography by Moses Wong

Endnotes

A Road Sign to Wellness Options

1. D. Ikeda, R. Simard, and G. Bourgeault, *On Being Human* (Montreal: University of Montreal Press, 2002).

Chapter 1

1. S.C. Rhind and P. Shek, "Stress, Immune System and Allergy," *WellnessOptions* (April/May 2001), 26–7.

Chapter 2

1. J. Denberg, "Allergy: Exploding into the 21st Century," *WellnessOptions* (April/May 2001), 11–12.

2. M. Castells, J. Boyce, C. Legendre, and S. Caillat-Zucman, "Transfer of Peanut Allergy by a Liver Allograft," *New England Journal of Medicine* 338 (1998), 232–8.

3. P. Vadas, Y. Wai, W. Burks, and B. Perelman, "Detection of Peanut Allergens in Breast Milk of Lactating Women," *Journal of the American Medical Association* 285 (2001), 1746–8; L. Frank, A. Marian, M. Visser, E. Weinberg, and P.C. Potter, "Exposure to Peanuts in Utero and in Infancy and the Development of Sensitization to Peanut Allergens in Young Children," *Pediatric Allergy and Immunology* 10 (1999), 27–32; S.H. Arshad and C. Grant, "Allergy to Nuts: How Much of a Problem Really Is This?" *Clinical & Experimental Allergy* 31 (2001), 5–7; F. Pucar, R. Kagan, H. Lim, and A.E. Clarke, "Peanut Challenge: A Retrospective Study of 140 Patients," *Clinical & Experimental Allergy* 31 (2001), 40–6; J.O. Warner, "Peanut Allergy: A Major Public Health Issue," *Pediatric Allergy and Immunology* 10 (1999), 14–20.

4. K. Ichikawa, E. Iwasaki, M. Baba, and M.D. Chapman, "High Prevalence of Sensitization to Cat Allergen among Japanese Children with Asthma, Living without Cats," *Clinical & Experimental Allergy* 29 (1999), 754–61.

5. M. Chan-Yeung, P.A. McClean, P.R. Sandell, A.S. Slutsky, and N. Zamel, "Sensitization to Cat without Direct Exposure to Cats," *Clinical & Experimental Allergy* 29 (1999), 762–5.

6. R. Ader, D.L. Felton, and N. Cohen (eds.), *Psychoneuroimmunology*, 3rd ed., vol. 1 and 2 (New York: Academic Press, 2001).

7. H. Selye, *The Stress of Life* (New York: McGraw-Hill, 1976).

8. William Osler, *The Principles and Practice of Medicine* (New York: D. Appleton, 1892).

Chapter 3

1. P. Slade, "What Is Body Image?" *Behavioural Research Therapy* 32 (1994), 497.

2. M. Griffin, "Building Blocks for Children's Body Image," *Body Image Task Force*, P.O. Box 360196, Melbourne, FL 32936, http://home.earthlink.net/ ~dawn_atkins/bitf.htm.

3. W. Erhardt, American Society of Plastic Surgeons, www.plasticsurgery.org

4. H.D. Posavac, S.S. Posavac, and E.J. Posavac, "Exposure to Media Images of Female Attractiveness and Concern with Body Weight among Young Women," *Sex Roles* 38 (1998), 187–201; H.D. Posavac, S.S. Posavac, and R.G. Weigel, "Reducing the Impact of Media Images on Women at Risk for Body Image Disturbance: Three Targeted Interventions," *Journal of Social and Clinical Psychology* 20 (2001), 324–40.

5. M.J. Tovee, P.J. Hancock, S. Mahmoodi, B.R. Singleton, and P.L. Cornelissen, "Human Female Attractiveness: Waveform Analysis of Body Shape," *Proceedings of the Royal Society of London B Biological Sciences* 269 (2002), 2205–13.

6. P.T. Katzmarzyk and C. Davis, "Thinness and Body Shape of Playboy Centerfolds from 1978 to 1998," *International Journal of Obesity* 25 (2001), 590; M.J. Tovee, S.M. Mason, J.L. Emery, S.E. McCluskey, and E.M. Cohen-Tovee, "Supermodels: Stick Insects or Hourglasses," *Lancet* 350 (1997), 1474–5; M.J. Tovee, S. Reinhardt, J.L. Emery, and P.L. Cornelissen, "Optimum Body-Mass Index and Maximum Sexual Attractiveness," *Lancet* 352 (1998), 548; M.J. Tovee and P.L. Cornelissen, "Female and Male Perceptions of Female Physical Attractiveness in Front-View and Profile," *British Journal of Psychology* 92 (2001), 391–402; M.J. Tovee, J.L. Emery, and E.M. Cohen-Tovee, "The Estimation of Body Mass Index and Physical Attractiveness Is Dependent on the Observer's Own Body Mass Index," *Proceedings of the Royal Society of London Series B Biological Sciences* 267 (2000), 1987–97; M.J. Tovee, K. Tasker, and P.J. Benson, "Is Symmetry a Visual Cue to Attractiveness in the Human Female Body?" *Evolutionary Human Behaviour* 21 (2000), 191–200; M.J. Tovee, D.S. Maisey, J.L. Emery, and P.L. Cornelissen, "Visual Cues to Female Physical Attractiveness," *Proceedings of the Royal Society of London Series B Biological Sciences* 266 (1999), 211–18; A. Furnham, M. Lavancy, and A. McClelland, "Waist-to-Hip Ratio and Facial Attractiveness: A Pilot Study," *Personality and Individual Differences* 30 (2001), 491–502; R. Henss, "Waist-to-Hip Ratio and Female Attractiveness. Evidence from Photographic Stimuli and Methodological Considerations," *Personality and Individual Differences* 30 (2001), 501–13.

7. F. Marlowe and A. Wetsman, "Preferred Waist-to-Hip Ratio and Ecology," *Personality and Individual Differences* 30 (2001), 481–9.

8. Ibid.

9. H. Katzen and R. Mahler (eds.), *Diabetes, Obesity and Vascular Disease, Advances in Modern Nutrition* vol. 2 (New York: Hemisphere, 1978).

10. P.T. Katzmarzyk and C. Davis, "Thinness and Body Shape of Playboy Centerfolds from 1978 to 1998," *International Journal of Obesity* 25 (2001), 590; M.J. Tovee, S.M. Mason, J.L. Emery, S.E. McCluskey, and E.M. Cohen-Tovee, "Supermodels: Stick Insects or Hourglasses," *Lancet* 350 (1997), 1474–5.

11. M.J. Tovee, K. Tasker, and P.J. Benson, "Is Symmetry a Visual Cue to Attractiveness in the Human Female Body?" *Evolutionary Human Behaviour* 21 (2000), 191–200; F. Marlowe and A. Wetsman, "Preferred Waist-to-Hip Ratio and Ecology," *Personality and Individual Differences* 30 (2001), 481–9.

12. M.J. Tovee, K. Tasker, and P.J. Benson, "Is Symmetry a Visual Cue to Attractiveness in the Human Female Body?" *Evolutionary Human Behaviour* 21 (2000), 191–200.

13. M.J. Tovee, D.S. Maisey, J.L. Emery, and P.L. Cornelissen, "Visual Cues to Female Physical Attractiveness," *Proceedings of the Royal Society of London Series B Biological Sciences* 266 (1999), 211–18; R. Hens, "Waist-to-Hip Ratio and Female Attractiveness. Evidence from Photographic Stimuli and Methodological Considerations," *Personality and Individual Differences* 30 (2001), 501–13.

14. M.J. Tovee, K. Tasker, and P.J. Benson, "Is Symmetry a Visual Cue to Attractiveness in the Human Female Body?" *Evolutionary Human Behaviour* 21 (2000), 191–200.

15. M.J. Tovee, S. Reinhardt, J.L. Emery, and P.L. Cornelissen, "Optimum Body-Mass Index and Maximum Sexual Attractiveness," *Lancet* 352 (1998), 548.

16. F. Neziroglu, *Psychiatric Times* 15, 1 (January 1998).

17. *Women's Own,* May 2001 issue.

18. D.M. Garner, "The 1997 Body Image Survey Results," *Psychology Today* (January/February 1997), 75–84.

19. "Anorexia Nervosa (Apepsia Hysterica, Anorexia Hysterica)," *Transactions of the Clinical Society of London,* 1874, 7: 22–8.

20. D.L. Braun, S.R. Sunday, A. Huang A, and K.A. Halmi, "More Males Seek Treatment for Eating Disorders," *International Journal of Eating Disorders* 25 (1999), 415–424.

21. D.B. Woodside, P.E. Garfinkel, E. Lin, P. Goering, A.S. Kaplan AS, D.S. Goldbloom, and S.H. Kennedy, "Comparisons of Men with Full or Partial Eating Disorders, Men without Eating Disorders, and Women with Eating Disorders in the Community," *American Journal of Psychiatry* 158 (2001), 570–4.

22. Ibid.

23. I. Schiff and M. Schiff M, "The Biblical Diagnostician and the Anorexic Bride, *Fertility and Sterility* 69 (1998), 8–10.

24. A. E. Andersen, "Progress in Eating Disorders Research," *American Journal of Psychiatry* 158 (2001), 515–17.

25. P. Slade, "What Is Body Image?" *Behavioural Research Therapy* 32 (1994), 497.

26. R. Olivardia, "Mirror, Mirror on the Wall, Who's the Largest of Them All? The Features and Phenomenology of Muscle Dysmorphia," *Harvard Review of Psychiatry* 9 (2001), 254–9.

27. H.G. Pope, R. Olivardia, A. Gruber, and J. Borowiecki, "Evolving Ideals of Male Body Image as Seen through Action Toys," *International Journal of Eating Disorders* 26 (1999), 65–72.

28. P. Slade, "What Is Body Image?" *Behavioural Research Therapy* 32 (1994), 497.

29. B. Taylor and J. Money, "Amputee Fetishism: An Exclusive Journal Interview with Dr. John Money of Johns Hopkins," *Maryland State Medical Journal* 25 (1976), 35–9.

30. S. Bratman, *Health Food Junkies: Overcoming the Obsession With Healthy Eating* (New York: Broadway Books, 2000).

31. P.T. Katzmarzyk and C. Davis, "Thinness and Body Shape of Playboy Centerfolds from 1978 to 1998," *International Journal of Obesity* 25 (2001), 590.

32. National Heart, Lung, and Blood Institute, "The Framingham Heart Study," www.nhlbi.nih.gov/ about/framingham

33. J.L. Hoeyberghs, "Fortnightly Review: Cosmetic Surgery," *British Medical Journal* 318 (1999), 512–16.

34. www.face.ca/fees.htm

35. www.plasticsurgery.org

36. D.M. Garner, "The 1997 Body Image Survey Results," *Psychology Today* (January/February 1997), 31–44, 75–84; D.M. Garner, "The 1997 Body Image Survey Results," *Psychology Today* (January/February 1997), 31–44, 75–84.

37. D. Cheung, "Smooth out Your Wrinkles," *WellnessOptions* (June/July 2001), 39.

38. Ibid.

39. Ibid.

40. R.A. Yoho and J. Brandy-Yoho, *A New Body In One Day. A Guide to Same-Day Cosmetic Surgery Procedures* (Pasadena, CA: Inverness Press, 1998).

41. J.V. Kohl and R.T. Francoeur, *The Scent of Eros: Mysteries of Odor in Human Sexuality* (New York: Continuun, 1995).

42. M.F. Filosa, J. Kellen, and L. Chan, "Where Is Fancy Bred? In the Nose?" *WellnessOptions* (September/October 2001), 24–5.

43. Ibid.

44. C. Wedekind, T. Seebeck, F. Bettens, and A.J. Paepke, "MHC-Dependent Male Preferences in Humans," *Proceedings of the Royal Society of London Series B Biological Sciences,* 260 (1995), 245–9.

Chapter 4

1. L. Chan and M. Zitney, "Mood: An Overview," *WellnessOptions* (June/July 2002), 10–11.

2. M.W. Radomski, "Food for Mood," *WellnessOptions* (June/July 2002), 54–5.

3. J.E. Prousky, "Treating Depression Naturally," *WellnessOptions* (June/July 2002), 20–1.

4. J.P. Cleary, "Etiology and Biological Treatment of Alcohol Addiction," *Journal of Orthomolecular Medicine* 2 (1987), 166–8.

5. M.R. Werbach and J. Moss, *Depression: Textbook of Nutritional Medicine* (Tarzana, CA: Third Line Press, 1999), 302–16.

6. R.W. Lam and A.J. Levitt (eds.), *Canadian Consensus Guidelines for the Treatment of Seasonal Affective Disorder* (Vancouver: Clinical & Academic Publishing, 1999).

7. S. Atezaz Saeed and T.J. Bruce, "Understanding Seasonal Affective Disorder," *American Family Physician* (March 15, 1998).

8. C.B. Nemeroff, "The Neurobiology of Depression," *Scientific American* 278 (1998), 42–9.

9. "Depression," www.mayoclinic.com.

10. World Health Organization, *The World Health Report 2001, Mental Health, New Understanding, New Hope* (October 2001), www.who.int/dsa/justpub/WHR2001ENGLISH.pdf.

11. Ibid.

12. Ibid.

13. "Depression," www.mayoclinic.com.

14. Statistic Canada, "Canadian Statistics—Hospitalizations for Mental Disorders, by Cause," http://www.statcan.ca/english/Pgdb/health56c.htm.

15. World Health Organization, *The World Health Report 2001, Mental Health, New Understanding, New Hope* (October 2001), www.who.int/dsa/justpub/WHR2001ENGLISH.pdf.

16. "Depression," www.mayoclinic.com; "Major Depressive Disorders; a Patient and Family Guide," *American Psychiatric Association Practice Guidelines*, www.psych.org/clin_res/MajorDepressive.pdf.

17. A.K. Ferketich, J.A. Schwartzbaum, D.J. Frid, and M.L. Moeschberger, "Depression as an Antecedent to Heart Disease among Women and Men in the NHANES I Study," *Archives of Internal Medicine* 161 (2000), 1725–30.

18. Harvard Health Publications, *Understanding Depression Special Report*, www.health.harvard.edu/page.cfm?name=shrDepression.

19. S. Garlow, D. Musselman, and C. Nemeroff, "The Neurochemistry of Mood Disorders: Clinical Studies," in D. Charney, E. Nestler, and B. Bunney (eds.), *The Neurobiological Foundation of Mental Illness* (New York: Oxford University Press, 1999).

20. *Antidepressants*, National Institute of Mental Health, Harvard Medical Schools Community Health Information, Sept. 6, 2001.

21. Ibid.

22. Ibid.

23. D. Bloch, *Healing from Depression, 12 Weeks to a Better Mood* (Ten Speed Press, May 2002).

24. "Risk of Important Drug Interactions between St. John's Wort and Prescription Drugs," Health Canada Warning 00-012891 (April 6, 2000), www.hc-sc.gc.ca/hpb-dgps/therapeut/zfiles/english/advisory/tpd/st_johns_wort_e.html; K. Linde, G. Ramirez, C.D. Mulrow, A. Pauls, W. Weidenhammer, and D. Melchart, "St. John's Wort for Depression—An Overview and Metaanalysis of Randomized Clinical Trials," *British Medical Journal* 313 (1996), 253–8.

25. *Health Canada*, www.hc-sc.gc.ca.

26. A. Dalfen, "Understanding Depression," *WellnessOptions* (June/July 2002), 16–17.

27. "Major Depressive Disorders; a Patient and Family Guide," *American Psychiatric Association Practice Guidelines*, www.psych.org/clin_res/ MajorDepressive.pdf.

28. C.I. Eastman et al., "Bright Light Treatment of Winter Depression: A Placebo-Controlled Trial," *Archives of General Psychiatry* 55 (1998), 883–889; A.J. Lewy et al., "Morning vs Evening Light Treatment of Patients with Winter Depression," *Archives of General Psychiatry* 55 (1998), 890–6.

29. K. Lam, "Oriental Perspective on Moods," *WellnessOptions* (June/July 2002), 23.

30. Huang Di Nei Jing, *Yellow Emperor's Manual of Corporeal Medicine* (Chinese), version complied by Yang Shang-shan, circa A.D. 656, and revised by Wang Ping, circa A.D. 672, as indexed and dated by J. Needham, *Science & Civilisation in China* 6, 6 (Cambridge: Cambridge University Press, 2000).

31. K. Lam, "Oriental Perspective on Moods," *WellnessOptions* (June/July 2002), 23.

32. G. Maciocia, *The Practice of Chinese Medicine* (New York: Churchill Livingstone, 1994); P. Pitchford, *Healing with Whole Foods* (Berkeley, CA: North Atlantic Books, 1993).

33. L. Chan and M. Zitney, "Mood: An Overview," *WellnessOptions* (June/July 2002), 10–11.

34. *Addiction Science Network, 2000*, "The Biological Basis of Addiction," www.addictionscience.net/ASNbiological.htm.

35. J.K. Rowlett, J.S. Rodefer, R.D. Spealman, "Self-administration of cocaine, alfentanil, and nalbuphine under progressive-ratio schedules," Experimental and Clinical Psychopharmacology (2002): 10(4), 367–375.

36. *Addiction Science Network, 2000*, "The Biological Basis of Addiction," www.addictionscience.net/ASNbiological.htm.

37. K. Blum, P.J. Sheridan, R. Wood, and E.R. Braverman, "Dopamine D2 Receptor Gene Polymorphisms in Scandinavian Chronic Alcoholics: A Reappraisal," *European Archives of Psychiatry and Clinical Neuroscience* 254 (1995), 50–2.

38. J.P. Connor, R.M. Young, B.R. Lawford, T.L. Ritchie, and E.P. Noble, "D(2) Dopamine Receptor (DRD2) Polymorphism Is Associated with Severity of Alcohol Dependence," *European Journal of Psychiatry* 17 (2002), 17–23.

39. S. Schenk, A. Valadez, C.M. Worley, and C. McNamara, "Blockade of the Acquisition of Cocaine Self-Administration by the NMDA Antagonist MK-801 (Dizocilpine)," *Behavioural Pharmacology* 4 (1993), 652–9.

40. L.H. Robins, J.E. Helzer, and D.H. Davis, "Narcotic Use in Southeast Asia and Afterward: An Interview Study of 898 Vietnam Returnees, *Archives of General Psychiatry* 32 (1975), 955–61.

41. *Brookhaven National Laboratory*, www.bnl.gov/bnlweb/pubaf/GVG/GVG.htm.

42. *CNET.com*, News, http://news.cnet.com/investor/news/newsitem/0-9900-1028-20536051-0.html.

Chapter 5

1. C. Northrup, *Women's Bodies, Women's Wisdom* (New York: Bantam Books, 1998).

2. *Gerontological Society of America*, www.geron.org/history.htm.

3. S.W.J. Lamberts, A.W. Van Den Beld, and A.J. Van Der Lely, "The Endocrinology of Aging," *Science* 278 (1997), 419–24.

4. J.A. Knight, *Free Radicals, Antioxidants, Aging and Disease* (Washington, DC: AACC Press, 1999).

5. S.G. Rhind. "Aging and the Immune System," *WellnessOptions* (March/April 2002), 30–2.

6. L. Hayflick, *How and Why We Age* (New York: Ballantine Books, 1996).

7. R. Cape, R. Coe, and M. Rodstein (eds.), *Fundamentals of Geriatric Medicine* (New York: Raven Press, 1983).

8. N.R. Poulter, K.T. Khaw, B.E.C. Hopwood, M. Mugambi, W.S. Peart, et al., "The Kenyan Luo Migration Study: Observations on the Initiation of a Rise in Blood Pressure," *British Medical Journal* 300 (1990), 967–72.

9. R.M. Worth, H. Kato, G.G. Rhoads, A. Kagan and S.L. Syme. "Epidemiologic Studies of Coronary Heart Disease and Stroke in Japanese Men Living in Japan, Hawaii and California: Mortality," *American Journal of Epidemiology* 102 (1975), 481–90.

10. R. Dubbelman, J.H.P. Jonxis, F.A.J. Muskiet and A.E.C. Saleh, "Age-Dependent Vitamin D Status and Vertebral Condition of White Women Living in Curacao as Compared with Their Counterparts in the Netherlands," *American Journal of Clinical Nutrition* 58 (1993), 106–9.

11. T.B.L. Kirkwood and S.P. Wolff, "The Biological Basis of Ageing," *Age and Ageing* 24 (1995), 167–71.

12. S.W.J. Lamberts, A.W. Van Den Beld, and A.J. Van Der Lely, "The Endocrinology of Aging," *Science* 278 (1997), 419–24.

13. Ibid.

14. D. Rudman. "Growth Hormone, Body Composition, and Aging," *Journal of the American Geriatric Society* 33 (1985), 800–7.

15. M.W. Radomski, "Shifting Hormonal Balances," *WellnessOptions* (March/April 2002), 14–18.

16. C. Northrup, *Women's Bodies, Women's Wisdom* (New York: Bantam Books, 1998).

17. D. Hinch-Moroz, "Train for Tomorrow," *WellnessOptions* (March/April 2002), 24–6.

18. M.W. Radomski, "Shifting Hormonal Balances," *WellnessOptions* (March/April 2002), 14–18; D. Rudman. "Growth Hormone, Body Composition, and Aging," *Journal of the American Geriatric Society* 33 (1985), 800–7.

19. D. Rudman. "Growth Hormone, Body Composition, and Aging," *Journal of the American Geriatric Society* 33 (1985), 800–7.

20. D. Hinch-Moroz, "Train for Tomorrow," *WellnessOptions* (March/April 2002), 24–6.

21. D.M. McLeod and P.A. White, *Doctors' Secrets: The Road to Longevity* (Summerland, BC: Valley Publishing, 2001).

22. "Risks and Benefits of Estrogen Plus Progestin in Healthy Postmenopausal Women: Principal Results From the Women's Health Initiative Randomized Controlled Trial," *Journal of the American Medical Association* 288 (2002), 321.

23. Ibid.

24. M.W. Radomski, "Shifting Hormonal Balances," *WellnessOptions* (March/April 2002), 14–18.

25. J.E. Morley, "Testosterone Replacement and the Physiologic Aspects of Aging in Men," *Mayo Clinical Proceedings* 75 (2000), S83–7.

26. J.E. Morley, "Testosterone Replacement and the Physiologic Aspects of Aging in Men," *Mayo Clinical Proceedings* 75 (2000), S83–7; F.J. Hayes. "Testosterone—Fountain of Youth or Drug of Abuse?" *Journal of Clinical and Endocrinological Metabolism* 85 (2000), 3020–3.

27. J.E. Morley, "Testosterone Replacement and the Physiologic Aspects of Aging in Men," *Mayo Clinical Proceedings* 75 (2000), S83–7.

28. J.E. Morley, "Testosterone Replacement and the Physiologic Aspects of Aging in Men," *Mayo Clinical Proceedings* 75 (2000), S83–7; F.J. Hayes. "Testosterone—Fountain of Youth or Drug of Abuse?" *Journal of Clinical and Endocrinological Metabolism* 85 (2000), 3020–3.

29. J.C. Prior, J.D. Wark, S.I. Barr, D. Coen, et al., "The Prevention and Treatment of Osteoporosis," *New England Journal of Medicine* 328 (1993), 65–6.

30. C. Northrup, *Women's Bodies, Women's Wisdom* (New York: Bantam Books, 1998).

31. Ibid.

32. Ibid.

33. "Risks and Benefits of Estrogen Plus Progestin in Healthy Postmenopausal Women: Principal Results From the Women's Health Initiative Randomized Controlled Trial," *Journal of the American Medical Association* 288 (2002), 321.

34. C. Northrup, *Women's Bodies, Women's Wisdom* (New York: Bantam Books, 1998).

35. M. Kalimi and W. Regelson, *The Biological Role of Dehydroepiandrosterone* (New York: Walter de Gruyter, 1990); F.L. Bellino, R.A. Daynes, P.J. Hornsby, D.H. Lavrin and J.E. Nestler, "Dehydroepiandrosterone (DHEA) and Aging," *Annals of the New York Academy of Sciences* 774 (1995), 1–342.

36. M. Kalimi and W. Regelson, *The Biological Role of Dehydroepiandrosterone* (New York: Walter de Gruyter, 1990); F.L. Bellino, R.A. Daynes, P.J. Hornsby, D.H. Lavrin and J.E. Nestler, "Dehydroepiandrosterone (DHEA) and Aging," *Annals of the New York Academy of Sciences* 774 (1995), 1–342; E.E. Beaulieu et al., *Proceedings of the National Academy of Sciences USA*, 97 (2000), 4279–84; L. Mazat et al., *Proceedings of the National Academy of Sciences USA* 98 (2001), 8145–50.

37. J.A. Knight, *Free Radicals, Antioxidants, Aging and Disease* (Washington, DC: AACC Press, 1999).

38. T. Harth, "The Aging and Nutrition Connection?" *WellnessOptions* (March/April 2002), 22.

39. Ibid.

40. J.A. Knight, "Free Radicals, Antioxidants and Aging," *WellnessOptions* (March/April 2002), 20–21.

41. S.G. Rhind. "Aging and the Immune System," *WellnessOptions* (March/April 2002), 30–2.

42. Ibid.

43. Ibid.

44. Ibid.

45. Ibid.

46. W.C. Dement, *The Promise of Sleep* (New York: Living Planet Press, 1999).

47. T.H. Monk, D.J. Buysse, J. Carter, B.D. Billy and L.R. Ross, "Effects of Afternoon Siesta Naps on Sleep, Alertness, Performance, and Circadian Rhythms in the Elderly," *Sleep* 24 (2001), 680–7.

48. T.H. Monk, D.J. Buysse, J. Carter, B.D. Billy and L.R. Ross, "Effects of Afternoon Siesta Naps on Sleep, Alertness, Performance, and Circadian Rhythms in the Elderly," *Sleep* 24 (2001), 680–7; A. Buguet and M.W. Radomski, "Sleep and Aging," *WellnessOptions* (March/April 2002), 44–5.

49. D. Hinch-Moroz, "Train for Tomorrow," *WellnessOptions* (March/April 2002), 24–6.

50. Ibid.

51. Ibid.

52. T. Harth, "The Aging and Nutrition Connection?" *WellnessOptions* (March/April 2002), 22.

53. *WellnessOptions* issue on aging (March/April 2002).

54. J.E. Williams, F.J. Nieto, C.P. Stanford, and H.A. Tyroler, "Effects of an Angry Temperament on Coronary Heart Disease Risk," *American Journal of Epidemiology* 154 (August 2001), 230–5.

55. L. Chan, "Longevity and Anti-Aging: An Oriental Perspective," *WellnessOptions* (March/April 2002), 28–9.

56. Ibid.

57. L. Chan, "Longevity and Anti-Aging: An Oriental Perspective," *WellnessOptions* (March/April 2002), 28–9; G. Maciocia, *The Foundations of Chinese Medicine* (London and New York: Churchill Livingstone, 1989).

58. G. Maciocia, *The Foundations of Chinese Medicine* (London and New York: Churchill Livingstone, 1989).

59. Ibid.

60. Ibid.

62. L. Chan, "Longevity and Anti-Aging: An Oriental Perspective," *WellnessOptions* (March/April 2002), 28–9; G. Maciocia, *The Foundations of Chinese Medicine* (London and New York: Churchill Livingstone, 1989).

62. L. So, "Interview with L. Jozsa, Forester, Forintek, British Columbia," *Maclean's* Chinese edition (October/November 1997), 56.

63. Ibid.

64. Ibid.

Chapter 6

1. F.T. Vertosick, *Why We Hurt: The Natural History of Pain* (Orlando, FLA: Harcourt, 2000).

2. Ibid.

3. M.W. Radomski and L. Chan, "Acute and Chronic Pain," *WellnessOptions* (January 2002), 14–17; D.B. Carr and L.C. Goudas, "Acute Pain," Lancet 353 (1999), 2051–8; J.D. Loeser and R. Melzack, "Pain: An Overview," *Lancet* 353 (1999), 1607–9.

4. J.D. Loeser and R. Melzack, "Pain: An Overview," *Lancet* 353 (1999), 1607–9.

5. M. McCaffery and C. Pasero, "Basic Mechanisms Underlying the Causes and Effects of Pain," in B. Bowlus (ed.), *Pain, Clinical Manual* (St Louis, MO: Mosby, 1989), 17.

6. J.J. Bonica, "Considerations of Chronic Pain," in: J.J. Bonica, J.D. Loeser, C.R. Chapman, and W.E. Fordyce (eds.), *The Management of Pain* (Philadelphia, PA; Lea & Febiger, 1990), 180–96; M. Wolff, H. Wittink, and T.H. Michel, "Chronic Pain Concepts and Definitions," in *Chronic Pain Management for Physical Therapists* (Boston: Butterworth-Heinemann, 1997), 1–26.

7. J.D. Loeser and R. Melzack, "Pain: An Overview," *Lancet* 353 (1999), 1607–9; M. McCaffery and C. Pasero, "Basic Mechanisms Underlying the Causes and Effects of Pain," in B. Bowlus (ed.), *Pain, Clinical Manual* (St Louis, MO: Mosby, 1989) 17; J.J. Bonica, "Considerations of Chronic Pain," in: J.J. Bonica, J.D. Loeser, C.R. Chapman, and W.E. Fordyce (eds.), *The Management of Pain* (Philadelphia, PA; Lea & Febiger, 1990), 180–96; M. Wolff, H. Wittink, and T.H. Michel, "Chronic Pain Concepts and Definitions," in *Chronic Pain Management for Physical Therapists* (Boston: Butterworth-Heinemann, 1997) 1–26; C.J. Woolf and R.J Mannion, "Neuropathic Pain: Aetiology, Symptoms: Mechanisms and Management," *Lancet* 353 (1999), 1959–64.

8. S.W. Mitchell, *Injuries of Nerves and Their Consequences* (Philadelphia: J.B. Lippincott, 1872).

9. R. Leriche, *La Chirurgie de la Douleur* (*The Surgery of Pain*; Paris: Masson, 1937).

10. M.W. Radomski and L. Chan, "Acute and Chronic Pain," *WellnessOptions* (January 2002), 14–17; D.B. Carr and L.C. Goudas, "Acute Pain," Lancet 353 (1999), 2051–8; J.D. Loeser and R. Melzack, "Pain: An Overview," *Lancet* 353 (1999), 1607–9.

11. J.J. Bonica, "Considerations of Chronic Pain," in: J.J. Bonica, J.D. Loeser, C.R. Chapman, and W.E. Fordyce (eds.), *The Management of Pain* (Philadelphia, PA; Lea & Febiger, 1990), 180–96; M. Wolff, H. Wittink, and T.H. Michel, "Chronic Pain Concepts and Definitions," in *Chronic Pain Management for Physical Therapists* (Boston: Butterworth-Heinemann, 1997), 1–26.

12. M. Wolff, H. Wittink, and T.H. Michel, "Chronic Pain Concepts and Definitions," in *Chronic Pain Management for Physical Therapists* (Boston: Butterworth-Heinemann, 1997), 1–26.

13. M.A. Ruda, Q.D. Ling, A.G. Hohmann, Y.B. Peng, and T. Tachibana, "Altered Nociceptive Neuronal Circuits after Neonatal Peripheral Inflammation," *Science* 289 (2000), 628–31.

14. T. Cheung, "How Do Painkillers Work?" *WellnessOptions* (January 2002), 22–3.

15. Ibid.

16. Y.M. Chan and M.W. Radomski, "Opioids," *WellnessOptions* (January 2002), 32–3.

17. Ibid.

18. M. Booth, *Opium, A History* (New York: St Martin's Press, 1996).

19. J.P. Rathmell and R.N. Jamison, "Opioid Therapy for Chronic Noncancer Pain," *Current Opinions in Anaesthiology* 9 (1996), 436–42.

20. W.E.M. Pryse-Phillips, D.W. Dodick, J.G. Edmeads, M.J. Gawel, R.F. Nelson, R.A. Purdy, G. Robinson, D. Stirling, and I. Worthington, "Guidelines for the Nonpharmacologic Management of Migraine in Clinical Practice," *Canadian Medical Association Journal* 159 (1998), 47–54 .

21. W.E.M. Pryse-Phillips, D.W. Dodick, J.G. Edmeads, M.J. Gawel, R.F. Nelson, R.A. Purdy, G. Robinson, D. Stirling, and I. Worthington, "Guidelines for the Nonpharmacologic Management of Migraine in Clinical Practice," *Canadian Medical Association Journal* 159 (1998), 47–54.

22. J. Sumner, *The Natural History of Medicinal Plants* (Portland, OR: Timber Press, 2000).

23. C. Ross, "Pain: A Naturopathic Medical Approach," *WellnessOptions* (January 2002), 24–5.

24. T. Cheung, "How Do Painkillers Work?" *WellnessOptions* (January 2002), 22–3.

25. "Acupuncture"(NIH Consensus Development Panel on Acupuncture), *Journal of American Medical Association* 280 (1998), 1518–24.

26. Y.M. Chan, "Acupuncture in the Management of Pain," *WellnessOptions* (January 2002), 26–8; G. Stux and B. Pomeranz, Acupuncture, *Textbook and Atlas* (Berlin and Heidelberg : Springer-Verlag, 1987).

27. Y.M. Chan, "Acupuncture in the Management of Pain," *WellnessOptions* (January 2002), 26–8.

28. C.K. Lo and S.K. Tsui, *Acupuncture in Clinical Practice* (Hong Kong: The Commercial Press, 1998).

29. C.K. Lo and S.K. Tsui, *Acupuncture in Clinical Practice* (Hong Kong: The Commercial Press, 1998); G. Stux and B. Pomeranz, Acupuncture, *Textbook and Atlas* (Berlin and Heidelberg : Springer-Verlag, 1987).

30. G. Stux and B. Pomeranz, Acupuncture, *Textbook and Atlas* (Berlin and Heidelberg : Springer-Verlag, 1987).

31. C.K. Lo and S.K. Tsui, *Acupuncture in Clinical Practice* (Hong Kong: The Commercial Press, 1998); G. Stux and B. Pomeranz, Acupuncture, *Textbook and Atlas* (Berlin and Heidelberg: Springer-Verlag, 1987).

32. G. Stux and B. Pomeranz, *Acupuncture: Textbook and Atlas* (Berlin and Heidelberg: Springer-Verlag, 1987).

33. Y.M. Chan, "Acupuncture in the Management of Pain," *WellnessOptions* (January 2002), 26–8; G. Stux and B. Pomeranz, Acupuncture, *Textbook and Atlas* (Berlin and Heidelberg : Springer-Verlag, 1987).

34. Y.M. Chan, "Acupuncture in the Management of Pain," *WellnessOptions* (January 2002), 26–8.

35. A.M. Rapoport, "Emerging Nonspecific Migraine Therapies: Targets and Unmet Needs," *Headache* 39 (1999), suppl. 2 S27–34;

N. Bogduk, and A. Marsland, "The Cervical Zygapophysial Joints as a Source of Neck Pain," *Spine* 13 (1988), 6; M.M. Braaf and S. Rosner, "Trauma of Cervical Spine as Cause of Chronic Headache," *Journal of Trauma* 15 (1975), 441–6.

36. C. Chan Gunn, *The Gunn Approach to the Treatment of Chronic Pain* (New York: Churchill Livingstone, 1989).

37. L. Chan, "Expanding Pain Threshold?" *WellnessOptions* (January 2002), 36–7.

38. Ibid.

Chapter 7

1. W.C. Dement, *The Promise of Sleep* (New York: Living Planet Press, 1999).

2. M. Filosa, "Sleeping with an Opened Eye?" *WellnessOptions* (February/March 2001), 31; I. Tobler, "Is Sleep Fundamentally Different between Mammalian Species?" *Behavioural Brain Research* 69 (1995), 35–41.

3. W.C. Dement, *The Promise of Sleep* (New York: Living Planet Press, 1999).

4. N.C. Rattenborg, C.J. Amlaner, and S.L. Lima, "Behavioral, Neurophysiological and Evolutionary Perspectives on Unihemispheric Sleep," *Neuroscience Biobehaviour Reviews* 24 (2000), 817–42.

5. Ibid.

6. J. Horne, *Why We Sleep* (New York: Oxford University Press, 1988).

7. Ibid.

8. W.C. Dement, *The Promise of Sleep* (New York: Living Planet Press, 1999); J. Horne, *Why We Sleep* (New York: Oxford University Press, 1988).

9. L. Chan, "The Sleep Mystery," *WellnessOptions* (February/March 2001), 10–13.

10. W.C. Dement, *The Promise of Sleep* (New York: Living Planet Press, 1999).

11. Ibid.

12. Ibid.

13. J. Horne, *Why We Sleep* (New York: Oxford University Press, 1988).

14. W.C. Dement, *The Promise of Sleep* (New York: Living Planet Press, 1999); J. Horne, *Why We Sleep* (New York: Oxford University Press, 1988).

15. K. Louie and M.A. Wilson, "Temporally Structured Replay of Awake Hippocampal Ensemble Activity during Rapid Eye Movement Sleep," *Neuron* 29 (2001), 145–56.

16. D.F. Kripke, L. Garfinkel, D.L. Wingard, M.R. Klauber, and M.R. Marler, "Mortality Associated with Sleep Duration and Insomnia," *Archives of General Psychiatry* 59 (2002), 131–6.

17. S. Coren, *Sleep Thieves* (New York: Simon and Schuster, 1997).

18. W.C. Dement, *The Promise of Sleep* (New York: Living Planet Press, 1999).

19. W.C. Dement, *The Promise of Sleep* (New York: Living Planet Press, 1999); M.W. Radomski, "Sleep Strategies and Military Effectiveness," *WellnessOptions* (February/March 2001), 25–7.

20. S. Coren, *Sleep Thieves* (New York: Simon and Schuster, 1997).

21. W.C. Dement, *The Promise of Sleep* (New York: Living Planet Press, 1999).

22. W.C. Dement, *The Promise of Sleep* (New York: Living Planet Press, 1999); J. Horne, *Why We Sleep* (New York: Oxford University Press, 1988); S. Coren, *Sleep Thieves* (New York: Simon and Schuster, 1997).

23. W.C. Dement, *The Promise of Sleep* (New York: Living Planet Press, 1999).

24. W.C. Dement, *The Promise of Sleep* (New York: Living Planet Press, 1999); S. Coren, *Sleep Thieves* (New York: Simon and Schuster, 1997).

25. Ibid.

26. Ibid.

27. Ibid.

28. M.W. Radomski, "On the Night Shift," *WellnessOptions* (September/October 2001), 48–9.

29. W.C. Dement, *The Promise of Sleep* (New York: Living Planet Press, 1999); S. Coren, *Sleep Thieves* (New York: Simon and Schuster, 1997); M.W. Radomski, "On the Night Shift," *WellnessOptions* (September/October 2001), 48–9.

30. A. Dalfen, "Insomnia," *WellnessOptions* (January/February 2001), 14–16.

31. *Diagnostic and Statistical Manual of Mental Disorders,* 4th ed. (Washington, DC: American Psychiatric Association, 1994).

32. W.C. Dement, *The Promise of Sleep* (New York: Living Planet Press, 1999); A. Dalfen, "Insomnia," *WellnessOptions* (January/February 2001), 14–16.

33. A. Dalfen, "Insomnia," *WellnessOptions* (January/February 2001), 14–16.

34. W.C. Dement, *The Promise of Sleep* (New York: Living Planet Press, 1999).

35. G. Maciocia, *The Practice of Chinese Medicine* (Churchill Livingstone, 1994).

36. W.C. Dement, *The Promise of Sleep* (New York: Living Planet Press, 1999); D.E. Ford and D.B. Kamrow, "Epidemiology Study of Sleep Disturbances and Psychiatric Disorders. An Opportunity for Prevention," *Journal of the American Medical Association* 262 (1989), 1479–84.

37. W.C. Dement, *The Promise of Sleep* (New York: Living Planet Press, 1999); A. Dalfen, "Insomnia," *WellnessOptions* (January/February 2001), 14–16.

38. Ibid.

39. W.C. Dement, *The Promise of Sleep* (New York: Living Planet Press, 1999).

40. W.C. Dement, *The Promise of Sleep* (New York: Living Planet Press, 1999); A. Dalfen, "Insomnia," *WellnessOptions* (January/February 2001), 14–16.

41. W.C. Dement, *The Promise of Sleep* (New York: Living Planet Press, 1999); S. Coren, *Sleep Thieves* (New York: Simon and Schuster, 1997); D. Cheung, "When Old Tricks Fail ..." *WellnessOptions* (February/March 2001), 22–4.

42. M. Tetley, "Instinctive Sleeping and Resting Postures: An Anthropological and Zoological Approach to Treatment of Low Back and Joint Pain," *British Medical Journal* 321(2000), 1616–8.

43. G. Maciocia, *The Practice of Chinese Medicine* (Churchill Livingstone, 1994).

44. E. Ebbel, "Sleep Positions," *WellnessOptions* (February/March 2001), 30.

45. W.C. Dement, *The Promise of Sleep* (New York: Living Planet Press, 1999); S. Coren, *Sleep Thieves* (New York: Simon and Schuster, 1997); G. Maciocia, *The Practice of Chinese Medicine* (Churchill Livingstone, 1994).

46. W.C. Dement, *The Promise of Sleep* (New York: Living Planet Press, 1999); S. Coren, *Sleep Thieves* (New York: Simon and Schuster, 1997).

47. D. Cheung, "When Old Tricks Fail ..." *WellnessOptions* (February/March 2001), 22–4.

48. M. Perlis, M. Aloia, A. Millikan, J. Boehmler, et al., "Behavioral Treatment of Insomnia: A Clinical Case Series Study," *Journal of Behavioral Medicine* 23 (2000), 149–61.

49. Ibid.

50. M.W. Radomski, "Sleep Strategies and Military Effectiveness," *WellnessOptions* (February/March 2001), 25–7.

51. Ibid.

52. Ibid.

Chapter 8

1. S. Margen and the editors of the University of California at Berkeley Wellness Letter, *The Wellness Encyclopedia of Food and Nutrition* (New York: Rebus, 1992).

2. Health Products and Food Branch, Health Canada, *Canada's Guide to Healthy Eating* (2002), www.hc-sc.gc.ca/hpfb-dgpsa/ onpp-bppn/ food_guide_rainbow_e.html.

3. L.A Bazzan, J. He, L.G. Ogden, C.M. Loria, S. Vupputuri, L. Myers, and P.K. Whelton, "Fruit and Vegetable Intake and Risk of Cardiovascular Disease in U.S. Adults: The First National Health and Nutrition Examination Survey Epidemiologic Follow-up Study," *American Journal of Clinical Nutrition* 76 (2002), 93–9.

4. K.A. Chevaux, L. Jackson, M.E. Villar, et al., "Proximate Mineral and Procyanidin Content of Certain Foods and Beverages Consumed by the Kuna Amerinds of Panama," *Journal of Food Composition and Analysis* 14 (2001), 553–63; C.L. Keen, G.F. Fletcher, and M.M. Engler, "Chocolate May Be Good for Your Heart," *American Heart Association Scientific Sessions,* Chicago (Nov. 17–20, 2000); M.G.L. Hertog and P.C.H. Hollman, "Potential Health Effects of the Dietary Flavonol Quercetin," *European Journal of Clinical Nutrition* 50 (1996), 63–71.

5. H.C. Lu, *Chinese Natural Cures* (New York: Black Dog & Leventhal, 1994), 31–2.

6. D.J. Jenkins, C.W. Kendall, C.J. Jackson, et al., "Effects of High- and Low-Isoflavone Soyfoods on Blood Lipids, Oxidized LDL, Homocysteine, and Blood Pressure in Hyperlipidemic Men and Women," *American Journal of Clinical Nutrition* 76 (2002), 365–72.

7. L.R. White, H. Petrovitch, G.W. Ross, et al., "Brain Aging and Midlife Tofu Consumption," *Journal of American College Nutrition* 19 (2000), 242–55.

8. A. Ohry and J. Tsafrir, "Is Chicken Soup an Essential Drug?" *Canadian Medical Association Journal* 161 (1999), 1532–3.

9. National Academy of Sciences–National Research Council, *Recommended Dietary Allowances* (1989).

10. L.E. Cleveland, A.J. Moshfegh, A.M. Albertson, and J.D. Goldman, "Dietary Intake of Whole Grains," *Journal of American College Nutrition* 19 (2000) suppl. 331–8S.

11. Ibid.

12. Health Canada, *Addition of Vitamins and Minerals Policy Review and Implementation* (November 2002).

13. D. Kritchevsky and C. Bonfield (eds.), *Dietary Fiber in Health and Disease* (St Paul, MN: Eagan Press, 1995); G.A. Spiller (ed.), *CRC Handbook of Dietary Fiber in Human Nutrition* (Boca Raton, FL: CRC Press, 1993).

14. Ibid.

15. Pesticide Residues Committee, British government, *Pesticide Residues Monitoring Report—4th Quarter Results* (October–December 2001).

16. Ibid.

17. Canadian General Standards Board, Public Works and Government Services Canada, "Organic Agriculture," CAN/CGSB-32.310-99.

18. J.A. Nordlee, S.L. Taylor, J.A. Townsend, L.A. Thomas, and R.K. Bush, "Identification of a Brazil-Nut Allergen in Transgenic Soybeans," *New England Journal of Medicine* 334 (1996), 688–92.

19. M.F. Filosa, "Fat Chance?" *WellnessOptions* (August/September 2002), 43.

20. Ibid.

21. M.F. Filosa, "Changes in Nutritional Needs," *WellnessOptions* (April/May 2001), 34–5.

22. Ibid.

23. J.P. Flatt, "Use and Storage of Carbohydrates and Fats," *American Journal of Clinical Nutrition* 61 (1995), suppl. 952–9S.

24. Ibid.

25. J.F. Balch and P.A. Balch, *Prescription for Nutritional Healing* (New York: Avery, 1997), 4–5.

26. M. Meydani and J. Mayer, "Omega-3 Fatty Acids Alter Soluble Markers of Endothelial Function in Coronary Heart Disease Patients," *Nutrition Reviews* 58 (2000), 56–9.

27. M.B. Katan, "Trans Fatty Acids and Plasma Lipoproteins," *Nutrition Reviews* 58 (2000), 188–91.

28. H.N. Munro and M.C. Crim, "The Proteins and Amino Acids," in M.E. Shils and V.R. Young (eds.), *Modern Nutrition in Health and Disease* (Philadelphia: Lea and Febiger, 1988) 1–37.

29. A. Ocana, "Food for Energy," *WellnessOptions* (August/September 2002), 12–14; www.healthsmith.com.

30. U.S. National Institute of Nutrition, "Statistics Related to Overweight and Obesity," www.niddk.nih.gov.

31. Ibid.

32. Statistics related to soft drinks, www.softdrink.ca.

33. Food consumption statistics, www.statscan.ca/english/Pgdb.

34. M.W. Radomski, "Tomato for Prostate?" *WellnessOptions* (September/October 2001), 58–9.

35. C. Gärtner, W. Stahl, and H. Sies, "Lycopene Is More Bioavailable from Tomato Paste than from Fresh Tomatoes," *American Journal of Clinical Nutrition* 66 (1997), 116–22; *ScienceNewsOnline*, "Looking for Lycopene" (July 1997), www.sciencenews.org.

36. E. Giovannucci, "Tomatoes, Tomato-Based Products, Lycopene, and Cancer: Review of the Epidemiologic Literature," *Journal of the National Cancer Institute* 91 (1999), 317–31; A.V. Rao, "Lycopene, Tomatoes, and the Prevention of Coronary Heart Disease," *Experimental Biology & Medicine (Maywood)* 227 (2002), 908–13.

37. A.R. Kristal and J.W. Lampe, "Brassica Vegetables and Prostate Cancer Risk: A Review of the Epidemiological Evidence," *Nutrition & Cancer* 42 (2002), 1–9; P. Talalay and J.W. Fabey, "Phytochemicals from Cruciferous Plants Protect against Cancer by Modulating Carcinogen Metabolism," *Journal of Nutrition* 131 (2001), suppl. 3027–33S.

38. S. Renaud and M. de Lorgeril, "Wine, Alcohol, Platelets, and the French Paradox for Coronary Heart Disease," *Lancet* 339 (1992), 1523–6.

39. R. Glahn, "Effects of Juices on the Ability of Intestinal Cells to Absorb Iron," *Journal of Agricultural and Food Chemistry* (Nov. 6, 2002).

40. M. Loewe, *Early Chinese Texts: a Bibliographical Guide* (Chicago: Society for the Study of Early China, 1993).

41. L. Koo, *Nourishment of Life* (Hong Kong: The Commercial Press, 1982); J. Needham, *Science and Civilization in China*, vol. 6 (Cambridge: Cambridge University Press 2000), 79.

42. M.F. Filosa and E. Ebbel, "Water, Life's Most Essential Nutrient" *WellnessOptions* (January/February 2003), 48–50.

43. Ibid.

44. Commission on Life Sciences, *Recommended Dietary Allowances*, 10th ed. (Washington, DC: National Academy of Sciences Press, 1989).

45. Commission on Life Sciences, *Recommended Dietary Allowances*, 10th ed. (Washington, DC: National Academy of Sciences Press, 1989).

46. Commission on Life Sciences, *Recommended Dietary Allowances*, 10th ed. (Washington, DC: National Academy of Sciences Press, 1989); S.M. Kleiner, "Water: An Essential but Overlooked Nutrient," *Journal of the American Dietetic Association* 99 (1999), 200–6.

47. S.M. Shirreffs, "Markers of Hydration Status," *Journal of Sports Medicine* 80 (2000), 80–4.

48. Ibid.

49. J.W. Gardner, "Death by Water Intoxication," *Military Medicine* 167 (2002), 432–4.

50. M.F. Filosa and E. Ebbel, "Water, Life's Most Essential Nutrient" *WellnessOptions* (January/February 2003), 48–50.

51. E.Davies, "Followers of Fashion," *Chemistry in Britain* 38, 11 (November 2002).

52. J.E. Alpert and M. Fava, "Nutrition and Depression: The Role of Folate," *Nutrition Reviews* 55 (1997), 145–9.

53. M.W. Radomski, "Food for Mood," *WellnessOptions* (June/July 2002), 54–7.

54. Ibid.

55. Ibid.

56. T. Decker, *Nutrition and Recovery* (Toronto: Centre for Addiction and Mental Health, 2002).

57. Ibid.

58. M.W. Radomski, "Food for Mood," *WellnessOptions* (June/July 2002), 54–7.

59. J.A. Knight, "Free Radicals, Antioxidants, and Aging," *WellnessOptions* (March/April 2002), 20–1.

60. M.W. Radomski, "Food for Mood," *WellnessOptions* (June/July 2002), 54–7; T. Decker, *Nutrition and Recovery* (Toronto: Centre for Addiction and Mental Health, 2002).

61. T. Harth, "The Aging and Nutrition Connection?" *WellnessOptions* (March/April 2002), 22.

62. W. Zheng and S.Y. Wang, "Antioxidant Activity and Phenolic Compounds in Selected Herbs," *Journal of Agriculture and Food Chemistry* 49 (2001), 5165–70.

63. M. Filosa and A.M. Ocana, "Fuel for Energy, Food for Life," *WellnessOptions* (August/September 2002), 12–14; A. Abdulla and F.H. Abdulla, "Sport Nutrition for Performance," *WellnessOptions* (August/September 2002), 40–1.

64. M.W. Radomski, "Energy Bars and Drinks," *WellnessOptions* (August/September 2002), 50–2.

65. Ibid.

Chapter 9

1. Canadian Fitness and Lifestyle Research Institute, *Physical Activity Monitor 2001*, www.cflri.ca.

2. Ibid.

3. D. Hinch-Moroz, "Compulsive Exercise," *WellnessOptions* (June/July 2002), 42–43.

4. J.S. Raglin, "Psychological Factors in Sport Performance: The Mental Health Model Revisited, *Sports Medicine* 31 (2001), 875–90.

5. M. Babyak, J. Blumenthal, and colleagues, *Health Psychology* 21, 6 (November 2002), 553–63.

6. Canadian Fitness and Lifestyle Research Institute, *Physical Activity Monitor 2001*, www.cflri.ca.

7. Canadian Fitness and Lifestyle Research Institute, *Physical Activity Benchmarks Report*, www.cflri.ca.

8. Canadian Fitness and Lifestyle Research Institute, *Physical Activity Monitor 2001*, www.cflri.ca.

9. J.A. Blumenthal et al., "Effects of Exercise Training on Older Patients with Major Depression," *Archives of Internal Medicine* 25, 159 (October 1999), 19.

10. W.C. Dement, *The Promise of Sleep* (New York: Living Planet Press, 2000).

11. Health Canada, *The Canadian Physical Activity Guide*, www.hc-sc.gc.ca/hppb/paguide.

12. S. O'Brien Cousins, "Belief about Exercise Benefits and Risks," *Journals of Gerontology Series B Psychological Sciences & Social Sciences* 55 (September 2000), 5.

13. C.M. Friedenreich and M.R. Orenstein, "Physical Activity and Cancer Prevention: Etiologic Evidence and Biological Mechanisms," *Journal of Nutrition* 132, 11(2002), suppl. 3456–64S.

14. A. Manuel, "Diabetes: Complications and Treatment," *WellnessOptions* (June/July 2001), 10–12.

15. G.D. Curfman, "The Health Benefits of Exercise," *New England Journal of Medicine* 328 (1993), 574–6; A. Young, "Exercise," in S. Ebrahim and A. Kalache (eds.), *Epidemiology in Old Age* (London: BMJ Publishing, 1996), 190–200.

16. Ibid.

17. S. O'Brien Cousins, "Belief about Exercise Benefits and Risks," *Journals of Gerontology Series B Psychological Sciences & Social Sciences* 55 (September 2000), 5.

18. Ibid.

19. L.G. Pelletier, K.M. Tuson, and N.K. Haddad, "Client Motivation for Therapy Scale: A Measure of Intrinsic Motivation, Extrinsic Motivation, and Amotivation for Therapy," *Journal of Personnel Assessment* 68 (1997), 414–35.

20. Ibid.

21. A.S. Abdulla, "Preparticipation Evaluation," *Patient Care Canada* 13 (2002), 5.

22. R.J. Shephard, T.J. Verde, S.G. Thomas, and P. Shek, "Physical Activity and the Immune System," *Canadian Journal of Sports Science* 16 (1991), 163–185.

23. Canadian Fitness and Lifestyle Research Institute, *Physical Activity Monitor 2001*, www.cflri.ca.

24. Sandia National Laboratories, "Physical Activity Readiness Questionnaire," www.sandia.gov; A.S. Abdulla, "Preparticipation Evaluation," *Patient Care Canada* 13 (2002), 5.

25. M.W. Radomski, "Sports Injuries," *WellnessOptions* (December/January 2002), 52–54.

26. Canadian Fitness and Lifestyle Research Institute, *Physical Activity Monitor 2001*, www.cflri.ca.

27. D. Jones, "Moving Your Body," *WellnessOptions* (September/October 2001), 52–53.

28. D. Hinch-Moroz, "Train for Tomorrow," *WellnessOptions* (March/April 2002), 24–25.

29. L. Strasberg, *Dream of Passion* (Boston: Little Brown, 1987).

30. D. Hinch-Moroz, "Compulsive Exercise," *WellnessOptions* (June/July 2002), 42–43.

31. *American College of Sports Medicine*, www.acsm.org.

32. G.A. Borg, "Perceived Exertion as an Indicator of Somatic Stress," *Scandinavian Journal of Rehabilitative Medicine* 2 (1970), 92–98.

33. C.Y. Lo, "Tai Chi: Beginner's Q&A," *WellnessOptions* (March/April 2002), 51–53.

Chapter 10

1. C.L. Ruffin, "Stress and Health—Little Hassles vs. Major Life Events," *Australian Psychologist* 28 (1993), 201–8.

2. H. Selye, *The Stress of Life*, 2nd ed. (New York: McGraw-Hill, 1978).

3. K.S. Kendler et al., "Causal Relationship between Stressful Life Events and the Onset of Major Depression," *American Journal of Psychiatry* 156 (June 1999), 837–41.

4. K. Ogawa, L. Tsuji, K. Shioni, and S. Hisamichi, "Increased Acute Myocardial Infraction Mortality Following the 1995 Great Hanshin-Awaji Earthquake in Japan," *International Journal of Epidemiology* 29 (June 2000), 449–55.

5. L. Moore, F. Meyer, M. Perusse, B. Cantin, G.R. Dagenais, I. Bairati, and J. Savard, "Psychological Stress and Incidence of Ischaemic Heart Disease," *International Journal of Epidemiology* 28 (1999), 652–8.

6. S.A. Stansfeld, R. Fuhrer, M.J. Shipley, and M.G. Marmot, "Psychological Distress as a Risk Factor for Coronary Heart Disease in the Whitehall II Study," *International Journal of Epidemiology* 31 (2002), 248–55.

7. H. Selye, *The Stress of Life*, 2nd ed. (New York: McGraw-Hill, 1978).

8. C. Tennant and L. McLean, "The Impact of Emotions on Coronary Heart Disease Risk," *Journal of Cardiovascular Risk* 8 (2001), 175–83.

9. D.B. Posen, "Are You Stressed?" *WellnessOptions* (February/March 2001), 72–3.

10. C.L. Ruffin, "Stress and Health—Little Hassles vs. Major Life Events," *Australian Psychologist* 28 (1993), 201–8.

11. L. Moore, F. Meyer, M. Perusse, B. Cantin, G.R. Dagenais, I. Bairati, and J. Savard, "Psychological Stress and Incidence of Ischaemic Heart Disease," *International Journal of Epidemiology* 28 (1999), 652–8.

12. J.E. Williams, F.J. Nieto, C.P. Sanford, and H.A. Tyroler, "Effects of an Angry Temperament on Coronary Heart Disease Risk: The Atherosclerosis Risk in Communities Study," *American Journal of Epidemiology* 154 (2001), 230–5.

13. Ibid.

14. D. Hevey , H.M. McGee , D. Fitzgerald, and J.H. Horgan, "Acute Psychological Stress Decreases Plasma Tissue Plasminogen Activator (tPA) and Tissue Plasminogen Activator/Plasminogen Activator Inhibitor–1 (tPA/PAI-1) Complexes in Cardiac Patients," *European Journal of Applied Physiology* 83 (2000), 344–8.

15. C.M. Stoney and T.O. Engebretson, "Plasma Homocysteine Concentrations Are Positively Associated with Hostility and Anger," *Life Science* 66, 23 (2000), 2267–75.

16. J.E. Williams, F.J. Nieto, C.P. Sanford, and H.A.Tyroler, "Effects of an Angry Temperament on Coronary Heart Disease Risk," *American Journal of Epidemiology* 154, 3 (August 2001), 230–5.

17. T.M. Sharpe et al., "Attachment Style and Weight Concerns in Preadolescent and Adolescent Girls," *International Journal of Eating Disorders* 23 (January 1998), 41–4.

18. M.W. Radomski, "Mental and Emotional Fatigue," *WellnessOptions* (August/September 2002), 16.

19. M.W. Radomski, "Mental and Emotional Fatigue," *WellnessOptions* (August/September 2002), 16; C. Maslach and S.E. Jackson, "Burn-out," *Human Behaviour* 5 (1976), 16–22.

20. M.W. Radomski, "Mental and Emotional Fatigue," *WellnessOptions* (August/September 2002), 16.

21. S. Radovic and H. Malmgrem, "Fatigue and Fatigability," *Proceedings of the National Correlates of Consciousness*, Bremen, Germany (June 1998).

22. S. Coren, "Bored and Tired of Life," *WellnessOptions* (August/September 2002), 17.

23. H. Selye, *The Stress of Life*, 2nd ed. (New York: McGraw-Hill, 1978).

24. C.L. Coe and G.R. Lubach, "Social Context and Other Psychological Influences on the Development of Immunity," in C.D. Ryff and B.H. Singer, *Emotions, Social Relationships, and Health* (London: Oxford University Press, 2000), 243–61.

25. C.B. Pert, *Molecules of Emotion: Why You Feel the Way You Feel* (New York: Simon and Schuster, 1999).

26. C.B. Pert, H.E. Dreher, and M.R. Ruff, "The Psychosomatic Network: Foundations of Mind-Body Medicine," *Alternative Therapy Health Medicine* 4, 4 (July 1998), 30–41.

27. M.J. Esplen, P.E. Garfinkel, M. Olmsted, R.M. Gallop, and S. Kennedy, "A Randomized Controlled Trial of Guided Imagery in Bulimia Nervosa," *Psychology Medicine* 28, 6 (November 1998), 134–57.

28. K.S. Seybold and P.C. Hill, "The Role of Religion and Spirituality in Mental and Physical Health," *Current Directions* 10 (2001) 21–4.

29. C.M. Beck et al., *Mental Health—Psychiatric Nursing: A Holistic Life-Cycle Approach* (St Louis, MO: Mosby, 1984).

30. P.G. Reed, "An Emerging Paradigm for the Investigation of Spirituality in Nursing," *Research in Nursing & Health* 15 (1992), 349–57.

31. C.S. Heriot, "Spirituality & Aging," *Holistic Nursing Practice* 7, 1 (1992), 22–31.

32. K.S. Kendler et al., "Religion, Psychopathology, and Substance Use and Abuse," *American Journal of Psychiatry* 154 (March 1997), 322–9.

33. A.N. Fabricatore et al., "Personal Spirituality as a Moderator of Stress & Well-Being," *Journal of Psychology & Theology* 28 (2000), 211–28.

34. D.A. Mathews, M.E. McCullough, D.B. Larson, et al., "Religious Commitment and Health Status: A Review of the Research and

Implications for Family Medicine," *Archives of Family Medicine* 7 (1998), 118–24; J.S. Levin and H.Y. Vanderpool, "Is Religion Therapeutically Significant for Hypertension?" *Social Science and Medicine* 29 (1989), 69–78; C.E. Thoresen, "Spirituality & Health: Is There a Relationship?" *Journal of Health Psychology* 4 (1999), 291–300.

35. D.A. Mathews, M.E. McCullough, D.B. Larson, et al., "Religious Commitment and Health Status: A Review of the Research and Implications for Family Medicine," *Archives of Family Medicine* 7 (1998), 118–24; D.B. Larson, J.P Swyers, and M.E. McCullough, *Scientific Research on Spirituality and Health: A Consensus Report*" (Rockville, MD: National Institute for Healthcare Research, 1998); J.S. Levin and H.Y. Vanderpool, "Is Religion Therapeutically Significant for Hypertension?" *Social Science and Medicine* 29 (1989), 69–78; J.S Levin and H.Y. Vanderpool, "Religious Factors in Physical Health and the Prevention of Illness," in K.I. Pargament (ed.), *Religion and Prevention in Mental Health* (New York: Haworth Press, 1992); M.E. McCullough, W.T. Hoyt, D.B. Larson, H.G. Koenig, and C.E. Thoresen, "Religious Involvement and Mortality," *Health Psychology* 19 (2000), 211-22; C.E. Thoresen, A.H.S. Harris, and D. Oman, "Spirituality, Religion and Health," in T.G. Plante (ed.), *Faith & Health* (New York: Guilford Press, 2001); C.E. Thoresen and A.H. Harris, "Spirituality and Health: What's the Evidence and What's Needed?" *Annals of Behavioral Medicine* 24 (2002), 3–13; C.E. Thoresen, "Spirituality & Health: Is There a Relationship?" *Journal of Health Psychology* 4 (1999), 291–300; K.S. Seybold and P.C. Hill, "The Role of Religion and Spirituality in Mental and Physical Health," *Current Directions* 10 (2001) 21–4.

36. S. Taylor et al., "Psychological Resources, Positive Illusions, & Health," *American Psychologist* 55 (2000), 99–109.

37. N.S. Goldman, "The Placebo & the Therapeutic Uses of Faith," *Journal of Religion & Health* 24 (1985), 103–16.

38. M. Poloma, "The Effects of Prayer on Mental Well-Being," *Second Opinion* 18 (1993), 37–51.

39. H. Benson, *Beyond the Relaxation Response* (New York: Berkley Books, 1992).

40. L. Dossey, *Healing Words* (San Francisco: Harper, 1993).

41. R.C. Byrd, "Positive Therapeutic Effects of Intercessory Prayer in a Coronary Care Unit Population," *Southern Medical Journal* 81 (1988), 826–9.

42. W.S. Harris, M. Gowda, J.W. Kolb, et al., "A Randomized, Controlled Trial of the Effects of Remote, Intercessory Prayer on Outcomes in Patients Admitted to the Coronary Care Unit," *Archives of Internal Medicine* 159 (1999), 2273–8.

43. K. Bakken and M. Hofeller, *The Journey towards Wholeness* (New York: Cross-Road, 1988).

44. L. Ching, R. Bell, and Y.J. Tso, "Meditative Movement for Energy," *WellnessOptions* (August/September 2002), 28–9.

45. H. Benson, T. Dryer, and L.H. Hartley, "Decreased VO2 Consumption during Exercise with Elicitation of the Relaxation Response," *Journal of Human Stress* 4 (1978), 38–42; H. Benson, T. Dryer, and L.H. Hartley, "The Relaxation Response: A Bridge between Psychiatry and Medicine," *Medical Clinics of North America* 61 (1977), 929–38.

46. G. Anderson, *Healing Wisdom* (New York: Penguin, 1994).

47. Chuang Chou, "Inner Chapters," *Chuang Tsu (The Book of Master Chuang)* (circa 320–200 B.C.), in Chinese language; dating reference: A.C. Graham, *Studies in Chinese Philosophy and Philosophical Life*.

Appendix

1. *Health Canada,* Natural Health Products Directorate, www.hc-sc.gc.ca/hpfb-dgpsa/nhpd-dpsn.

2. R. Imrie and D. Ramey, *Complementary Therapies in Medicine* 8 (2000), 123.

3. C. Bartlett et al., *British Medical Journal* 325 (2002), 81.

4. L. Schwartz et al., *Journal of the American Medical Association* 287 (2002), 2859; S. Woloshin and L. Schwartz, *Journal of the American Medical Association* 287 (2002), 2856.

5. T. Bodenheimer, *New England Journal of Medicine* 342 (2000), 1539.

6. T. Greenhalgh, *British Medical Journal* 315 (1997), 243; M. Winker et al., *Journal of the American Medical Association* 283 (2000), 1600; D. Hunt et al., *Journal of the American Medical Association* 283 (2000), 1875; K. Patterson, *The New York Times* (published May 5, 2002), www.nytimes.com/2002/05/05/magazine/05EVIDENCE.html.

7. PubMed link: www.ncbi.nlm.nih.gov/PubMed.

8. X. Chen and L. Siu, *Journal of Clinical Oncology* 19 (2001), 4291.

Index

Italicized numerals denote charts and illustrations.

A

academic–industry arrangement, 255–256

acetaminophen, 107, *112*

acetylsalicylic acid (ASA), 28, 107, 111, *112*

acupressure, 5, 114, 136, 144

acupuncture, 6, 66, 82, 110, 111, 113–117 (*See also* electro-acupuncture; moxibustion; sonopuncture)

adaptive theory, sleep, 128

addiction: behavioral roots, 68; biochemical aspects, 66–67; case study, 69–70; defined, 66; feel-good, 66–67; neurological basis, 55, 68; recovery, 69; treatment, 67, 68, 110 (*See also* alcholism; drug abuse)

adenosine triphosphate (ATP), 168

adjustment sleep problems, 141

adolescents: obesity/overweight, 44; and physical fitness, 195

Adonis complex, 41

adrenal glands, 56, 86

adrenal medulla, 100

adrenaline, 117, 130, 143, 226

adrenopause, 86

adult-onset growth hormone deficiency, 80

aerobic exercise, 90, 198, 199, 207; FIT formula, 209–210

after-nap sleep inertia, 146–147

ages: percentage age groups, *76*; world median, *76*

aging: chronic disease related to, *77*; and diet, 156, 168; and exercise, 89–90, 198; and hormone changes, 77–78, 86; lifestyle factors and, 86–90; and negative mindset, 91–92; onset of, 79; Oriental perspective, 92–94; physiological basis of, 75, *78*; and sexual desire, 83–85; and sleep patterns, 88–89, *129*; symptoms, 75, 77, 79–80; wellness concept, 75; world trends, *76* (*See also* anti-aging industry; hormone replacement therapy; populations, youngest/oldest; male menopause; menopause)

agoraphobia, *60*

Agriculture Minister's Collection of

Medicinal Herbs, 155, 156

AIDS/HIV, 58, 109

alcohol consumption, 56, 66, 90, 143–144, 184

alcoholism, 67 (*See also* substance abuse)

alert–sleepy windows, *135–136*

allergens, 23, 24, 164

allergies, 8, 17, 23–26

Alzheimer's disease, 139, 156

American College of Sports Medicine (ACSM), 209–210

American Journal of Psychiatry, 40, 41

American Psychiatric Association, 40

American Psychological Association, 198

American Society of Plastic Surgeons, 36

amino acids, 56, 117, 153, 171, 183–184

amphetamines, 67

amputations, voluntary. *See* apotemnophiles

amputees, phantom pain, 102–103

anabolic steroids, 41, 42

anabolism, 86

anaerobic exercise, 207

analgesics, 106–107 (*See also* opioids)

anallergic reaction, 23

anaphylaxis, 17

Anderson, Greg, 239

androgen: DHEA/DHEAs conversion, 86; supplement. *See* testosterone supplemention

andropause, 78, 80 (*See also* male menopause)

anemia, 42 (*See also* iron-deficiency anemia)

anger, 65, 91–92, 101, 198, 226, 228–29

anorexia nervosa, 40, *60*

anti-aging industry, 79 (*See also* growth hormone replacement; hormone replacement therapies)

antibiotics, overprescription, 24

anti-cancer drugs, 61

anti-convulsants, 107

anti-depressants, 54, 61–62, 107, 140

antigens, 17, 87

antioxidants, 86, 153, 156, 174, 185, 187

anti-psychotic medications, 61

anxiety disorders, *60*, 138, 139

apotemnopiles, 42

appreciation, sense of, 19, 91, 122, 239, 241–242, 243

aromatherapy, 113, 146

arthralgia, 80

arthritis, 58, 61, 104, 105, 140, 199

ASA. *See* acetylsalicylic acid

Aspirin, 28, 111

asthma, 113, 139

atherosclerosis, *81*

athletes: and cross-training; 208; and training diet, 187–89; water consumption, 179–180

attraction, unconscious, 47–48

attractiveness: and body measurements, 36–39; facial, 38; and fluctuating asymmetry, 38; and social position, 39; stereotypes, 36; and success, 39 (*See also* body image)

"Authorization to Possess" (marijuana), 109

autoimmune diseases, 61, 87

"awake" hemisphere, 127

awareness, total, 241 (*See also* moment, appreciation of)

awe, sense of, 16

B

balance, 5: and body image, 49; Oriental perspective, 92, 93–94 (*See also* qi; yin-yang)

balanced diet, 43, 90, 153, 159, 173 (*See also* Canada's Food Guide to Healthy Eating)

basal metabolic rate (BMR), 166

beauty, media image of, 35, 36, 38–39, 43 (*See also* attractiveness; body image; body-image obsession)

Bell, Charles, 99

Benson, Herbert, 237

benzodiazepines, *145*

Bergman, Stephen, 68

beriberi, 158

beta-carotene, 185

beverage industry, 182 (*See also* soft drinks)

bihemispheric sleepers, 127

bingeing and purging, 40, *60*

biofeedback, 146

bioflavonoids, 87

biological clock, 133, 137 (*See also* circadian rhythms)

biomedical research, 254–56

bipolar (manic-depressive) disorder, *60*; stats., 59

birth sequence, 23

bisphosphonates, *83*

blame, 2, 85, 92

Blum, Ken, 67

body: and complementarity, 175–178; ideal, 36, 39, 42; measurements, 36–39; mechanistic view, 16, 22; odors, 47–48, *47*

body dissatisfaction, 42; stats., 45 (*See also* Adonis complex; apotemnophiles; eating disorders; muscle dysmorphia)

body-emotion-mind connection, 231–232

body image, 9; defined, 35; media-promoted, 35, 36, 38–39, 43, 49, 165

body-image obsession, 34–36, 39–43 (*See also* attractiveness; cosmetic surgery)

body mass index (BMI), 36–37, *37*, 44

body odor attractions, 47–48, *47*

body pictures (studies), 36–38

body shape. *See* hip/waist ratio; waist/chest ratio

body size. *See* body mass index (BMI)

body temperature, 128, 135–136

Bonaparte, Napolean, 47, 48, 132

Bonica, John J., 105

boredom, 231

botanical medicines, 111, *112*

Bougeault, Guy, 4, 239

brain: and addiction, 66–67; aging process, *78*; and pain, 99, 100, 101; and physical activity, 195; physiology of, 53–55; and prayer, 235; psycho-neuro-immunological aspect, 17, 25–26, 231–232; and psychosomatic network, 232–233; re-uptake process, 54, 55; and sex appeal, 39; and sleep, 126–127, 133, 135

brain chemicals, 54–55 (*See also* neurotransmitters)

brain control center, 53

brain stem, 53

Bratman, Steven, 42

breakfast, menu, 185, 186

breast augmentation, 35–36, 45; case study, 46

breast cancer, *83*

breast-feeding, 24, 63

breast reduction, 45

breathing: exercises, 221; meditation, steps, 237–238; techniques, 237

British Medical Journal, 45

broccoli, 174

Building Blocks for Children's Body Image (Griffin), 35

bulimia nervosa, 40–41, *60*, 233
burnout, 229
burns, 121
Bushnell, Catherine, 101, 121
B vitamins, 183
Byrd, Randolph, 236

C

caffeine consumption, 56–57, 184
calcium, *84*, 160, 187
calisthenics, 207
calcitonin, *83*
calories: burning, 168, 210;
    counting, 35; daily requirements,
    166, 168, 172 (*See also* fat, burning)
camphor, *114*
*Canada's Food Guide to Healthy
    Eating*, 154, 187
Canadian Fitness and Lifestyle
    Research Institute, 197–198, 203
cancer, 75, 81, 87, 104, 109, 140, 169,
    173, 199
capsicum/capsaicin, 111, *112*
carbohydrate/fat/protein ratio, 173
carbohydrates, 56, 169, *171*, 185,
    186, 188, 189, 210 (*See also*
    complex carbohydrates)
carpal tunnel syndrome, 80, 113
case-control studies, 250
case reports, 251
catabolism, 86
cat allergens, 24
cataracts, 77
causalgia, 103 (*See also* phantom
    pain)
cell metabolism, 86
central nervous system (CNS), 25–26,
    56, 99, 102, 104, 111, 231–232
Centre for Addiction and Mental
    Health (Toronto), 185
cerebral cortex, 54, 101, 121
chanting, 6–7
chicken soup, 157
children: and allergies, 24;
    emotional environment, 229;
    obesity/overweight in, 44
Chinese medicine. *See* traditional
    Chinese medicine
chiropractic, 113
chocolate, health benefits, 155–156
choice, and wellness, 4, 5, 7, 197
cholesterol, 170
chronic fatigue syndrome, 61
chronic obstructive pulmonary
    disease, 200

chronic pain, 61, 105; cause of,
    99–100; cost of, 105; and
    depression, 100, 105; managing,
    106; and posture, 118; treatment
    106 (*See also* pain control)
chronic stress, 226; symptoms, 227
Chuang Tsu, 240, 243
circadian rhythms, 133, 135–136
clinical trials, 249–250
cocaine, 55, 67, 68, 69–70
codeine, 107, 108
coenzymes, 159
cognitive-behavioral therapy (CT),
    41, 64, 146
cohort studies, 250
colon, 161, 179, 198, 199
commuting, 224, 225
compassion, 49, 120
compassion fatigue, 229
complementarity: evidence for,
    251–252; principles, 175–177
complex carbohydrates, 136, 143, 184
conditioned predisposition, 53
contemplation, 65, 202
contentment, 4, 71, 235
continuous positive airway pressure
    (CPAD), 140
contract-research organizations
    (CROS), 256
conventional medicine, efficacy of,
    253
cooking, spiritual aspect, 181
Coren, Stanley, 133
corticosteroids, 117
cortisol, 56, 130, 199, 226, 237
cosmetic surgery, 35–36, 44–47;
    preferences by gender, *46*
cravings: addictions, 67, 68; food, 57,
    184
creativity, 49, 233
cross-medication, 28, 62, 63, 144, 188
cross-training, 207–208
cytokines, 231, 232

D

daily value (DV), 159
da Vinci, Leonardo, 132
darkness, 135, *135*, 137 (*See also*
    circadian rhythms; SAD)
death: confronting, 122; risk of, and
    sleep, 131–132
de Beauvoir, Simone, 49
Decker, Trish, 185
dedicated neural pain pathway
    principle, 99

dehydration, 179–180, 187
della Mirandola, Pico, 16
Dement, William C., 132
dementia, 75, *83* (*See also*
    Alzheimer's disease; senility)
D-phenylalanine, 111
depression: and addiction, 66; case
    study, 69–70; Chinese medicine
    approach, 65–66; concurrent
    disorders, 60, 61; and chronic pain,
    100, 105; and diet, 183–85; and
    emotional environment, 229;
    episodic nature of, 57, 59; and
    exercise, 89, 110, 195, 198; genetic
    predisposition to, 59; and
    insomnia, 138, 139; and lifestyle
    habits, 56–57; medications, 61–62;
    natural remedies, 62–63;
    neurological basis of, 53–55; stats.,
    58–59; and substance abuse, 61;
    symptoms, 59, *60*; treatment, 64;
    types, *60* (*See also* dysthymia;
    major depression; SAD)
Descartes, Rene, 99
desire discrepancy, 84–85
desynchronization, 136–37 (*See also*
    sleep disorders)
DHEA (dehydroepiandrosterone), 62,
    78, 86
DHEAs (sulfate ester), 86
diabetes, 37, 58, 61, 75, 77, *81*, 82,
    89, 169, 198, 199, 226
diet: anti-aging, 90; antioxidant
    sources, 87; balanced; 43, 90, 153,
    159, 173; carbohydrate/fat/protein
    ratio, 173; Chinese medicine
    approach, 66; high-carb, 187; high-
    fat, 169; immune system–building,
    26, 87; and mood disorders, 56;
    sample menu, 186; serving sizes,
    154, 187; and sleep, 143, 185, 186;
    vegetarian, 171 (*See also* eating
    styles; eating well; genetically
    modified foods; meal patterns;
    organic foods)
diet industry, 43
digoxin, 63
disharmony, (Oriental) perception
    of, 92
dissimilarity, subconscious
    recognition of, 48
distraction, and pain control, 120, 121
DNA (deoxyribonucleic acid), 117
doctor/patient relationship, 258–259
dopamine, 54, 55, 61, 63, 66, 67, 68,
    184
double-blinded randomized trials,
    250
dreaming, 131, 137
drug abuse, 55, *60*, 110, 111 (*See also*

opioid [abuse]; substance abuse)
dynorphins, 108
dysthymia, *60*

E

eating disorders, 40–44, *60*, 110,
    229, 232–233 (*See also* anorexia
    nervosa; bingeing and purging;
    bulimia nervosa; food obsession;
    orthorexia nervosa)
eating styles, 180–181
eating well, guidelines, 177
Edison, Thomas, 132
eggs, 153
Einstein, Albert, 132, 242
electro-acupuncture, 116
electro-convulsive therapy (ECT), 64
emotional disturbances, 228–229
    (*See also* mood changes)
emotional fatigue. *See* burnout
emotionally coded peptides, 232
emotion-mind-body connection,
    231–232
emotions: Chinese medicine
    approach to, 65–66, 92; link to
    illness, 228; negative, 91–92, 119;
    positive, 120, 242; repressed, 209,
    238; triggers, 53
sympathy, 49
emptiness, concept of [Tao], 94
encouragement, impact of, 8
endocrine system, 25–26, 231, 232
endometrial cancer, *83*
endogenous opioids, 109
endorphins, 63, 108, 109, 116, 195
endurance activities, 206
energy nutrition, 187–189
enkephalins, 108
enlightenment, 237
ennui, 231
environmental sensory cues, 232–233
epilepsy, 109
erectile dysfunction, *80*, *81* (*See also*
    libido; sexual function)
ergonomics, 212–213
Erhardt, Walter, 36
estradiol, 78, 83
estrogen, 82, 83, 86, 140;
    benefits/risks, *83*
evening person, *135–136*, 137
everyday events, emotion-arousing
    aspects, 224–225; uplifts, 228
evidence-based medicine (EBM), 251
evolution: and attractiveness
    measures, 36, 37; and dissimilarity,
    48; and exercise, 194

exercise, 9, *84*; and aging, 89–90; and curing/managing disease, 199–200; duration of, 210; evolutionary link, 194; excessive, 40, 41, 209, 211; frequency of, 210; fun sports/activities, 205; health benefits of, 194, 195, 197–198, 204; and immune system, 26, 202; intensity of, 210; moderate activity, 204, 211; and mood, 57, 110, 195; most popular activities, *196*; motivation to, 200–201; obstructions to, 196; and pain control, 109–110, 120; readiness for, assessing. *See* PAR-Q questionnaire; safety, 203–204 (*See also* aerobic exercise; cross-training; FIT formula; fitness, activity groups; flexibility training; isometric exercise; meditative movement exercises; mind-body exercise; overexercising; relaxation exercise; training diet; working out)

exercise equipment, 204

exercise guide, 212–221

existential pain, 119,122

external analgesics, 106–107, *112*

extrinsic motivation, 201

eyelid surgery, 45

F

facelifts, 45; case study, 46

facial attractiveness, 38

fad diets, 42–43

family therapy, 64

fast foods, 164, 165–166

fat, 169–170

fat burning, 166–167, 210

fatigue: emotional. *See* burnout; mental, 230

fat reserves, 168–169

fat-soluble vitamins, 159

feel-good addiction, 66–67

feel-good neurotransmitters, 55, *55* (*See also* dopamine, norepinephrine, serotonin)

feeling spectrum, 53 (*See also* mood changes)

fertility, 36, 37, 38, 41

fetal position, sleep, 142

fibre, 161, 189

fibromyalgia, 61, 113, 140

fight or flight response, 226

FIT formula (exercise), 209–210

fitness, activity groups, 206

5-HTP, 63

flavonols, 155

flavorings market, 182

flexibility training, 90, 206, 207

flu, 88

fluctuating asymmetry, 38

folic acid, 183

follicle-stimulating hormone, 78

food allergies, 24, 26

food-body compatibility, 175–177

food consumption stats., 172–173

food cravings, 57, 184

food flavor and fragrance (F&F) industry, 182

food fortification, 160–161

food groups, 153, 173

food labels, 170

food-medicines, 155

food metabolism, 160

food obsession, 34, 42

food trends, 164–165

forgiveness, 92, 235

fractures, 79, 83, 84 (*See also* osteoporosis)

Framingham Heart Study, 44

free radicals, 75, 86–87, 174, 185

free testosterone, 81 (*See also* testosterone supplementation)

frontal cortex, 54

fructose, 188

frustration, 91–92, 101

Funk, Casimir, 157

G

Galen, 99

gall-bladder disease, 37

Gardner, Randy, 127

Garner, D.M., 45

gastric ulcers, 61

gate control theory (pain), 99, 116

genetically modified foods, 163–164

genetics: and alcoholism, 67; allergies, 25; and depression, 59; and feelings, 53; and "non-self," 48; and pain signals, 100

Gerontological Society of America, 75

gingko biloba, 62, 63, *84*

Gionet, Normand, 197–198

glycogen, 210

glucose (blood sugar), 169

glucose polymers, 188

glucose tolerance, 78

glutamate, 67

glycogen, 169

Good, Robert, 25

grape juice, 174

Griffin, Marius, 35

Grocery Manufacturers of America (GMA), 163

group therapy, 64

growth hormone (GH), 80; and exercise, 199; and sleep, *88*, 130

growth hormone replacement, 79–80

guilt, *60*, 92

Gull, Sir William, 40

GVG (gamma-vinyl GABA), 68

H

hair transplants, 45

half-awake sleep, 127

hamburgers, 165–166

harmony, 4, 114 (*See also* balance; qi; ying-yang)

Harris, William, 236

Harrison Act (1914), 108

headaches, 105, 113 (*See also* migraine headaches)

healing: defined, 3; and prayer, 235–236; therapies, 113

Healing (Lawrence), 22

Health Canada, 63, 252

health: defined, 4; levels of, 3; and optimal well-being, 4, 5

health articles, sources, 247

Health Food Junkies (Bratman), 42

health foods obsession. *See* orthorexia nervosa

health information, evaluating, 246–259

heart attack, 61, 89, 174, 224, 228

heart disease, 37, 61, 75, 77, *81*, 82, 169, 174, 197, 198, 225, 226, 228–229

heart failure, 44, 77

helplessness, 2, 100

herbal remedies, 5, 6, 62, 66; evidence for, 252; menopause, 82; sleep, 144, *145*

herbs, 155, 156, 187

heroin, 55, 68, 108

Hippocrates, 98–99

histamine, 26

Hobson, J. Allan, 131

home dining, 181

homeopathy, 82

homosexuality, and eating disorders, 41

hope, 120, 235, 238

hormonal fluctuations (sleep disorders), 140

hormonal system disorder, 61

hormone deficiencies, 77–78

hormone replacement therapy (HRT), 79; risks/benefits, *83, 84* (*See also* growth hormone replacement)

hot flashes, *60, 83, 84*, 140

human studies, 249

hydrocortisone drugs, 61

hydrogenation, 170

hypersomnia, 57

hypertension, 58, 61, 75, 77, *81*, 110, 198, 224, 226, 229

hypnosis, 25, 121

hypnotics, 144; benefits/risks, *145*

hypoglycemia, 56

hypogonadism, 80

hypothalamus-pituitary system, 75, 116

hysterectomy, 83

I

ibuprofen, 107

ideal body, 36, 39, 42 (*See also* attractiveness; body image; body-image obsession)

Ikeda, Daisaku, 239

immune gland. *See* thymus

immune system, 8; aging of, 75, 87–88; and allergies, 17, 23–25; default setting, 23, 24; and emotional/mental health, 22; and exercise, 202; and free radicals, 185; functions of, 17–18; imbalance, 23–24, *24*; and lifestyle, 26; Oriental perspective, 93; psycho-neurological aspects, 25, 231–232; and sleep, 127–128, 130; and spirituality, 235; and stress, 25–26, 224–225, 231; subsystems, 17

immunosenescence, 87

implants (breast), 46

indomethacin, 107

industry-academic relationship, 255–256

infants: rec. fluid intake, 179; water intoxication in, 180

infectious diseases, 23, 24

infertility, 37

information (medical), evaluating, 246–259

insomnia, 9, 89, 137–140; caused by medical conditions, 139–140; Chinese medicine approach, 138–139; and mood disorders, 138, 139

insulin, 199

insulin resistance, 78, *81*

integrated health care, 7, 8, 23, 26–29

integration: medical disciplines, 7, 8, 23, 26–29; wellness conditions, 9, 23

internal analgesics, 107, *112*

International Association for the Study of Pain, 99, 105

International Journal of Epidemiology, 225

Internet searches, health information, 256–257

interpersonal therapy (IPT), 64

interrelatedness, 71

intervention studies, 249–250

intrinsic motivation, 201

in vitro studies, 248–249

iodization, 161

iron, 174, 187

iron-defiency anemia, 140, 174

ischemia, 102

isoflavone, *84*

isometric exercise, 207

J

jet lag, 136–137, 146

jing [acupuncture], 114

jing [energy, aging], 92, 93

joy, 49, 65, 84, 243

juices, 174

junk food, 172

K

kidney stones, 179

Kim Bong Han, 117

Krauchi, Kurt, 133

Kripke, Daniel F., 131

L

laudanum, 108 (*See also* opiodes)

Lawrence, D.H., 22

Lavoisier, Antoine Laurent, 157

Lenfant, Claude, 44

Leriche, RenÈ, 103

L-5-hydroxytryptophan (5-HTP), 62, 63

libido, 57, 58, *80*, 81, 82, 83–85, 237

life elements, Oriental perspective, 92–94

life expectancy: Japanese, 156; Russian men, 225; women, 82

life force, 236–237 (*See also* qi; qi gong)

lifespans: longest recorded, *76*, 94–95; Oriental perspective, 92

lifestyle: and aging, 86–90; and immune response, 26; impact on mood, 56–58, *56*; sedentary, 194, 195, 197, 198, 199

light, 57, 89, 135, *135*, 137 (*See also* SAD)

light therapy, 64

liposuction, 36, 45

Livingston, William K., 103

love, 49, 68, 69, 84, 85, 120, 122, 235

low-carbohydrate diet, 56

lower back pain, 104, 113, *117*

lung disease, 199–200

lungs, aging process, *78*

luteinizing hormone, 77–78

lycopene, 174

lympocytes, 25, 87, 231

M

McQuay, Henry, 110

Magendie, Francois, 99

major depression, 59, 71, 139, 195

major histocompatibility complexes (MHC), 48

male menopause, 80–82 (*See also* andropause; testosterone supplementation)

maltodextrins, 188

manic-depressive disorder. *See* bipolar manic-depressive disorder

marijuna, 67, 109

Marijuana Medical Access Regulations, 109

massage, 6, 113

masturbation, 85

meal patterns, 184–185; sample menu, 18

media: and body images, 35, 36, 38–39, 43, 49, 165; and medical information, 253–254

medical disciplines, integration of, 7, 8, 23, 26–29

medications: and addictions, 67, 68; analgesics, 106–107; anti-depressants, 54, 61–62; cause of depression, 61; cause of insomnia, 140; cough & cold, 62, *145*; and health communication, 28; hypnotics, 144, *145*; overdoses, 144, *145*; sleeping pills, 144; and stress, 225 (*See also* botanical medicines; cross-medication; herbal remedies; hormone replacement therapies; natural remedies; non-steroidal anti-inflammatory drugs; over-the-counter drugs; painkillers; psychedelic drugs)

meditation, 92, 93, 146; techniques, 236–238

meditative movement exercises, 208–209 (*See also* mind-body exercise)

melatonin, 57, 78, 135, *135*, 136, *145*

Melzach, Ronald, 99, 116

memory, 54, 57, 131 (*See also* pain memory)

menopause, 78, 82, 140 (*See also* andropause; male menopause)

mental disorders, statistics, 59

mental fatigue, 230

meridians, 93, 114, 115–116, 117

meta-analysis, 251

metabolism, 86, 114, 168–169, 235 (*See also* basal metabolic rate; catabolism; food metabolism; resting metabolic rate)

mircosleep, 132–133

migraine headache, 61, 102, 105

mind-body exercise, 207, 208–209, 216–221

mind-emotion-body connection, 231–232

mind, training, 241

mirrors, 34–35, 49 (*See also* body-image obsession)

Mitchell, Silas Weir, 103

MK-801 (experimental drug), 67

models, male, 42–43

Mogie, Jeffrey, 100

Moldofsky, Harvey, 129

Molecules of Emotion (Pert), 232

moment: appreciation of, 18, 91, 239, 241–242, 243; external, 2; totality of, 16

monounsaturated fats, 170

mood, defined, 52

mood changes: elements of, 53, 71; and exercise, 57, 195, 198; and lifestyle habits, 56–57; neurological basis of, 53–55; and nutritional deficiencies, 56, 183, *185*; and testosterone supplementation, *81*

mood disorders, defined 58

morning person, *135–136*, 137

morphine, 107, 108

mortality, confronting, 122

Morton, Richard, 40

motivation, 58, 200–201

moxibustion, 116

Mueller, Johannes, 99

multiple sclerosis (MS), 109

muscle dysmorphia, 41

muscle relaxation exercises, 219–221

muscles, aging process, *78*, 79

muscularity, preoccupation with, 41

N

naloxone, 108

napping, 88–89, 132, 146

naproxen, 107

National Food Processors Association (NFPA), 163

natural disasters, 224, 226 (*See also* post-traumatic stress disorder)

natural health products (NHP), 252; defined, 253

Natural Health Products Directorate, 252

natural killer cells. *See* T-cells

natural remedies, 62–63, 110–111, 113–122

neck, shoulder pain, stats., *117*

nerve cells (neurons), 54, 55

nerve endings, 54, 55

nerve fibers, 54, 55

neural pathways, 100, 101

neuroadaptation, 67

neuromatrix, 100

neuropathic pain, 99–100

neuropeptides, 232

neurotransmitters, 54–55, 232

New England Journal of Medicine, 24, 44, 82, 164

news releases, medical information, 254

night shift paralysis, 137

nociceptive pain, 99

nociceptors, 100, 104 (*See also* pain receptors)

non-benzodiazepines, *145*

"non-self," genetic recognition of, 48

non-steroidal anti-inflammatory drugs (NSAIDS), 107, 111, *112*

norepinephrine, 54, 55, 61, 184, 199

Northrup, Christine, 74, 82

nose reshaping, 36, 45

NREM (non-rapid eye movement) sleep, 129, 133 (*See also* REM [rapid eye movement] sleep)

nutrient fortification, 160

nutritional products industry, 158

O

obesity, 37, 44, 77, 89, 90, 164, 172, 226

observational studies, 250

obsessive-compulsive disorder, *60*, 67, 138

odors, body, 47–48, *47*

Olivardia, Roberto, 41

omega-3 oils, 62

opioides, 67, 105, 107–110; abuse, 111; history of, 108; how they work, *112*

optimal living/wellness, 3–4

oral contraceptives, contraindications, 63

oregano, 187

organic farming, 162–163

organic foods, 161–163

orthorexia nervosa, 42

Osler, William, 18, 22, 28

osteoarthritis, 77, 113, 199, *200*

osteoporosis, 42, 79, 82, *83, 84,* 89, 199, 206

ovarian cancer, 86

overexercising, 40, 41, 209, 211

over-the-counter drugs, 62, *145*; diet aids, 43; sleeping aids, 43, *144*

overweight, 44, 164, 172 (*See also* obesity)

oxidation, 86

oxycodone, 107

P

PABA (para-aminobenzoic acid), 110–111

pain, 9: checklist, 118; concepts, 99–100; definition, 99; and genetics, 100; historical views of, 98–99; influences on, 98; levels of, 119; neurological basis of, 100, 101; and posture, 118; types of, 99–100, 102–106; vs. suffering, 101; working in, *117* (*See also* chronic pain; existential pain; phantom pain; referred pain)

pain control, 106–122

pain memory, 100, 101, 103

Pain Paradox Theory, 107

pain receptors, 99, 100

painkillers, how they work, *112*

pain threshold, 98, 109, 119; expanding spiritual, 122; expanding total, 120

pancreas, aging process, *78*

panic disorder, *60,* 61

Paracelsus, 108

paranoia, 59

Parkinson's disease, 61, 139

PAR-Q (Physical Activity Readiness Questionnaire), 203–204

Paxil, 62

peanut allergy, 24

peer review process, 253

Pelletier, Luc, 200

peptides, 232

Pert, Candace B., 232

pesticides, 161–162

phantom pain, 102–103

pheromones, 48

Phillips, Barbara, 89

Physical Activity Benchmarks Report (1997), 197

Physical Activity Guide, 199

physical education classes, 195

physiology, mechanistic view, 22

physiotherapy, 113

Pilates, 207

pineal gland, 57, *145*

pituitary gland, 77–78, *78,* 80, 108, 116

placebo effect, 235

plastic surgery, 35–36, 44–47

Plato, 98

playing, 205

polyphenols, 174 (*See also* antioxidants)

polyunsaturated fats, 170

Pomeranz, Bruce, 116

populations, oldest/youngest, *76*

positive thinking, 239

post-natal qi, 93

post-traumatic stress disorder (PTSD), *60,* 139

posture: at desk, 213; and pain, 118; sleep, 142

power naps, 88–89, 146

prayer, 235–236

pregnancy, 24, 63, 140, 142, 179

pre-natal qi, 93

primary insomnia, 138

Principles of Correct Diet, The (Hu Ssu-Hui), 175

Principles and Practice of Medicine, The (Osler), 28

Prior, J.C., 82

processed foods, 184

professions, high-risk, and burnout, 229

progesterone, 82, 83, 140

progestins, benefits/risks, *83*

prostaglandins, 100

prostate: cancer, 174; enlargement, 81

protein, 170–171, 184, 185, 186, 189; daily requirement, 187; sources of, *171*

protein-bound testosterone, 81

Prozac, 62, 140

psychedelic drugs, 67, 109

psycho-neuro-immunology, 25–26, 231, 224

Psychology Today, 40

psychosomatic network, 232–233

psychotherapy, 64

Q

qi (energy), 65, 66, 92, 93, 114, 237 (*See also* post-natal qi; pre-natal qi)

qi gong, 208, 209, 237; breathing, 221

R

Raglin, Jack, 195

randomized clinical trials (RCT), 249–250, 251, 253

Rating of Perceived Exertion (RPE) scale, 210

recommended daily allowance (RDA), 159

Records of Celebrated Physicians, 156

referred pain, 102

regret, 91, 101

relaxation exercise, 209, 219–221

relaxation techniques, 120, 146, 225

religion: defined, 234; health benefits of, 234–36; role of, 122; unhealthy, 234 (*See also* spirituality)

REM (rapid eye movement) sleep, 129, 130–131, 133

repair theory, sleep, 128

research, communicating results, 253

resistance exercise training, 89

restaurants, 180–181

resting metabolic rate, 166

restless leg syndrome (RLS), 140

restraint, 92, 94

re-uptake process, 54, 55

Robins, Lee, 68

S

Sabril, 68

SAD (seasonal affective disorder), 57, *57, 60,* 64

St. John's wort, 62, 63

salicylates, *112*

salicylic acid, 111

SAM-e (S-adenosylmethioninel), 62, 63

saturated fat, 169, 170

schizophrenia, 138, 139

sciatica, 102

sedative-hypnotic drugs, 144, *145*

sedentary lifestyle, 194, 195, 197, 198

selective estrogen receptor modulators, *83*

selective serotonin re-uptake inhibitors (SSRIs), 55, *55,* 62

self-acceptance, 238

self-awareness, 34, 69, 233, 238

self-direction, 238

self-esteem, 58, 84, 198, 229

self, loss of, 49

self-perception, 34, 49

self-worth, 36

Selye, Hans, 25, 224, 226, 231

senility, 89 (*See also* Alzheimer's disease; dementia)

sensory pain neurons, 102

sequoia trees, 94–95

serotonin, 54, 55, *55,* 56, 57, 61, 62, 63, 64, 111, 143, 183, 184

Serturner, Friedrich, 108

sex appeal, 39 (*See also* attractiveness)

sex hormones, 86

sexual arousal, and body odor, 47–48 (*See also* libido)

sexual desire, 83–95

sexual function, aging, *80, 81, 81,* 82

shape, body. *See* waist/chest ratio; waist/hip ratio

shen (spirit), 92, 93

Sherrington, Charles S., 99

shift work, 137, 146

single-blinded randomized trials, 249–250

skin cancer, 90

skin laser treatment, 45

Slade, Peter, 35

sleep: and aging, 88–89, *129*; and alcohol consumption, 143–144; amount required, 131–132; average hours of, by species, *126*; and diet, 143, 185, 186; and exercise, 198; and growth hormones, *88,* 130; and immune system, 26; and intelligence, 132; light exposure and, 89; measuring, *128*; memory and learning, 130, and mood disorders, 53, 59; neurological aspects of, 126–127, 133, 135; physiological aspects of, 127–131; and risk of death, 131–132; stages of, 129; strategies, 141–147; theoretical basis of, 128; unihemispheric, 127 (*See also* napping)

sleep apnea, 81, *81,* 140, 144

sleep cycle, 129

sleep debt, questionnaire, *134*

sleep deprivation, 127–128, 132–133

sleep disorders, 137–141 (*See also* sleep problems)

sleep inertia, 146–147

sleep positions, 142

sleep problems, categories, 136–137

sleep rhythms, 133, 135–136

sleep spindles, 130

sleeping aids, 144, *145*

slow-brain-wave sleep (SWS), 129, 130, 147

Smith, David, 66

smoking, 56, 90, 200, 225, 226

snacks, healthy, 185, 186

SnowWorld, 121

social phobia, *60*, 61

soft drinks, 172, 173

somatic pain, 102

somatopause, 79–80 (*See also* growth hormone replacement)

sonopuncture, 116

sorrow, 65

soybeans, 155, 156

soy products, *84*

spinal cord, 99, 100, 102, 111

spinal cord injury, 109

spiritual fitness, reflections, 238–242

spiritual pain, 119, 122

spirituality: defined, 233–234; and eating, 181; health effects, 234, *234*; positive impact of, 235–236; role of, 122; unhealthy, 234

sport drinks, 188

steroids, 41, 42

Strasberg, Lee, 209

strength activities, 206, 207

streptococcal pneumonia, 88

stress: causes of, 224–225, 226; defined, 226; and exercise, 194; good, 226; harmful, 226, 228; and heart problems, 225; and immune system, 25–26, 231; impact on health, 61, 224; and injury, 100; managing, 225, 226, 228; risk factors, 226; and spirituality, 234; symptoms, 226–227 (*See also* chronic stress; fight or flight response; uplifts)

stress hormones, 100, 108, 226, 237, 238

stretching, 90, 207, 209, 237

stroke, 37, 61, 75, 82, 113, 154, 169, 228

studies, types, 248–251

substance abuse, 55, 58, 61, 66–67 (*See also* alcoholism; drug abuse; opioid [abuse])

substance P, 111

suffering vs. pain, 101

sugar, 184

sugar metabolism, aging, *81*

suicide, 58, 59, 71, *60*

sulphorafane, 174

supplements industry, 158

suprachiasmatic nucleus (SN), 135

synapses, 54, 55

Systematic Treasury of Medicine (Chang Chi), 175

T

tai chi, 146, 207, 208, 209, 218–219, 237

talk therapy, 64

Tao, 152, 240

Taoism, 94

T-cells, 23, 25, 130, 199, 231

team sports, 204, 205

telemeres, 75

testosterone, 78, 80, *83* (*See also* free testosterone)

testosterone supplementation, 81–82, *81*

tetanus, 88

Tetley, Michael, 142

textbooks, human physiology, 258

TH1 cells/TH2 cells, 23–24; immune imbalance, *24*

theophylline, 63

thermoregulation, 128

thinness, 35, 39, 42, 43, 164

thorax, 23

thymus, 23, 25, 79, 231

tofu, 156, 171

tomatoes, 174

total pain, 119

toys, 42, 205

traditional Chinese medicine, 7: aging, 92–94; depression, 65–66; food-body compatibility, 175–177; principles of, 92–93, 113–114, 138–149; sleep, 138–139, 142, 143

training diets, 187–189

tranquillizers, 106, 144

transcendence, 16 (*See also* enlightenment)

trans-fatty acids, 170

transient pain, 102

trauma, reaction to. *See* post-traumatic stress disorder

triglyceride, 169

tryptophan, 56, 111, 143, 183, 184

tummy tucks, 45

tyrosine, 184

U

unconscious attractions, 47–48

unihemispheric sleep, 127

uplifts, 228

urban living, link to stress, 224–225

urinary tract cancers, 179

U.S. Department of Agriculture (USDA), 163, 187

U.S. National Cattlemen's Beef Association, 165

U.S. National Heart, Lung & Blood Institute (NHLBI), 44

U.S. National Institutes of Health (NIH), 83, 113

V

vaccinations, preventive, 87–88

valerian, *145*

vasodilation, 102

vegetable consumption, 154–155

vegetarians, protein for, 171

Vernejoul, Pierre, 117

Vertosick Jr., Frank T., 98

vigabatrin, 68

virtual games, and pain control, 121

visceral pain, 102

vitamin A, 87, 159, 185

vitamin B1, 158

vitamin C, 87, 160, 161, 185

vitamin D, *84*, 159, 160, 161

vitamin E, 87, 159, 185

vitamin K, 159

vitamin supplementation, 87, 158, 159

vitamins/minerals, 111, 157–159 (*See also* nutrient fortification)

vomeronasal organ (VNO), 48

W

waist/chest ratio (WCR), 38

waist/hip ratio (WHR), 36–37

Wall, Patrick, 99, 116

walking, 195, 197, 200, 204, 206

warfarin, 63

water consumption, 18, 177–179

water intoxication, 180

water recipes, 190

water-soluble vitamins, 159

weighlifting, 90, 207

Wedekind, Claus, 48

weight management, 166–167 (*See also* obesity; overweight)

weight management obsession, 42–43 (*See also* eating disorders)

Wellness Options: goals, 19; steps, 29

WellnessOptions magazine, 8, 10

white blood cells. *See* lymphocytes

whole-grain foods, 154, 160

Williams, J.E., 228

Wilson, Matthew, 131

wine, health benefits, 155–156

wisdom, 5, 27–28, 71, 98

Wittink, Harriet, 106

Women's Health Initiative Study (2002), 83

Women's Own magazine, 39

working out: around the house, 204–205, 212; FIT formula, 209–210; safety tips, 204; at work, 205, 212–215

World Health Organization (WHO), 4, 58, 104–105, 113

Y

Yellow Emperor's Manual of Corporeal Medicine (Huang Di Nei Jing), 65, 92, 114

yin-yang, 92–93, 113–114, 139, 176 (*See also* complementarity [principles])

yoga, 146, 207, 208, 209, 237; exercises, 216–218

Yoho, Robert, 36–47

youth suicide, 59

Z

zinc, 87

Zoloft, 62

Reader Response and Trial Subscription

Enjoy this book? Want to share your comments?
Fill out this questionnaire to receive a six-month trial subscription to
WellnessOptions magazine at no charge. If you already subscribe to
WellnessOptions magazine, please designate the trial subscription
as a gift from you to a friend.

HOW DO YOU RATE "The Wellness Options Guide to Health"?

5=Excellent 4=Good 3=Average 2=Below average 1=Poor

Content:	☐ 5	☐ 4	☐ 3	☐ 2	☐ 1
Design:	☐ 5	☐ 4	☐ 3	☐ 2	☐ 1
Overall:	☐ 5	☐ 4	☐ 3	☐ 2	☐ 1

YOUR COMMENTS:

_____

_____

_____

Topics you would like us to cover in future publications:

_____

Design elements you would like us to include:

_____

On average, how many health and wellness publications do you read each year?

Books _____   Magazines _____   Journals _____

On average, how many books do you read each year?   _____

ABOUT YOU:

Gender: ☐ Male ☐ Female

Age: ☐ < 25 ☐ 25–34 ☐ 35–49 ☐ 50–64 ☐ 65+

Household income: ☐ < 50K ☐ 50K-75K ☐ 75K-100K ☐ > 100K

Occupation: Health-care related? ☐ Yes ☐ No

If health-care related: ☐ Professional ☐ Technical ☐ Administrative ☐ Other

Highest education level attained:
☐ High-school graduate ☐ College or university graduate
☐ Masters degree ☐ Doctoral degree

WellnessOptions magazine trial subscription:

Do you subscribe to **WellnessOptions** magazine? ☐ Yes ☐ No

Do you want to receive a trial subscription? ☐ Yes ☐ No

Do you want to send your trial subscription to a friend? ☐ Yes ☐ No

---

SEND A SIX-MONTH TRIAL SUBSCRIPTION TO WELLNESSOPTIONS MAGAZINE TO:

Name
_____

Address
_____

_____

City
_____

Province/State
_____

Postal code
_____

Telephone
_____

E-mail
_____

Do you what to know about future
publications from Lillian Chan
and/or **WellnessOptions**?

☐ Yes ☐ No

If "yes," please provide address
and contact information (if
different from above):

Name
_____

Address
_____

_____

City
_____

Province/State
_____

Postal Code
_____

Telephone
_____

E-mail
_____

Please send completed form with
original proof of purchase by mail to:
WellnessOptions magazine
250 Consumers Road, Suite 505
Toronto, Ontario, Canada M2J 4V6

WellnessOptions
www.wellnessoptions.ca